# VIOLENCE
# IN THE HOME:
## *Interdisciplinary*
## *Perspectives*

# *VIOLENCE IN THE HOME:*
## *Interdisciplinary Perspectives*

*Edited by*

## Mary Lystad, Ph.D.

**BRUNNER/MAZEL,** *Publishers* • *New York*

**Library of Congress Cataloging-in-Publication Data**
Main entry under title:

Violence in the home.

  Includes bibliographies and index.
  1. Family violence—United States.  2. Family
violence—United States—Prevention.  3. Problem
families—Counseling of—United States.  I. Lystad,
Mary
HQ809.3.U5V57  1986      362.8′2      85-25450
ISBN 0-87630-416-1

*Published by*
BRUNNER/MAZEL, INC.
19 Union Square
New York, New York 10003

# Interdisciplinary Perspectives on Family Violence: An Overview

## *Mary Lystad*

### INTRODUCTION TO THE PROBLEM

Family violence is not a unique product of our time and our place. Research on infanticide, the most widely studied form of family violence, documents its presence in many human and nonhuman societies. Kellum (1974) discusses the existence of massive infanticide in Europe during the Middle Ages. Langer (1974) notes that, except among Christians and Jews, infanticide has from time immemorial been an accepted procedure for disposing not only of deformed or sickly infants, but of newborns who might strain the resources of the individual family or the larger community. Langer reports that infanticide is employed now by some nonindustrialized societies in an effort, however unsuccessful, to keep the population in reasonable adjustment to available food supply.

In America, concern over family violence began with concern not for infanticide per se but for a broader spectrum of child abuse and neglect. In the nineteenth century, the Society for the Prevention of Cruelty to Animals succeeded in removing a maltreated child from her parents on the grounds that she was a member of the animal kingdom and entitled to protection under the laws against animal cruelty. This action precipitated the formulation of the Society for Prevention of Cruelty to Children (Radbill, 1968). Recent interest in the battered-child syndrome has its origins in the discipline of pediatric radiology, begun in 1906. X rays make it possible to document repeated injuries to a child over time and to confirm suspicions of abuse (Radbill, 1968).

More current attention to family violence has turned to another form of family violence, namely that of husband to wife. The substantial achievements of women in obtaining social justice and social equality over the last decade have prompted analyses of women's relationships inside and outside the home. Wife battering and rape have been identified as forms of violence and the beliefs that a man's home is his castle and a man's wife is his property have been identified as myths and not as licenses to do physical harm. Studies of these forms of violence documents its existence in all social classes and ethnic and racial groups in this country (Straus, Gelles, & Steinmetz, 1980).

The women's movement is also partly responsible for special attention in the last ten years to sexual abuse of adults and children. Studies in this country have shown that sexual abuse occurs most often in the home; the definition of such abuse has been broadened to include not only oral and vaginal penetration but also, for the child, fondling of her or his sexual organs and encouraging her or his fondling of the sexual organs of others. That such abuse occurs to boys as well as girls is now well documented (Finkelhor, 1979, 1984). Furthermore, while the prevailing evidence shows that violence is primarily perpetrated by men on women and children, the incidence and situation of women and children as perpetrators must be addressed in order to understand the problem more clearly and to cope with it more effectively.

This book uses a broad definition of violence in the home. "Violence" refers to behavior that involves the direct use of physical aggression against other household members which is against their will and detrimental to their growth potential. This includes behaviors of homicide, beatings, and forced sex.

Despite their societal significance, situations of population management that affect life at extreme ends of the continuum of the life cycle are not the subject of this book. Hrdy and Hausfater (1984) reason that infanticide is but one point in a continuum of contraception, abortion, direct killing of an infant, or nutritional neglect of a child; these acts differ only in the stage of the reproductive cycle at which curtailment of parental investment occurs. At the far end of the life cycle emerge other issues that relate to care of the severely disabled elderly for whom technology extends life far longer than before by expending far more of society's resources. There is little research on abuse of the elderly and little societal agreement on right-to-die issues. These emotional and political subjects must be noted, however, because they have become social concerns which stimulate intense public discussion and which will be a subject of debate over public policy for decades to come.

Data on the incidence of violence in the home are hard to come by. Few offenders admit to committing such crimes, few victims are willing to say they have been assaulted, and few family onlookers will discuss family dysfunction. Family members are afraid of the social and emotional consequences of destroying the family group through public disclosure.

A number of studies of physical and sexual violence in American society show that a large proportion of victim/offender pairs are members of the same family. For example, studies of homicide indicate that between 30% and 70% of the involved persons are family members (Boudouris, 1971; Field & Field, 1973; Wolfgang, 1969). Studies of less violent acts show significant occurrences of physical abuse between husbands and wives; in a national sample of 2,143 husbands and wives, Straus et al. (1980) found that 16% reported abuse during the year studied. Physical and sexual abuse of women, furthermore, appear to be correlated; interviews by Walker (1979) with 120 battered women reveal that 59% of them felt they had been raped by their battering partners.

Estimates of the incidence of abuse of children vary widely. Zalba (1971) estimates that 200,000 to 250,000 children in the United States, 30,000 of them badly hurt, need protection against abuse each year. Gil and Noble (1967) argue that reported cases are only a fraction of the real number of abused children, which they estimate at between 2.5 and 4.1 million per year. The National Center on Child Abuse and Neglect (1981) conservatively estimates that 100,000 children are sexually abused each year and that a high proportion of the cases involve parents or other persons familiar to the child. According to Kempe (1979), sexual abuse is as damaging as physical abuse to the long-term development of children.

The ones most vulnerable to violence in the home are the least powerful in the family and in the society, that is, women and children. Gelles and Straus (1979) and Steinmetz (1980, this volume) point to the traditional superordinate-subordinate relationships of men and women, and adults and children, which hold not only in the American family situation but in other societal groups as well. These relationships allow for and condone the use of power by those of superior status. Further, men are socialized to play hard, work hard, and treat others in a rough manner. Women and children are expected to react submissively and silently. Women are not only victimized, they are also blamed for their victimization and they do not have the socioeconomic supports which would enable them easily to leave the abusive relationship.

The most likely perpetrators, recent studies have shown, are those who were themselves victimized as children. Steinmetz (Chapter 3, this volume) points to the intergenerational cycle of abuse, with persons who were abused as children more often than not abusing their own children and/or spouses. Groth and Hobson (1983) write that particularly significant in the developmental histories of persons who commit sexual abuse is the high incidence of their having been sexually victimized themselves as children by parents. For the sexually victimized young male by whom sex is experienced as a way of being controlled, a method of combating the experience of helplessness as the victim is to be the more powerful victimizer.

An area of family violence that has had very little study is the relationship between nonphysical psychological aggression and physical aggression. Is male physical aggression sometimes provoked by psychological aggression of women and children? Is male physical aggression sometimes countered by psychological aggression of women and children? Does psychological aggression by the victim increase the physical aggression of the offender? The developmental progression of the violent social situation must be addressed in order to understand adequately the extent as well as the nature of the problem.

Lack of good incidence data is a serious disadvantage in understanding the problem of family violence and in educating the public about its severity and about the need for prevention and intervention. There isn't enough information on how often abuse occurs, and what subpopulations are more prone to the occurrence. Also unknown is to what extent one type of abuse, i.e., physical assault, increases the likelihood of another, i.e., sexual assault, in a family. Unclear is the extent to which normal developmental changes in the family trigger such events. While spousal violence and violence of parent to child have been addressed, the frequencies of brother-sister, child-parent, close friend or lover-family member violence have not been examined closely. What is clear, though, is that the problem is significant enough to require immediate public health attention.

Part I of this volume looks at American society itself and at the forces which encourage or discourage violent behaviors in all institutions, but particularly in the institution of the family. Part II analyzes the psychological, social, and cultural causes of violence as gleaned from the research literature.

Part III turns to clinical interventions for individuals and families; exemplary clinical programs in health, mental health, and legal settings are discussed. Finally, Part IV looks at far-reaching intervention/prevention programs focused more on social institutions than on individual behaviors. These programs involve neighborhood groups, schools, and the court system.

## VIOLENCE AND AMERICAN SOCIETY

Through stories, plays, and film, American society glamorizes the violence in its history. The Western cowboy image of a well-armed man riding tall in the saddle is a stereotype that American society views with pride. Cowboy movies extolling this image are viewed all over the world, and persons in industrialized and nonindustrialized countries alike learn about and enjoy this stereotype of the American male.

American society places value on individualism and success in competition. It emphasizes winning. It emphasizes this for children in Little League and for adults in big business. The goal of getting to the top is clear, although rules for achieving the goal are not at all clear. And the pressure is considerable for Americans, particularly men, to be aggressive, to move up. Violence is a form of aggression which can be used to obtain the goal or to compensate for failing to obtain the goal.

Daniel Glaser, in Chapter 1, uses a symbolic interactionist approach to look at violence in American society. He asks the question: What prompts the rise or decline of violence whether it occurs in homes, work places, political demonstrations, or military battles? His simple answer is "words." Words can incite or placate; they can be instigators to violence or alternatives to it.

Glaser provides evidence of traditional subcultures in American society that show higher rates of physical violence. Both the killer and the killed come from these groups, which are disproportionately male, poor, and of Latin American origin or from the South. He states further that a large proportion of murders result from quarrels between acquaintances, relatives, or friends. Research on the events preceding these killings supports the view of victim precipitation in a substantial number of the murders since in about a third of them the initial physical assault was by the one killed.

The author also points out that the great cultural equalizer, television, depicts physical violence in the majority of its programs, averaging seven violent incidents per hour. Of particular concern are the effects of television violence on children. Studies show that children tend to copy aggression when they see this behavior on the screen by persons with whom they identify; that after children see violence in films, they become less likely to call on adults to intervene when they observe aggression by other children; that the more children watch violence on television, the less they regard such behavior as misconduct.

Glaser warns that the increased grouping of human activity into large scale organizations, and the mobility of persons through many organizations in the course of their careers, increases the extent to which life is highly routinized and formalized. The American society's approval of violence in many situations, the subcultures of violence that seem to characterize portions of it, and the models of aggression appearing on American television clash with the requirements for restraint in today's work world. The school and the home are major sources of preparation for adult employment and for other activities in formal organizations that are intolerant of violence by the rank and file. When school and home are inadequate for the task, the society must provide special programs to compensate for their inadequacies.

Glaser contends that the tendency of violence to escalate and spread is evident in interpersonal, intergroup, and international relations. The accelerating rate of technological change, furthermore, makes it more urgent that organizations as well as individuals be prepared to cope rationally with new kinds of problems as they emerge. Rationality, he argues, requires the replacement of physical strife with nonviolent methods of dispute resolution; the fate of the world depends on how well humans can develop verbal alternatives to physical violence.

If the family is not performing the necessary functions of reducing violence, why is it not doing so? What is the present American family like? First of all, it is changing dramatically. The most significant social change in the last decade has been the shift of the wife from the home to the work place. The U.S. Department of Labor (1984a) reported that labor force participation of mothers with young children had quadrupled since 1950; about six of every ten mothers with preschool or school-age children were in the labor force in March 1984.

Another important change is the rapid rise of single-parent households. In 1960, according to the U.S. Department of Commerce (March, 1983), 88% of all children lived in families with both parents present. In 1975 this had dropped to 80%, and in 1983 only 75% of all children under age 18 lived with two parents.

Still another significant change is the leveling off of the birth rate. Since 1940, but especially over the last decade, families have become substantially smaller and the variety of living arrangements has increased (U.S. Department of Labor, 1984b). Today's school-age and preschool children are more likely to be living with one parent or a stepparent and are more likely to have a working mother.

In Chapter 2, Laura Lein addresses the implications of these changes. She points out that the public frequently blames families for the strains on individuals engendered by working women and marital breakup. The public blames women far more often and more strongly than men. Service workers, most often women, who provide direct services to families, are also under increased pressure and are also blamed for family disorders. Lein emphasizes that the most frequent sources of family disorder are, in actuality, lack of adequate income, heavy responsibilities for spouses, and lack of expertise. These deficiencies may make it difficult or impossible for families to fulfill all the responsibilities for which society holds them accountable.

Lein argues that any effective effort to reach out to families in stress requires more knowledge about the stresses that occur rather than a simplistic placing of blame on family members or family service workers. She views the family as an integrated economic, political, and social institution, and asks how the responsibilities of the family in each of these domains can be fulfilled in today's world. Her response is to advocate a helping rather than a judgmental approach to family problems.

Several schools of thought deal with the role of the family in modern society, and particularly with the role of women in the family. Carl Degler (1980) is representative of those historians who view women as trapped in a special dilemma. Only a woman can carry, bear, and breast-feed a child in infancy, and mother/child bonding occurs in the early years of a child's life. Degler and others see these demands placed on women and the values that justify them as incompatible with the values of equality, individualism, and merit which operate outside the family.

Feminist social scientists, such as Nancy Chodorow, challenge such a view. Chodorow (1978) does not regard women as either the oppressors or the victims in family life. She argues that women mother because they have been mothered by women and that men, because they are mothered by women, have thereby reduced capacities to carry out a parenting role. Recognizing that the present sex-role system has created widespread discomfort and resistance in American society, Chodorow's solution for social equity is the elimination of the present organization of parenting in favor of a system of parenting in which both men and women are held responsible.

A more tempered view of the tensions between persistent family commitment and important social values is expressed by the sociologist Mary Jo Bane (1976). Bane asserts that the facts about marriage, child rearing, and family ties in the United States today provide convincing evidence that family commitments are likely to persist in our society. Bane does not see family ties as archaic remnants of a disappearing traditionalism, but rather as persistent manifestations of human needs for stability, continuity, and affection. While acknowledging that at the present time these family commitments generate persistent stress between traditional parenting values and the more contemporary values of sexual equality and equality of opportunities for women and children, Bane argues that the historical trend has long been toward greater equality and that the trend is unlikely to change. She urges recognition of the stress and of the need to design creative ways to live with both sets of values.

In Chapter 3, Suzanne Steinmetz provides an overview of the extent of violence in the modern American family. She reports that recent studies show that between one-half and three-fourths of all women have probably experienced physical violence from partners at least once in the relationship. In terms of violence to children, spanking is reported in between 84% and 97% of all families, and a nationwide study finds that 8% of children have been kicked, bitten, or punched and 1% beaten each year. Sibling violence is reported to occur in 63 to 73% of homes. Only now are studies beginning to appear on violence to elderly kin, who increasingly will be living in the home due to the increase in longevity and in cost of nursing home care.

Steinmetz systematically explores the evidence in the literature for some of the factors commonly associated with family violence: mental illness, substance abuse, and socioeconomic status. Analysis of research findings shows that mental illness is comparatively unimportant as a factor. Few batterers show mental illness or personality characteristics very different from a cross section of the general population. Actual relationships between alcohol and violence appear to be controversial. In some societies the use of alcohol is associated with considerable violence; in some, no relationship is found; and in others, violence is associated with alcohol under certain conditions. By comparison, income level appears to be consistently related to violence. Violence decreases as income levels increase. Unemployment and part-time employment of the male head of household is predictive of family violence, with the male using violence as a mechanism of social control at a time when he is unable to perform expected social responsibilities.

## CAUSES OF FAMILY VIOLENCE

If the function of the family is to love, to nurture, and to support its members, then violence in the family is incompatible with its function. Why does it occur? Theories of the causes of family violence have changed considerably over time. In some of the early clinical discussions of the problem, the female victim and her vulnerabilities were blamed: She fantasized the attack, wished for the attack, enjoyed the attack, and was too weak to protect herself from it. Only recently has the offender been looked at carefully as an individual person and also as a collective of persons who aggress against those in less powerful positions because they view this behavior as their right. The sociocultural factors in this justification of large-scale victimization of women and children is just beginning to be studied in depth.

Those anthropologists and biologists who have studied infanticide in animals and humans have provided some important insights into evolutionary aspects of family violence. Over the past decade, the intellectual pendulum in behavioral biology and related disciplines has swung from the earlier view, that infanticide could not possibly represent anything other than abnormal and maladaptive behavior, to the current view that in many populations infanticide is a normal and individually adaptive activity.

Dickemann's (1984) critique of current research on human infanticide in both industrialized and nonindustrialized societies provides concepts and classifications for systematic analyses. Dickemann notes the occurrence in human populations of all four of the hypothesized functions of infanticide in animals identified by Hrdy and Hausfater (1984): exploitation of the infant as food resource by consumption of the young or by birth spacing; reduction of competition for available societal resources; reduction of competition for breeding mates; and more effective parental management of the family as a social group.

Hrdy and Hausfater (1984), in reviewing ethnographic and historical sources, conclude that the most reliably documented cases of infanticide in humans involve parents and are best described as parental manipulation or reproductive management of their progeny. In contrast to other primates, but similar to some birds and fish, close relatives tend to be the perpetrators. Among humans, one or both parents appear to make conscious or unconscious appraisals of the cost of the infant, probable current and future demands on parental resources, alternative uses to which those resources might be used, and future breeding options. The infant's own survival and breeding or marriage prospects may also be taken into account in decision making.

Whiting, Bogucki, Kwong, and Nigro (1977), using materials on ethnographies encoded in the Human Relations Area Files, examined infanticide for 84 societies in which reliable data on the behavior were available. They found that in one-third of the societies infanticide is reported as a means of eliminating defective offspring. Birth spacing is another frequently mentioned reason for infanticide. In 72 societies for which it was possible to make a judgment, 36% reported the practice of killing an infant born too soon after its older sibling. The likelihood of this event was greatest in hunting-gathering-fishing societies, which tend to be nomadic, and relatively low in settled pastoral and agricultural ones. Such cross-cultural findings have led to a fairly general consensus among anthropologists that infanticide by parents has deep roots in human history, and has probably been a part of human adaptive processes since Pleistocene times.

In this volume, three behavioral causes of family violence are examined in detail. The first cause involves psychological needs and motives, which are reflected in interpersonal violence between individuals. The second cause involves societal needs and those social structures, statuses, and roles which encourage or discourage family violence. The third cause involves cultural values which legitimize violence in the family and in all societal institutions.

Lenore Walker, in Chapter 4, reviews major psychological theories of domestic violence. Early psychological theories of wife abuse presented women as masochistic and as provocative of their own abuse; thus, psychological counseling was directed at persuading women to stop behaving in such dysfunctional ways. This "blame the victim" interpretation is unsupported by empirical evidence. Attribution theory postulates that battered women are more likely to attribute causation of events to powerful others and uncontrollable forces. Contradictory results of studies of battered women's perceptions of the locus of control, however, suggest that attribution theories require further testing. Another psychological theory, that of cognitive dissonance, postulates that battered women begin to doubt their own reality and substitute a male world view for their own in an attempt to reduce conflict. This theory is yet to be tested. Aggression theorists have examined whether the interaction between victims and aggressors can stimulate further aggressive behavior. In her own research, Walker has found that while battered women may contribute to reinforcing their own abuse, they usually do so unwittingly in their attempts to stop the violence.

According to Walker, social-learning theories yield the most information consistent with available empirical and clinical findings. In these theories, violence is seen as learned aggressive behavior that is continually reinforced, because punishment for the behavior is not consistently applied.

Walker also finds sociological and cultural theories of violence helpful to the understanding of domestic battering. McCall and Shields, in Chapter 5, employ largely sociological theories in their systematic analysis of seven forms of domestic violence, each of which may be either nonsexual or sexual in expression: husband to wife; wife to husband; father to child; mother to child; sibling to sibling; younger to elder; and date to date (courtship).

McCall and Shields interpret the evidence of each form in terms of 11 theories: feminist; cultural; subcultural; family organization; systems; resource/exchange; interactionist; sex role; intergenerational transmission; victim precipitation; and stress/isolation. Except in the case of nonsexual abuse of husband to wife, these theories unfortunately have been tested on only one or two forms of abuse at most. The incidence and nature of three forms of abuse (sibling to sibling, younger to elder, and date to date), furthermore, are largely undocumented in the research literature.

These authors conclude that the research findings about various specific forms of family violence do not add up to an adequate understanding of the overall phenomenon. In addition, they point out that attention devoted to the principal theoretical problem within the sociology of family violence—i.e., to explain how family violence is even thinkable—has deflected attention away from the key questions asked in applied or policy-oriented research. These questions concern variations among groups in the approval of violence and identification of those aspects of family functioning which promote or constrain the direct use of physical force within families.

In Chapter 6, David Gil looks not at the group dynamics of the family itself but at the culture in which the family exists. His thesis is that violence in human relations, including violence in the family, is rooted in institutionalized inequalities of status, rights, and power between the sexes, and among individuals, ages, classes, races, and peoples. These inequalities violate the individual development of persons and brings forth violent reactions from oppressed individuals and groups. Furthermore, the inequalities in human relations and social institutions are not the result of freedom of choice by individuals and groups who are victimized. Rather they are the consequences of the more powerful social groups' use of coercion, which has become institutionalized into legal systems and justified through mythology, religion, philosophy, ideology, and history.

Gil's thesis contends that the coercive processes by which social inequalities are established tend to induce violent responses from individuals and groups who are exploited. In turn, violent reactions from oppressed groups tend to lead to intensified repressive reactions on the part of dominant groups, and to vicious circles of ever-escalating violence and repression, consonant with Glaser's view mentioned earlier.

Gil maintains that the only way to overcome these violent interactions on every level of society is to transcend socially originated and maintained inequalities. His analysis concludes that life in the United States involves frustration of fundamental human needs. To overcome family violence, particular needs must be addressed by the society so that all families within it can benefit.

By and large the various psychological, social, and cultural theories of family violence discussed in these chapters appear to be compatible. Their general consistency leads to the conclusion that a comprehensive theory of violence at home must take into account factors at these several levels, placing individual functioning within the social group and within the cultural norms by which the group operates. Violence at home occurs when social and psychological needs and expectations of the individual are unsupported by either the family or by other social institutions, and when violent modes of expression seem to be both eminently available and legitimate to the individual.

## CLINICAL INTERVENTION PROGRAMS

In this section some exemplary clinical interventions, along with their conceptual underpinnings, are described by medical personnel experienced in providing services to those affected by family violence. Clinical interventions with adult and child victims and with child witnesses to violence in the home are presented. These programs are not limited to medical settings; they involve other settings in which medical personnel work closely with personnel from social service and legal agencies and with the family and the school.

In Chapter 7, Carol Nadelson and Maria Sauzier report that violence in a family usually takes several forms: physical abuse of a wife is often accompanied by physical abuse of a child; physical abuse of either is often accompanied by sexual abuse. Not only are individuals who are abused in childhood more likely to abuse as adults, but individuals who see abuse in childhood are more likely to abuse as adults.

The impact of abuse on battered women, according to these authors, involves somatic symptoms of asthma, gastrointestinal upset, and chronic pain, as well as psychiatric histories of depression, drug overdose, and suicide attempts. An important point made by Nadelson and Sauzier is that, although abused women often have multiple medical contacts over many years, they tend not to discuss the abuse with their physicians nor do their physicians ask about possible cause of their problems.

According to Nadelson and Sauzier, intervention usually involves short-term and issue-oriented crisis counseling with the goal of restoring the victim to her or his previous level of functioning as soon as possible. Counselors, however, must also consider the possibility of long-term symptoms such as are seen in post-traumatic stress disorders, since the onset of symptoms may be delayed for months to years after the abusive situation.

These authors report on a model family crisis program for sexually abused children which draws on classic crisis theory. The goal of the intervention is both to relieve the individual's current distress and to strengthen his or her capacity to withstand future stresses. Crisis theory suggests that these goals are best met by intervening soon after the crisis situation develops; the objective is to engage the client in therapeutic work while she or he is most accessible to change.

This model program involves a four-pronged approach to the problem: 1) investigation, substantiation, and case management, performed by the state agency responsible for child welfare; 2) clinical services, which may be necessary at any stage of contact with sexually abused children and their families; 3) judicial system involvement, with the decision about whether to prosecute made at a multidisciplinary conference which includes the mental health worker caring for the child and family; and 4) advocacy in various forms, including (a) consciousness raising with the public, the legislature, and health care and human service providers, on the prevalence of the problem of sexual abuse of children; (b) education of the public, especially parents and health care providers, on presenting symptoms, elucidation of suspicions, and the most helpful responses to revealed abuse; and (c) prevention programs in schools, health care systems, and the mass media.

The authors emphasize that therapy with an incest or sexual-abuse victim and his or her family does not exist in a vacuum. Cooperation and consultation with other agencies involved are crucial and include work with child protective personnel investigating the allegations of sexual abuse and offering services after substantiation, and work with the judicial system in providing testimony and in providing guidance and support to those victims and families who are testifying.

In Chapter 8 Howard Levy, Stephen Sheldon and Jon Conte present a systems approach to intervention in child-abuse cases. They describe the system as a composite of professional groups which include health and mental health, social service, and judicial and law enforcement agencies, each of which has a specific community role to play in responding to violence. The authors describe ways in which each of these services do or do not work, and then provide a theoretical basis for community intervention utilizing factors that are known to increase an individual's vulnerability to abuse.

Levy et al. cite the multiplicity of descriptions in the literature of risk and vulnerability factors for family violence and child abuse. They note that no one factor, or combination of factors, has been proven to be an absolute predictor of abuse. They see abuse as an interactional event, combining risks and vulnerabilities of the host, agent, and environment. Upon the conceptual foundation of vulnerabilities as early determinants of child maltreatment, they have developed a theoretical matrix to assess the likelihood of abuse in a given family over time.

Child vulnerabilities are defined in physical, emotional, and behavioral terms, including prematurity, congenital defects, hyperactivity, emotional unresponsiveness, tantrums, nightmares, and sleep disturbances. Parental vulnerabilities are defined in physical, emotional, and behavioral terms as well, but also include social situations which can cause stress (e.g., marital strife or job instability) and poor parenting skills (e.g., lack of knowledge of child development or incompatibility of their own needs with those of the child).

Environmental vulnerabilities are defined by these authors in social-structural and cultural terms. The social-structural variables include unemployment, poverty, and lack of family and community supports; the cultural variables include the sanctioning of corporal punishment in the home and the use of force throughout societal groups.

This theoretical framework assumes the family to be composed of three interacting and overlapping spheres (child, parents, and siblings), affected by and existing within a neighborhood, town, society, and culture (the ecological unit). The spheres are constantly changing, resulting in a dynamic interaction of variables. With the use of this framework, the matrix of child, parent, and environmental vulnerabilities to child abuse provides clues for identification of the risk of abuse as well as actual occurrence. Such data should be of value to community support systems which need to direct scarce resources to those most in need.

In Chapter 9, Robert Pynoos and Spencer Eth consider intervention programs for child victims of family violence who, although not abused themselves, witness the abuse of loved ones usually by other loved ones. Large numbers of children are at risk because they have seen violent actions in the home, such as the murder of a parent, the rape of a mother, or a parent's suicide. In the uninjured child witnesses they have studied, almost 80% have shown symptoms of post-traumatic stress such as the perceived presence of a traumatic event, reexperience of the occurrence, psychic numbing, and/or incident-specific phenomena that were previously not present, such as sleep disturbances, startle reactions, and avoidance behavior linked to trauma-specific reminders.

Pynoos and Eth have developed child-interviewing techniques to assist a child to talk about a recent, extreme act of violence. The initial phase of the consultation with the child allows him or her to express the impact of the trauma in play and fantasy and through metaphor by use of free drawing and storytelling tasks. In the second or trauma phase, the interviewer shifts attention to the actual traumatic episode and supportively encourages a thorough exploration of the child's experience. In the third phase the consultant assists the child to address current life concerns with an increased sense of security and competence.

These authors report that, properly conducted within a few weeks of the violent act, this consultation can facilitate the child's acceptance of continued psychotherapy, if it is needed. This psychotherapeutic treatment makes use of three of the child's support groups: the family, the school, and the judicial system. The authors recommend that the parents or guardians carefully report the child's words and behavior. The therapist then advises the family members of ways to elicit more verbal meaning from the child about his or her responses and suggests steps they can take to ameliorate continued stress.

Liaison with the child's school, according to these authors, is essential to a successful intervention program for children exposed to violent acts. Children commonly exhibit changes in school behavior and cognitive performance that serve as indicators of the traumatic course. The behavioral change most noticed by teachers is the appearance of aggressive behavior that may progress to a conduct disorder. Cognitive performance difficulties relate to an inability to concentrate on academic tasks because of intrusive recollections and associations to the violent event.

Child victims or witnesses of crimes routinely become involved with the judicial system. Pynoos and Eth have found a continuing interaction between the course of a child's response to a violent crime and subsequent criminal proceedings. The child's efforts to master the trauma of witnessing violent acts can either be enhanced or impeded by required judicial participation. As part of their consultation, therefore, these authors follow children from the initial police investigation through testimony in open court to the sentencing of the defendant.

In each of the chapters in this section, clinicians emphasize the need to join forces with professionals in other disciplines and to work with social institutions in an effort to assist the victim and the victim's family. They speak further of the need for change in social systems themselves, particularly the legal system, which will protect the individual's physical and emotional well-being. Changes within the individual alone are not enough; social institutions must also change so that individuals may be free to pursue their goals and make full use of their skills.

## COMMUNITY INTERVENTION PROGRAMS

In addition to clinical intervention programs which focus on individual family members, particularly those who have been victimized, community intervention programs attempt to assist the social institution of the family and other social institutions (educational, legal, and medical) that support the family. These programs include public education efforts directed to parents and teachers, and innovative changes in legal and medical procedures for assisting the family in need.

In Chapter 10, Carolyn Swift describes family-focused programs in which human service workers and their agencies intervene with families at the microcosmic or individual level. Since human service workers generally have little control over the life stresses to which their clients are exposed, their efforts are usually focused on increasing the social supports and coping skills that contribute to increasing the self-esteem of the people they serve.

Swift emphasizes the importance of social supports for the individual's healthy functioning and their role in buffering the destructive effects of stress. Self-help groups and early intervention programs for parents expecting a first child exemplify this strategy. Educational interventions, such as parenting courses and workshops for the unemployed, are also useful because they usually involve meetings with groups of peers and professionals in leadership roles. In addition to standard sources of social support, Swift notes two supportive processes, each of which involves families in different ways: the process of parent-infant bonding, and the legislative process and related enforcement practices.

Most intervention programs for families include some sort of skill component. Swift points out that the incidence of family violence in the society at large will be little affected by skill-building programs targeted only to specific families, since sex-role stereotyping and discriminatory laws and customs, if unchanged, will continue to contribute to intrafamilial violence. However, skill building with individual family members may reduce their personal risk for victimization. Community workshops, parenting courses, and other similar interventions are designed to increase the capacity of family members to resolve stressful situations, such as unemployment and parenting problems. Skill-building interventions are useful in facilitating normal developmental passages from one life stage to another. Such interventions may also reduce risk status in individual situations. Arming individual women and children with escape, avoidance, or physical defense techniques may well reduce the risk status they occupy because of their sex or age.

Swift focuses on a skill that is critical to the prevention of family violence, namely the control of anger and aggressive behaviors. Anger has received comparatively little attention from researchers. Although anger and aggression are not the same, Swift argues that the arousal of anger increases the probability of aggression. A prevention approach for individuals at risk for developing abusive behavior is training in anger and conflict management (Novaco, 1977). The first phase of this approach is cognitive preparation, in which participants begin learning to identify the situational cues that arouse their anger. These cues include perceptions of others' intentions, imminent pain, or personal injury or loss.

The second phase of this approach is that of skill acquisition, involving the ability to reinterpret the anger-arousing situation in ways that reduce or eliminate the angry response. Applied to families, this skill means that parents learn to hold in check their anger responses long enough to realize that their child's misbehavior may be accidental, due to hunger, fatigue, or something else over which the child has little control.

The third phase is that of application and practice, and the procedures used are essentially those of desensitization. The learner is exposed to situations that have aroused anger in the past, and the newly learned skills are tested in these familiar situations.

The most powerful intervention and prevention programs take place at the macrocosmic, or social-institutional level, with interventions designed to change social institutions which assist or impede family functioning. Lisa Lerman's Chapter 11, on innovations in the criminal justice system, deals specifically with the prosecution of wife-beaters; a parallel analysis of programs focused upon the prosecution of child-beaters remains to be done.

Lerman points out that in the last several years, experimental programs and demonstration projects have increased the use of formal criminal charges in domestic assault cases, while there has been a move away from mediation, crisis intervention, and similar informal procedures used in family violence cases during the early 1970s. Through close coordination with mental health agencies, and through the development of extensive victim services, prosecution has become an appropriate and a desirable legal remedy for many battered women. Innovative programs emphasize the importance of enforcement of court orders, penalties, and rehabilitative measures.

Lerman states a number of reasons why prosecution may be the appropriate course in domestic abuse cases. First, failure of the criminal justice system to enforce the law against abusers contributes to the perpetuation of violence within families. Battering can no longer be regarded as an individual problem; it must be viewed as perpetuated in part by the inadequate responses of legal institutions. Second, some prosecutors have made changes in policy and procedure that demonstrate that the criminal courts can protect victims of abuse and can require batterers to change their behaviors. Third, if family violence becomes a priority for prosecutors, police response to battered women may be greatly improved. And last, unless prosecutors change their policies and take a more active role in protecting battered women, they may be subject to civil liability for denial of equal protection to battered women or for the wrongful death of battered women who have sought assistance from prosecutors and have been refused help.

Lerman also views diversion or deferred prosecution as a viable alternative to traditional criminal case processing. In such instances, prosecution is suspended while a defendant completes a counseling program. Successful completion of the program results in dismissal of charges. Diversion of domestic violence cases provides a means of obtaining control over a group of defendants who have largely eluded criminal justice intervention. The leverage obtained over batterers admitted to a diversion program may be used to require participation in a mental health counseling program focused on stopping violence and/or alcohol abuse. Few batterers voluntarily participate in counseling, but they may accept treatment ordered by the courts.

Diversion programs can be established by statute, by court rule, or by administrative policy. While statutory authority is not needed to set up a diversion program, implementation of statewide programs can be facilitated by legislation which lays out procedures for diversion. Comprehensive legislation on diversion of domestic violence cases has been passed now in several states.

Public concern at the present time focuses particularly on intervention programs intended to control or prevent violence toward children. In Chapter 12, David Finkelhor reviews educational programs designed to prevent child sexual abuse. Finkelhor reports that prevention activities in this area relate to a broad spectrum of children. This strategy has been encouraged by two important facts emerging from contemporary research on sexual abuse. First is the fact that boys are subject to victimization as well as girls in an estimated ratio of one to three (Finkelhor, 1984). Thus, prevention education is usually conducted in mixed classrooms, and both boys and girls are used as models in the media. Second is the fact that children are victimized at a very early age; estimates from some research indicate that a quarter of all abuse occurs before age seven (Finkelhor, 1984). This highlights the need to bring prevention to very young children.

Finkelhor mentions special populations of children who need special approaches, particularly children who are handicapped or who have already suffered victimization. Prevention curricula, specifically intended for disabled adolescents, take account of the fact that parents and the rest of society give less basic sex information to them. Children who have already suffered victimization are at high risk for reabuse, and treatment programs emphasize prevention skills as excellent vehicles for restoring their sense of security and self-esteem.

In addition to direct approaches to children, some current prevention programs are aimed at parents. Finkelhor writes that education from parents themselves or from other trusted sources provides children with learning experiences that classroom presentations cannot equal. However, Finkelhor's own research shows that parents do not provide such information in an accurate and useful way. Some of the inadequacies of current parental handling of sexual-abuse prevention are apparent from his survey in the Boston area in which only a minority of parents said they had ever had a discussion with their children specifically related to the topic of sexual abuse. Even when such discussions occurred, they often failed to mention the possibility of abuse by an adult acquaintance (Finkelhor, 1984).

In his analysis of the difficulties that parents have in teaching their children about sexual abuse, Finkelhor concludes that some parents do not visualize sexual abuse as a serious risk to their children. They are afraid of unnecessarily frightening them and/or they have a difficult time talking to their children about sexual topics of any kind.

Finkelhor identifies the organizational concerns that inhibit community education for children and their parents. He feels that the successful prevention programs define their goals not merely in terms of developing a teaching unit, but in terms of community organization. They have thought through political and organizational issues, and although their ultimate goal may be the education of children, much of the initial effort is directed to the community. Successful programs generally attempt first to create the proper climate for gaining entrée into a community by developing a cadre of influential people who support the use of the program and who can lobby on its behalf.

The last decade has given rise to a considerable number of innovative community programs for both victims and offenders. These intervention programs usually entail cooperation among several institutions: community organizations, schools, the legal system, and the mental health system. There have also been exemplary uses of public education directed particularly to children, who should learn of their rights, and to persons in the community, who will stand behind their rights. These programs deserve analysis which will reveal the degree of their effectiveness among various populations and community groups.

## DISCUSSION

Each of the chapters in this volume provides insights into the need for further research, innovative services for victims, and specific social policies related to the prevention of family violence. All of the chapters emphasize both the complexity of this public health problem and the absolute necessity of interdisciplinary work to address it effectively. Some specific research, service, and social policy implications are presented here. These and others are discussed more fully in the ensuing text.

## Research

The analysis of violent behavior in the family should begin with a consideration of the biological and psychological needs of individuals. What role does the family play in responding to these needs, and what is the interplay, or lack of interplay, between the family and other social groups?

From such perspectives there emerge further questions about an individual's frustrations and stresses resulting from factors such as malnutrition, illness, economic insecurity, overwork, and community isolation, and how they impact on the individual to contribute to spouse and child abuse. What are the ways in which a society's values and beliefs permit, condone, and institutionalize such behavior? Interrelationships between victim vulnerabilities, family dynamics, and community beliefs as they contribute to violence in the home deserve study as do the nature of family strengths and coping mechanisms which allow persons successfully to withstand stresses and misfortunes.

Attention should be given to the evaluation of health, mental health, and legal services to victims and offenders. Crisis and long-term treatment and service delivery modes, as well as integrative services among health and mental health, social, and legal agencies, demand more investigation. Studies of prevention strategies focused on interpersonal situations and/or institutional arrangements are also important.

Difficult methodological issues are encountered in researching family functioning. While it is relatively easy to obtain basic demographic data on families, especially those which are not functioning well and have become clients of public agencies which collect records, it is more difficult to obtain data on interpersonal relationships, attitudes, and values among a community sample of families. Important to such research is the analysis of data by class, occupation, and racial and ethnic groups, because such groups receive different societal opportunities and rewards, and they share different social beliefs and goals. Clear definitions of what constitutes violent behavior, particularly with regard to child abuse, are required of all such research. Sensitive instrument measures that achieve both reliability and validity, and adequate measures for protecting human subjects in this research, still must be devised.

Despite the methodological problems, it is essential that researchers continue to investigate family functioning and family violence as a major form of dysfunction. This research is important not only for theoretical reasons but for the humane reasons of defining and evaluating services that the society should be providing to all families as well as to those families in distress.

## Services

The provision of services for victims was spearheaded in the last ten years by the women's movement, which first expressed public outrage at family violence and which established rape crisis centers and shelters for battered women throughout the nation. The general consensus of mental health practitioners is that these women's centers have been highly beneficial to abused women and children. They provide victims with access to counselors and an environment of safety, dignity, and understanding. Close networking with other community agencies usually provides women with a choice of options. Although research evaluation of such programs is weak, detailed descriptions of exemplary programs are available.

Services to victims afford them social supports and coping skills. The value of supportive relationships for healthy functioning and their role in buffering the destructive effects of stress have been extensively documented and have demonstrated that skill building among individual family members can reduce their personal risk for victimization.

In addition to social services which aid the individual in handling his or her situation more adequately are legal programs which ensure the individual's enforceable right not to be beaten or raped. By taking the firm stand that battering is a punishable crime against society, prosecutors have been able to protect individuals from repeated attack. They have also been able to communicate to abusers that family violence will no longer be treated as a private matter.

Of special concern are services for children who may be victims or witnesses to victimization. Professionals working with children emphasize the need to allow them to express the impact of trauma in play and fantasy. They also emphasize the need to interconnect their services to children with the children's families, schools, and communities. For children who experience court proceedings, support throughout this additional trauma must be provided.

Because of limited funds for those in need, it is imperative that more efficient and compassionate methods of selecting clients and of ensuring them access to the health and welfare system be developed. This requires the cooperation of a number of community support groups and provisions for the training of health, mental health, and legal personnel in understanding and responding to the problems.

## Social Policy

Researchers and service providers alike have pointed out the great need for institutional intervention in family violence. The society, however, has not really addressed adequately in this century norms regulating the use of force. It is ambivalent about the uses of capital punishment, police brutality, and corporal punishment. It is also reluctant to adopt any well-defined, coherent family policy for the American population, which is composed of many racial, ethnic, and religious groups.

Substantive changes in social institutions are needed in order to provide equal rights for women and children, rights which are basic to the reduction of domestic violence. Women and children must be viewed and treated as persons entitled to the full protection of the Constitution, including protection of their minds and bodies. These rights, valid for all persons in the society, should include eligibility for treatment of physical and emotional ill health. They should include access to education according to his or her individual capacities. They should also include opportunities for meaningful participation in work.

The criminal justice system has successfully experimented with new methods of prosecution which show that certain procedures can reduce case attrition and increase conviction rates in domestic violence. The relative uniformity in the outcomes of these experiments form the basis for several recommendations. In order to reduce case attrition, prosecutors should adopt a policy that denies a victim's request for dismissal of an abuse case once charges have been filed. Prosecutors should relieve the battered adult victim of the obligation to file complaints. Prosecutors should sign the complaints and subpoena victims prior to trial. To prevent intimidation of the battered adult victim who becomes a complaining witness, prosecutors should request that the pretrial release of suspected batterers be conditioned on a no-contact order. Where violence has been serious and chronic, prosecutors may have no choice but to recommend incarceration.

Women's advocacy groups in the area of child abuse, sexual abuse, and battering can be looked to as models for the development of a victims' rights movement in this country. The President's Task Force on Victims of Crime (1982) and the Attorney General's Task Force on Family Violence (1984) are recent, important examples of federal and local attempts to define the problems and identify effective ways in which they can and should be addressed. There is a need for more groups to provide public education which speaks not only to the negative outcomes of family violence but to the positive effects of proper family interaction and conflict resolution.

While there is ample evidence to show that more research, services, training of service workers, and innovative social programs are needed to combat this major public health problem, these activities alone will not make a decisive difference. As long as girls and boys are treated differently from the time of birth in terms of the cultural artifacts given to stimulate them (i.e., guns for boys and rag dolls for girls) and later on in terms of the demands made of them (active competition in sports for boys and passive, polite, or subordinate roles for girls), there will be male offenders and female victims within the family, and outside of the home. As long as the society condones adult sex-role discrimination, awarding males far more opportunities and freedom than those afforded females, it will have violence.

The glorification of violence in the mass media, popular magazines, comic books, etc., and the constant presentation to children through television of adult combat and crime and cartoon violence, only legitimize violence. Crimes of violence are presented as permissible and exciting ways of controlling people; retribution through violence is also extolled.

What will make a substantial difference in the amount of family violence is the commitment of people to dignity, respect, and justice for all individuals. The public and private, professional and lay efforts described in this book demonstrate such commitment. Collectively they provide a basis for optimism that the problem of violence in the home is not unsolvable, that American society is able to effect change.

## REFERENCES

Awad, G. (1976). Father-son incest: A case report. *Journal of Nervous and Mental Diseases,* 162(2), 135–139.

Bane, M. J. (1976). *Here to stay: American families in the twentieth century.* New York: Basic Books.

Boudouris, J. (1971). Homicide and the family. *Journal of Marriage and the Family, 33*(4), 667–676.

Chodorow, N. (1978). *The reproduction of mothering: Psychoanalysis and the sociology of gender.* Berkeley: University of California Press.

Degler, C. (1980). *Women and the family in America from the Revolution to the present.* New York: Oxford University Press.

Dickemann, M. (1984). Infanticide in human populations: Societal and individual concerns. In G. Hausfater & S. Hrdy (Eds.), *Infanticide: Comparative and evolutionary perspectives.* New York: Aldine.

Elmer, E. (1971). Child abuse: A symptom of family crisis. In E. Pavenstedt (Ed.), *Crisis of family disorganization*. New York: Behavioral Publications.

Field, M. & Field, H. (1973). Marital violence and the criminal process: Neither justice nor peace. *Social Service Review, 47*(2), 221–240.

Finkelhor, D. (1979). *Sexually victimized children*. New York: The Free Press.

Finkelhor, D. (1984). *Child sexual abuse: Theory and research*. New York: The Free Press.

Fontana, V. (1971). Which parents abuse children? *Medical Insight, 3*(10), 16–21.

Gelles, R. & Straus, M. (1979). Determinants of violence in the family: Toward a theoretical integration. In W. Burr (Ed.), *Contemporary theories about the family, Vol. 1*. New York: The Free Press.

Gil, D. (1970). *Violence against children: Physical child abuse in the United States*. Cambridge, MA: Harvard University Press.

Gil, D. & Noble, H. (1967). Public knowledge, attitudes and opinions about physical abuse in the U.S.; No. 14, Papers in Social Welfare. Waltham, Massachusetts, Florence Heller Graduate School for Advanced Studies in Social Welfare, Brandeis University.

Groth, A. N. & Hobson, W. F. (1983). The dynamics of sexual assault. In E. Revitch (Ed.), *Sexual dynamics of anti-social behavior*. Springfield, IL: Charles C Thomas.

Hrdy, S. & Hausfater, G. (1984). Comparative and evolutionary perspectives on infanticide: Introduction and overview. In G. Hausfater & S. Hrdy (Eds.), *Infanticide: Comparative and evolutionary perspectives*. New York: Aldine.

Kellum, B. (1974). Infanticide in England in the later Middle Ages. *History of Childhood Quarterly, 1*(3), 367–389.

Kempe, C. H. (1979). Recent developments in the field of child abuse. *Child Abuse and Neglect, 3*, 9–15.

Langer, W. (1974). Infanticide: A historical survey. *History of Childhood Quarterly, 1*(3), 353–367.

Lystad, M. (1982). Sexual abuse in the home: A review of the literature. *International Journal of Family Psychiatry, 3*(1), 3–31.

Lystad, M. (1984). Family violence: A mental health perspective. *Emotional First Aid, 1*(2), 48–57.

National Center on Child Abuse and Neglect (1981). Child sexual abuse: Incest, assualt and sexual exploitation. DHHS Publication No. (OHDS) 81-30166. Washington, DC: National Center on Child Abuse and Neglect.

National Institute of Mental Health (1982). Television and behavior: Ten years of scientific progress and implications for the eighties. Washington, DC: DHHS Publication No. (ADM) 82-1195.

Novaco, R. (1977). A stress inoculation approach to anger management in the training of law enforcement officers. *American Journal of Community Psychology, 5*(3), 327–346.

President's Task Force on Victims of Crime: Final Report (1982). Washington, DC.

Radbill, S. (1968). A history of child abuse and infanticide. In R. E. Helfer & C. H. Kempe (Eds.), *The battered child*. Chicago: University of Chicago Press.

Steinmetz, S. K. (1977). *The cycle of violence: Assertive, aggressive, and abusive family interaction*. New York: Praeger.

Steinmetz, S. K. (1980). Women and violence: Victims and perpetrators. *American Journal of Psychotherapy, 34*(3), 334–350.

Straus, M. A., Gelles, R. J., & Steinmetz, S. K. (1980). *Behind closed doors: Violence in the American family*. New York: Doubleday.

Swift, C. (1977). Sexual victimization of children: An urban mental health center survey. *Victimology, 2*(2), 322–327.

Swift, C. (1979). The prevention of child sexual abuse: Focus on the perpetrator. *Journal of Clinical Child Psychology, 8*, 133–136.

U.S. Attorney General (1984). Task Force on Family Violence: Final Report, Washington, DC.

U.S. Department of Commerce. Bureau of the Census (1983). Marital Status and Living Arrangements. Washington, DC, Series P-20, No. 389.

U.S. Department of Labor, Bureau of Labor Statistics (1984a). News Bulletin, USDL 84-321. Washington, DC.

U.S. Department of Labor, Bureau of Labor Statistics (1984b). *Families at work: The jobs and the pay*. Bulletin 2209. Washington, DC.

Walker, L. E. (1979). *The battered woman*. New York: Harper & Row.

Whiting, J., Bogucki, P., Kwong, W-Y, & Nigro, J. (1977). Infanticide. Society for Cross-Cultural Research Newsletter, No. 5.

Wolfgang, M. (1969). Who kills whom. *Psychology Today, 3*(5), 54–56, 72–75.

Zalba, S. (1971). Battered children. *Transaction, 8*(9/10), 58–61.

# VIOLENCE IN THE HOME:
## *Interdisciplinary Perspectives*

# Part I

# VIOLENCE AND
# AMERICAN SOCIETY

# 1

# *Violence in the Society*

## Daniel Glaser

Just as violence committed by any individual cannot be well understood without knowing the violence in that person's home and other life situations, these settings are only well comprehended by taking into account the social and cultural influences upon them. This chapter discusses the interrelationships of violence in small and large groups, as well as at local, national, and international levels.

### INTRODUCTION: COMMON FEATURES IN
### ALL HUMAN VIOLENCE

What prompts the rise or decline of violence wherever it occurs, whether in homes or in work places, in political demonstrations, or in military battles? *Words*. Words that incite, words that placate, words that create or dissolve agreements, words said and unsaid, as well as physical actions that are perceived as expressions of attitudes as though they were words.

Verbal ability is what most distinguishes human mentality from that of other animals, and makes possible the development and accumulation of scientific knowledge and literature over the centuries to characterize what is called civilization. Yet humans demonstrate their similarity to other animals when a sudden and unexpected loud noise startles them. People are physiologically activated for fight or flight by the noise, as any dog, cat, bird, or other animal in the vicinity would be. In all of these creatures, adrenalin is automatically released into the bloodstream, and muscles are reflexively tensed. Humans, however, soon use this aroused energy to try to tell themselves what happened. This search for words to describe and explain, and hence to guide and justify conduct, distinguishes human reactions from those of other animals. The words with which we react to an experience, both those with which we talk to ourselves to interpret events or circumstances, and those with which we communicate to others, can be either instigations to violence or alternatives to it.

Some acts of physical aggression against other people are impulsive outbursts while some are planned and dispassionate, or as we say, some are "hot-blooded" and some "cold-blooded." These extremes of emotion or reason reflect the mixing in variable proportions of the two sources of violence indicated above:

1) physiological activation that humans share with other animals in reacting to whatever startles, disrupts, frustrates, angers, or otherwise arouses them; and
2) verbally expressed ideas to justify the use of violence, ideas communicated overtly to others or only covertly to oneself, and distinctive of humans.

Of course, everyone also has ideas about the impropriety of violence in certain circumstances, ideas that usually prompt them to inhibit impulses to act violently. Furthermore, people differ greatly in how immediately and how completely they superimpose on their purely physiological arousal their interpretation of their situation, and their ideas on what conduct is proper there. However, all types of physical assaults among humans also share two other features:

1) violence tends to evoke counterviolence; and
2) violence in one setting or relationship tends to spread to others.

These two features characterize all types of violence, whether between individuals or among groups of any size, including nations. They imply that unless it is interrupted and replaced by other methods of dispute resolution, violence tends to escalate and to become more widespread.

The foregoing minitheory will be the basis for analyzing more elaborate theories and observations summarized in this chapter. The above perspective is grounded in the symbolic interactionism approach to social psychology (Blumer, 1969; Mead, 1934), but it is compatible with both symbolic interactionist and psychophysiological theory on emotions (Hochschild, 1979; Mednick, 1977), as well as with behavioral formulations of social learning theory (Baldwin & Baldwin, 1978; Bandura, 1971).

The future of humanity depends on how well the two sources and two features of violence summarily listed above can be controlled. The problem of reversing escalation and spread of violence, whether between individuals or among groups or nations, is basically the same everywhere: How can physical force be replaced by verbal interaction? Achieving purely nonviolent resolutions of disagreements in all settings requires adequate and sufficiently widespread development of appropriate 1) cultural environments, 2) social controls, 3) dispute resolution procedures, and 4) personal skills. Filling each of these requirements is difficult, but progress in accomplishing any of them will facilitate achievement of the others.

## CULTURES AND SUBCULTURES OF VIOLENCE

The term "culture," as used by anthropologists and sociologists, refers to the shared contents and habits of thought that humans acquire from their elders and associates, and pass on to their progeny. Its principal component is the language that members of a society share, but also important are its ideas on science, art, religion, and morality, and its preferences in food, clothing, and manners. It is a nonbiological inheritance transmitted by communication and example to everyone reared or living long and intimately in a society. It changes from small modifications by many people, but few, if any, individuals alone can alter it greatly.

Broad ideas of good and bad conduct shared in a society are called its cultural values. Specific ideas of proper conduct that do not have strong moral implications, such as men's and women's hair styles or people's eating habits, are called norms. Culture includes words, ideas, values, and norms, but not the people who share and transmit them (although it is often carelessly used to refer to a people as well as to their shared thought).

### National, Tribal, or Ethnic Cultures of Violence

Marked and persistent differences in rates of violence among societies are often presumed to reflect contrasts in their cultural values regarding assaultive conduct. For example, killing is morally obligatory in certain circumstances in some societies, as a defense of one's honor or of that of one's family, while in other societies this would be morally condemned as an extremely evil act. Ruth Benedict's *Patterns of Culture* (1934), which contrasted the peacefulness of the Zuni Indians in New Mexico with the hostility and violence among natives of the Island of Dobu in Melanesia, did much to revive scientific status in anthropology and psychology to the study of relationships between culture and personality, a field that has long been beset by unscientific expressions of ethnic stereotyping and prejudice.

The United States, and the 13 colonies that preceded it, was a land of immigrants whose living conditions fostered more lethal violence than England had or any of the other countries from which they had come. Gun ownership was a monopoly of the aristocracy in Europe, but colonial America was unique in averaging at least one gun for every adolescent or adult male. These weapons were used for hunting since wild game was the principal source of meat, and hides and furs were used for clothing or export, but guns were also kept for protection from marauders (Kennett & Anderson, 1975).

The settlers feared the native Indians, and they especially feared the African slaves whom they imported, primarily in the South. Also evoking fear were the thousand or more British convicts sentenced each year during the colonial era to transportation to America. To recoup the cost of passage the sea captains were authorized to sell the convicts as indentured servants for a term of labor, but many of these ex-convicts then escaped and fled into the wilderness (Rusche & Kirchheimer, 1939). The successive influx of new immigrant groups, as well as ethnic group migration within the country, has repeatedly aroused in American communities fear of people who seemed different, and violence against them.

Throughout the eighteenth and nineteenth centuries, and even in the twentieth century, the prevalence of guns, especially in frontier areas, frequently prompted Americans to take the law into their own hands. Vigilante groups were organized, and ruthless mobs often developed, expressing their anger or prejudice against alleged offenders. They claimed to be seeking justice, but their objectives often seemed to be to rob and plunder, particularly when their targets were ethnic minorities who were newer immigrants. Also, the European custom of dueling to settle differences was maintained, especially in the South, and on the frontier it evolved into the quick-draw gun fights celebrated in today's television and movie Westerns (Brown, 1969a, 1969b; Frantz, 1969; Hofstadter & Wallace, 1970; Lane, 1976).

During the nineteenth century in the largest and oldest cities, especially New York, slum areas developed where the poorest and newest immigrants were concentrated. Here the law was especially weak, and violence was used for political and economic domination. From the 1870s on it could also be said that "the United States has had the bloodiest and most violent labor history of any industrial nation in the world" (Taft & Ross, 1969, p. 270). Throughout its history this country has had recurrent individual and group assaults on people because of their ancestry, their economic or political strivings, or for some combination of these reasons. For many decades it has repeatedly been estimated (with statistics of variable precision but improving in recent years) that this country has the highest murder rates of any of the technologically advanced nations.

While the United States thus appears to have always been a nation with norms and values encouraging violence, it should be noted that this allegation has often been made also against other nations, as well as against separate tribal groups within some countries. Mexico, Colombia, Guatemala, and some other Latin American nations have usually had higher homicide rates than the United States. This is often ascribed to an emphasis in their cultures on *machismo*, or manliness, which for males means attaching virtue to toughness, physical strength, daring, and dominance over females, as well as emphasizing the preservation of one's honor, which is deemed a justification for violence in response to insult (Heller, 1966). Bohannon (1960) described African tribal cultures with extreme contrasts in norms and values on killing.

One easily supported criticism of charges that an entire nation or tribe has a violence-supporting culture is the fact that there are always some segments in every society with relatively less violence than others. Thus, Wolfgang and Ferracuti (1967), while explaining the readiness to commit murder in Mexico as due to a "fatalistic acceptance of death," assert that both this resignation to what they presume is their destiny and the high homicide rates are found only in the lower socioeconomic classes in Mexico.

The term "subculture" refers to a pattern of thought and custom that is shared and transmitted only within a particular group in a society, a group that also shares other aspects of the dominant culture, such as the language. Cultures are always changing, and they are spread only by contact and communication among peoples who have different cultures. Consequently, if a group of people are largely isolated from others with the same culture, the isolated people are likely, in time, to develop some variation of the original common culture. For example, they may still speak the same language but with local accents or dialects.

A basic principle of anthropological and sociological theory that this author calls the Law of Sociocultural Relativity is that social separation fosters cultural differentiation. This explains not only the many different languages, foods, clothing styles, and other components of cultures that differentiate total societies, but also the subculture variations within each large nation, such as regional dialects, and local cooking or clothing styles. Several types of subcultures of violence that have been said to characterize parts of the population of the United States, therefore, should be considered separately.

## The Alleged Southern Subculture of Violence

The southeastern corner of the United States that formed the Confederacy in the Civil War has long had higher rates of homicide and aggravated assault known to the police than any other major segment of the country, although it has lower rates of property crimes than the national averages (FBI, 1935–1984). That there is a regional subculture in the South is indicated by the Southern accent in speech, and by the particular foods that comprise Southern cooking.

The South's cultural distinctiveness can be largely accounted for by the fact that from the end of the Civil War through World War II, it was the poorest area of the country and had the highest birth rate. Therefore, migration was predominantly out of the region rather than into it, so that its residents maintained and evolved their culture little affected by the rest of the country. This has largely changed since World War II, however, with Florida and Texas especially becoming relatively prosperous states, many people moving to the South from elsewhere in the country, national mass media reducing differences in local cultures, and regional rates of violent crime becoming less dissimilar although by no means disappearing.

Much has been written supporting the thesis that norms and values fostering violence became more prevalent in the Southern subculture than in most other parts of the country:

> . . . the image of the violent South confronts the historian at every turn: dueling gentlemen and masters whipping slaves, . . . lynching mobs, country folk at a bear baiting or a gander pulling . . . , panic-stricken communities harshly suppressing real and imagined slave revolts, robed night riders engaged in systematic terrorism, unknown assassins, church burners. . . . The image is so pervasive that it compels the attention of anyone interested in understanding the South. (Hackney, 1969, p. 479)

Until the post-World War II expansion of its highways, the South retained much more of a frontier atmosphere in its rural areas than did the northeastern or north central states because travel in the South was impeded by mountains, woods and swamps. However, its cities and their hinterlands were linked because most of the Southern economy was based on rural products and on the replenishment of its urban labor supply from the rural population.

Southern whites often blame the regional violence rates on blacks, but Hackney (1969) shows that in all years for which data are available, homicide rates were higher for whites in the South than in other regions of the country, and they were also higher in Southern rural areas than in rural areas elsewhere. In addition, he shows that the percentage of families owning firearms is much higher in the South than in other areas of the nation. He demonstrates by partial correlations that a Southern location is more predictive of a state's homicide rate than is its percentage of population urban, median age, median years of school completed, per capita income or unemployment rate.

Gastil (1971) also shows that not only did the South have the highest murder rates in the country throughout the nineteenth century, but that its penalties for murder were less extreme than those elsewhere. With more recent data he assigned an index of "Southernness" to all states based mainly on the percentage of their population that was of Southern origin, and demonstrated that this index accounts for more variance in state homicide rates than median income, percentage of population urban, and median age.

One of several types of challenge to subcultural explanations for Southern violence rates is the claim that homicide is determined more by "structural poverty" than by regional differences in cultural values. Loftin and Hill (1974) showed that if states are classified by their rates of *extreme* poverty, for which the percentage of the population with annual incomes under $1000 was one of several indexes, extreme poverty accounted for variations in state homicide rates as well as Southernness. The Blaus (1982) showed that an index of inequality in income, the Gini Coefficient, and also an index of income differences between races accounted more adequately than Southernness for variations in homicide rates in the 125 largest metropolitan areas of the United States. Williams (1984) pointed out errors in the work of some critics of the Blaus' findings, but also found that with the Blaus' data there was still some increase in homicide rates with Southernness that was not fully accounted for by the income inequality in the South.

Responses to survey research questions have been compiled by Erlanger (1975) to challenge the Southern violence subculture thesis, but they also give it some support. A 1966 survey in Milwaukee found that northern-born black men reported having had more fistfights as adults than did those born in the South who had the same amount of education. Both black and white men in rural North Carolina report less of such combat than did men of the same racial groups in Milwaukee. A 1965 national survey that asked whether anyone in the household over 13 years old had been assaulted seriously in the past year received a smaller percentage of affirmative answers in the South than in other regions.

Erlanger also notes that a few years later a national survey asked men between 21 and 65 years old if they could imagine situations in which they would approve any of six types of violence, for example, a teenage boy punching another boy of his age, a husband slapping his wife, or a husband shooting his wife. The percentages of positive answers to these questions were the same or lower in the South as in other regions. On the other hand, Erlanger reports that the same survey found that men in the South more often than men elsewhere said that they had been threatened or cut with a knife as adults. Southerners also led the rest of the country in approving the spanking of one's children, corporal punishment in schools, and gun ownership.

Doerner (1978) found from a national questionnaire that "lifelong residency in the South increases both the probability of owning a gun and being opposed to gun control" (p. 52), but is not significantly related to having "ever been threatened with a gun, or shot at," "ever been punched or beaten by another person," or asserting that you can imagine situations "in which you would approve of a man punching an adult male stranger" (pp. 51, 56). In comments published with this Doerner article, Loftin and Hill point out a so-called ecological fallacy that also applies to their article (1974), and that is that one may readily get erroneous results in applying aggregate data for areas to the "microlevel processes" implied in subcultural explanations for individual violence. Also, in his comments published with the Doerner article, Gastil questions whether the "brawling" to which the survey questions refer can be equated with homicide.

One can only speculate on the reasons for such diversity of response patterns in surveys, and for their deviance from the fact that the South has led in rates of actual homicides and aggravated assaults recorded by the police. One possible answer may be that the average Southerner more often than most other Americans accepts values justifying an attempt to kill someone in some circumstances of serious insult or challenge to one's honor, and believes in rigid discipline for children, but also maintains norms of greater courtesy and consideration than prevail elsewhere, and consequently does less fistfighting.

The anthropologist Lundsgaarde (1977), investigating all deadly assaults reported to the Houston police during an extensive period, found that when there was what the police regarded as legitimate provocation, such as adultery, the crime was not classified as murder and sometimes was not prosecuted at all. It may also be pertinent that while the South has had both the highest rates of murder and the highest rates of capital punishment in the years for which records are available in the United States, for the well over 90% of its convicted murderers whom it did not execute, it had the shortest terms of imprisonment (Glaser, 1979; Glaser & Zeigler, 1974). Possibly this ostensible contradiction expresses a prevalence of less outrage at murder or reverence for life in the South than elsewhere, at the same time that it has stronger norms than prevail in the rest of the country on kindly gestures, courtesy, and respect for the property of others.

Perhaps the strongest indication that Southern rates of homicide are a function of learned subcultural values is some old evidence that Southerners maintain such lethal violence even after they move out of the South. Pettigrew and Spier (1962) show that state rates of death from homicide for blacks in the Midwest during the 1950s could be predicted with a significant degree of accuracy by the homicide rates for whites in the states in which the blacks were born. About 95% of murders then were found to be by people of the same race as their victim, so the black murder victims in the Midwest then were probably killed by other blacks: however, the Pettigrew and Spier data strongly suggest that the black murderers share a subculture justifying homicidal violence with the whites in the states from which they came.

## *The Alleged Subculture of Poverty*

Both for Mexico and for the southern United States, evidence was cited that the high rates of homicide distinguishing these areas was concentrated in the poorest segments of their populations. The anthropologist Oscar Lewis, from studies of very poor people in Mexico, Puerto Rico, and elsewhere, concluded that with poverty there is " . . . a subculture with its own structure and rationale, as a way of life which is passed down from generation to generation . . . that transcends regional, rural-urban, and national differences" (1966, p. xliii). According to Lewis, people from this subculture acquire a fatalistic view of their experiences, as well as authoritarianism and justifications for violence.

Lewis also claimed that this subculture of poverty fosters female domination of child rearing. Therefore, he contended, boys reared in this subculture, controlled almost entirely by females but seeing adult men use violence to dominate their women, emphasized masculine toughness by violence during adolescence and young adulthood as a means of asserting their independence from their mothers and other females. A similar explanation has been given for violence by boys in black slum communities of the United States (Hannerz, 1969; Liebow, 1967), where nearly half the households with children have no resident fathers. Horowitz and Schwartz (1974) report the same emphasis on manliness among boys in Mexican-American slums where most of the homes have both parents present, but the Lewis thesis of maternal domination of child rearing in the Mexican culture of poverty might explain their "masculine protest" behavior.

One type of critique of subculture of poverty theory is the claim that the behavior of the poor that Lewis describes is not due to a subculture but to the circumstances of extreme poverty, such as the absence of savings and frequently even of food, as well as the absence of political power (Valentine, 1968). With such desperate helplessness, it is contended, people lose all stake in conformity to whatever happen to be the dominant values of their society, and simply live for immediate gratification, from day to day. Such critics view violence, in the short run at least, as a rational way of coping with the circumstances of extreme poverty. That this view is too simple, however, is suggested by the many poor communities that have much less violence than others which are not as poor.

Merton (1968) contended that it is not the absolute degree of poverty that generates discontent, but relative deprivation, that is, having much less than what the cultural norms of one's community define as appropriate. Such deprivation fosters what Merton, following Durkheim (1897), called "anomie," a state of weakened influence of cultural norms that fosters nonconforming conduct. That relative deprivation is associated with violence is suggested by the studies of the Blaus (1982) and of Williams (1984) showing that inequality of income in a metropolis is highly predictive of homicide rates. An earlier study found that all types of crime rates in metropolitan areas could be predicted by the ratio of people with over $10,000 annual income to those with income less than $3000, as well as by the extent to which the percentage of blacks in white-collar jobs was below the national average (Eberts & Schwirian, 1968).

Durkheim (1893) ascribed the rigidity of a society's "collective conscience"—his term for cultural values—to the uniformity and homogeneity of roles and relationships in its people. He ascribed anomie, or the weakening influence of these values, to the loss of such traditional and uniform relationships (Durkheim, 1897). During the 1960s in Kampala, Uganda, before that country was taken over by the dictator Idi Amin, sociologists Clinard and Abbott (1973, 1976) found much lower homicide rates in the poorest neighborhood, in which almost all residents were of the same tribe, had few incomplete families, and visited neighbors frequently, than in a neighborhood of much higher median income in which residents were of several different tribes and there were many transient and incomplete families who kept aloof from each other. Similarly, in American slum areas the neighborhoods settled by Oriental groups, such as the Chinese, Japanese, and Koreans, always had lower rates of violence than slum neighborhoods without the family and community cohesiveness of these Oriental groups, even when the median income of the Orientals was less than that of the residents of the higher crime-rate slum areas.

Lewis (1966), who also studied poor populations in India, asserted that deprivation does not generate the culture of poverty in caste societies, in which each group accepts its lot as divinely ordained and improvable in an afterlife or reincarnation by being accepted in this life. He sees the values of the culture of poverty as an adaptation to deprivation in a competitive society with highly individualistic ideologies that encourage efforts at self-betterment.

One may infer that great poverty relative to the standards of income achievement in one's community weakens cultural regulation of personal conduct, hence fostering violence. One may also conclude that such an influence of relative poverty may be effectively countered by close social bonds among people with the same cultural background whose shared beliefs make them more accepting of their circumstances. These bonds may also foster considerable mutual aid, both economic and in the supervision of childrens' conduct. The thesis that there is a culture or subculture of poverty, however, implies that people in communities where economic conditions are much worse than prevails in the rest of their society develop and share behavioral norms and values that they can meet. This could help them to think well of their daily achievements, hence of themselves and each other.

Rodman (1963) asserted that in the United States the lower socioeconomic classes share the values of the middle class as to the kinds of behavior that are desirable, but "stretch" these values to tolerate a larger range of conduct, including violence, than the middle class will accept. By this stretch, Della Fave (1974) pointed out, the poor gain more satisfaction in life than they could otherwise attain. The stretched values are cultural traits, rather than a mere adaptation to momentary circumstances, insofar as the people who acquire these values tend to maintain them collectively even when their economic conditions improve.

## Violence as Masculine Subculture

In most human, as well as in most other mammalian societies, violent behavior is reported to be more frequent in the male than in the female of the species. This gender difference is usually ascribed to a division of labor made necessary by the female's long periods of incapacitation for violence when pregnant or with nursing infants. For the species to survive during these periods, the male has to do most of whatever fighting is necessary for a mixed gender group's defense or food procurement. Such gender specialization and its contribution to species survival are enhanced by secondary sex traits that endow males with greater development of those muscles and types of hormones that aid in violent behavior.

In humans, of course, there is much variation in physical strength and agility within each gender, with some women certainly more capable of interpersonal violence than many men. In addition, one "contribution" of human cultural development is the gun, which has appropriately been nicknamed an "equalizer" because it reduces the significance of differences in physical strength for capacity to inflict lethal violence.

That differences in the behavior between men and women is more than a product of biology becomes evident when one observes how children are reared. Toy guns and other weapons are provided primarily for boys, with girls receiving dolls and other toys that cast them in maternal and housekeeping roles. The most violent sports, especially boxing, wrestling, and football, are organized almost exclusively for boys even in these days when girls participate more extensively and more diversely in sports than they formerly did. In general, boys are expected to respond physically to being pushed around or challenged to a fight by their peers, while girls are encouraged to be dignified and ladylike.

Gender contrasts in conduct norms are especially evident in one-sex schools and camps. Indeed, it is in all-male communities, such as traditional armed forces units, prisons, and merchant ships, that competition in expressing masculinity by violence, if necessary, seems most evident. In these settings and elsewhere, however, males are expected to become much more polite and genteel when girls or women are present. During the late 1970s and the 1980s, when most traditionally one-sex organizations became co-ed, a decline in violence was often reported.

Although the proportion of females in the United States who were arrested for homicide doubled between 1935 and 1965 according to the F.B.I.'s annual *Uniform Crime Reports* (1935–1984; in later years renamed *Crime in the United States*), and continued to rise thereafter, the proportion of males arrested for these lethal acts increased by about the same percentage. Therefore, for several decades almost 7 out of 8 arrestees for homicide have been males. The proportion of men among arrestees for robbery—the taking of property by force or threat of force—has only diminished slightly in this period, remaining about 12 out of 13. As societal evolution reduces differences in our culture's prescriptions for behavior by males and females, the correlation of violence with masculinity should diminish, but thus far this is not evident in official reports on rates of extreme violence.

A major reason for the great differences in violent crime rates between males and females is the different ways they express their emerging independence as young adults. The highest crime rates occur in the teens and early twenties, which is for both genders a period of striving for a sense of adulthood and of independence from parents or other adult figures. Boys can gain this sense of adult autonomy by violence, as well as by property crimes and other offenses, but for rebellious girls the easiest way to feel like an independent adult is to attract the company and attention of males. Therefore, adolescent delinquency and adult crime by females are primarily in sexual pursuits; the complaints against them in juvenile courts are mostly "incorrigibility," which usually means that their parents cannot keep them home at night, and in the courts for adults it is prostitution, but most heterosexual activity by young women does not involve lawbreaking. Males have their peak rates of violence as juveniles or young adults, and the earlier they began, the greater is the probability of their being again violent at any later age.

Insofar as contrast between males and females in norms and values on violent behavior are accepted by both sexes, these differences are part of the societal culture rather than of a masculine subculture.

## *Discussion*

That much homicide in the United States reflects shared subcultural values is suggested by the fact that the killer and the killed come from the same high-violence rate groups, which are still disproportionately poor and of Latin American or southern United States origin.

Further support for subcultural explanations of violence comes from investigation of the large proportion of murders that result from the escalation of quarrels between acquaintances, relatives, or friends. Reports on the events that precede these killings indicate that all who are involved in the quarrels share the same values that regard it as obligatory to respond by physical force to insults or to challenges to one's manhood. Indeed, in about a third of the murders in which the person who struck the first blow is known, the murder has been called "victim-precipitated" because the initial physical assault was by the one who was killed (Curtis, 1974; Voss & Hepburn, 1968; Wolfgang, 1958). Chance alone or quicker access to a lethal weapon often determines who is the killer and who is killed.

Violence also appears to be more frequent in situations where all cultural influences are weak, so that norms and values that might inhibit aggression are weak. This appears to be quite imperfectly correlated with poverty, but most closely associated with the absence of close personal ties with people who maintain cultural values proscribing violence. In urban and transient populations, especially where people of the same cultural background do not comprise the bulk of the population of a neighborhood and maintain close-knit families or other institutions of their own, the social control of individual behavior by a group's culture is diminished.

In the United States today, the majority share values opposing violence in most interpersonal relations. This may explain why: 1) only a small proportion of a random sample of the adult population will admit engaging in violence, 2) a still smaller proportion will express approval of violent conduct, and 3) the correlation between admitting violent behavior and approving such behavior is weak (Ball-Rokeach, 1973).

A culture's components, the shared ways of thought that guide behavior, change at variable rates and in unpredictable ways that cannot be ascribed to the influence of any separate person. An individual's maintenance of cultural traits may be altered by new learning experiences, but until this occurs, they tend to become habitual, and thus are not changed immediately when one moves to a different setting. Learning results from the communication of ideas, yet much of the communication that may affect thought today is not received in face-to-face interaction, but by other means.

## THE MASS MEDIA AS SOURCE OF VIOLENCE

Many people were disturbed when the National Commission on the Causes and Prevention of Violence (1969) reported that about 8 of 10 fictional programs on television depict physical violence. They average about 7 violent incidents per hour, and about 6 out of 10 of these incidents involve the use of weapons, but in only about 2 out of 10 of these incidents are there indications that the violence is followed by lawful punishment of the aggressor. The most violent programs were reported to be children's cartoons, which average 20 incidents of physical aggression per hour. More recently, a study that monitored the 109 most viewed programs in British Columbia, of which 76% originated in the United States, found that they averaged 9 acts of physical aggression per hour, 7.8 incidents of what was called ''verbal aggression'' per hour, and rarely any other method of dispute resolution, with only about 2% of the physical violence being accidental (Williams, Haertel, & Welberg, 1982).

Despite such evidence of the persistently frequent display of physical aggression on television, there has been much controversy as to its impact on the behavior of viewers. It has been pointed out that Grimm's *Fairy Tales* and innumerable other children's stories from time immemorial, as well as Shakespeare's plays and most of the other classics of literature, are filled with violence. As Aristotle pointed out in his *Poetics* (McKeon, 1941), the "tragic pleasures" of fear and pity are the most moving emotions evoked by drama, and of course, violence arouses such feelings most intensely. On the other hand, it has been contended that motion pictures, especially now that they are intimately viewed on home television, present violence much more vividly and realistically than can be done in literature or even in stage dramas.

Scientific research and theory by psychologists and others has produced somewhat contradictory evidence and inference. The *catharsis theory*, which goes back to Aristotle but is related to psychoanalytic perspectives, contends that everyone has aggressive impulses which they tend to express, but that they can satisfy these impulses vicariously by identifying with people whom they watch acting violently on the screen or in athletic contests, and they will then be less aggressive in their own behavior. Research that was interpreted as supporting this theory found that seeing violent films did not change the answers that college students gave on questionnaires which probed for evidence of aggressiveness in word associations or in attitude scales (Feshbach, 1961; Feshbach & Singer, 1971).

Critics have questioned the measurement procedures of these studies supporting catharsis theory. They have found increased aggressiveness in responses by college students after seeing physical assaults on films (Berkowitz, 1962), and especially in the changed responses of lower-class boys after seeing violent films (Liebert, Neale, & Davidson, 1975). Others had shown much earlier that allowing aggression by children under controlled circumstances, which catharsis theorists had assumed would reduce their aggression in other settings, reduced only the inhibition of aggression (Nighswander & Mayer, 1969). Indeed, there is much evidence to support a *modeling theory*, that children tend to copy aggression when they see it done on the screen by persons with whom they identify. For example, Bandura (1973, Chapter 2) found that after seeing violent films, children were more assaultive towards a plastic punching bag, and in a controlled experiment inmates in cottages of a youth correctional institution were found to be significantly more aggressive after seeing violent than after viewing nonviolent films (Leyens, Camino, Parke, & Berkowitz, 1975).

These short-run results of viewing violence are called *cueing* or *trig-gering* effects. They are also indicated when certain movies depicting youths in an orgy of violence are found by theater managers and police to be followed regularly by outbreaks of vandalism and fighting among adolescents in the audience. Phillips (1983) showed that a short-run spurt in homicide followed each heavyweight boxing championship fight in the United States between 1973 and 1978.

A *desensitization* theory contends that the long-term effects of exposure to violence in the mass media is indifference to aggression, and hence more tolerance of its occurrence. Evidence supporting this theory includes the fact that physiological arousal, as measured by the galvanic skin response (GSR), frequently occurs when people see violent events on the screen, but that this arousal declines and remains at a low level the longer they watch such violence (Howitt & Cumberbatch, 1975). Also, controlled experiments showed that after children saw violence in films, they became less likely to call on adults to intervene when they observed aggression by other children that was staged by the researchers (Thomas & Drabman, 1975).

Support for a desensitization view of the impact of television watching on children is also provided by a Dutch study (van der Voort, Vooijs, & Bekker, 1982). Its data showed that the more that children watch violence on television, the less they regard such behavior as misconduct. Also, those who watched more "realistic" television violence have more difficulty distinguishing between television and "real life" violence. These effects, as well as fright from television violence, diminished as children became older.

There is still general acceptance of the conclusions from an early British study (Himmelweit, Oppenheimer, & Vince, 1958) that children are least disturbed by violence in movies if 1) it is stylized or done in a manner or setting very different from real life, as occurs in cartoons and in Westerns; 2) it is done against obviously very bad people; and 3) the events are clearly make-believe, but not eerie or spooky. On the other hand, modeling of violent events in movies, television, or the news seems to be reported most often when the people portrayed are ordinary, they are in familiar settings, both the good and the bad are struck from behind or otherwise completely victimized and are unable to resist a violent attack, or the crimes are committed very easily and successfully wtih a gun or by pretending to have a gun or a bomb.

Of course, most people do not become violent when they see, hear, or read about aggressive behavior by others; it is generally presumed that most people triggered to violence by the media are disturbed individuals who are already inclined to delinquent or criminal activity. The correlation between violence rates and poverty may be supported by the fact that teenagers from low-income homes, as well as their parents, watch more television than children or adults in middle-class homes, and are more likely to say that what they watch depicts life as it "really is" (Greenberg & Dervin, 1970). This type of evidence supports the arguments by many that people accept from the mass media only the ideas and attitudes that are consistent with what they already feel and believe, and consequently their behavior is not affected much by what is available on the screen.

On the other hand, billions are spent by advertisers and propagandists on television because they have objective evidence that they thereby influence how people think, purchase, and vote. It seems unlikely that nothing on the screen except the commercials affects behavior. Furthermore, there is evidence that television viewing in excess of 10 hours per week impedes schoolwork, especially in girls and in high-IQ children (Williams et al., 1982), and it has long been established that poor schoolwork is associated with all types of delinquency, including violence (Hirschi, 1969; Polk & Schafer, 1972). Yet television viewing of up to 10 hours per week was correlated with improved schoolwork (Williams et al., 1982), and it is obvious that there is much that is instructive in the media. While the prospect of censorship of the screen by the state is distasteful in a free society, more control of viewing in the home and more private as well as government support for superior educational television might well be endorsed as a means of staving off violence.

## SOCIAL CONTROLS AND PROCEDURES TO REDUCE VIOLENCE

The results of a controlled experiment in police reactions to domestic violence has contradicted the belief common in the caring professions that reaction to aggression by physical coercion is likely to be less effective than purely verbal interventions (Sherman & Berk, 1984). Researchers trained Minneapolis police in three alternative methods of response in cases of domestic violence: arrest, advice, including informal mediation, and ordering the suspected aggressor to leave the house for eight hours (to avoid arrest). Calls for police assistance in such cases were then randomly assigned to police instructed to use only one of these three modes of reaction.

A six-month follow-up of this experiment showed less violence following the arrest than following the other alternative responses. These results were consistent whether the results were measured by subsequent reports to the police of violence in these households during these six months, or by self-report of the alleged victim when interviewed six months after the initial complaint. Only 3 of the 136 arrestees were formally punished by the courts, but most were detained for over eight hours before being released, and apparently the fact of arrest and the prospect of a more severe penalty if rearrested sufficed to deter recidivism.

Because most of the alleged offenders against whom action was taken in this experiment had had prior domestic violence and other delinquency and crime records, and because there may be other unique features in the sample or in police procedures in Minneapolis, it would be inappropriate to conclude from this experiment that arrest is always likely to be the most effective government intervention in violence.

Nevertheless, there have been many instances where government use or threat of coercion has been necessary as a first step to getting people who dominate others by physical force to develop alternative procedures for dispute resolution. In the histories of most countries, some organizations at one time had used physical force to pursue their political, economic, religious or ethnic interests, and their violence tended to escalate until firm action was taken, usually by government, to require their use of verbal procedures to resolve their quarrels.

Labor strife was once violent in virtually every country, and it still is in many. It usually begins with assaults on organized workers or their leaders by a company's or the government's armed personnel, and this evokes counterviolence by labor groups. The escalation of such conflict was most intense everywhere when the disputed issue was the workers' right to organize and to bargain collectively, rather than issues of pay, hours or working conditions. In all of the developed democracies and some other countries, the frequency and intensity of violence in labor disputes have now been greatly reduced, if not eliminated, as a result of firmly established collective bargaining, mediation or arbitration procedures.

The tendency for violence to spread is indicated by the evidence that in those unions in which violence by or on behalf of employers was most used, not only was there the most counterviolence by the unions against employers or strikebreakers, but there was also the most violence over the years in struggles for power within the union. In the United States the Teamsters, the United Mine Workers, and some of the construction craft unions have had this history of much external and internal violence. They contrast with the histories of the more democratic unions, such as those in the printing and clothing industries, and in recent years, the United Auto Workers. Routinely peaceful labor relations seem to require a commitment to democratic and legal procedures by both labor and management. This commitment may grow now that there is a trend in the United States, following prior developments in Scandinavia and West Germany, to have interpenetrating democracies, that is, union representatives on company governing boards and company representatives in union organizations.

The tendency of violence in one relationship to spread to others is also illustrated in the history of many countries by organizations that initially conducted guerrilla warfare and terrorism in pursuit of their ideals, but eventually used it instead to rob, extort and kidnap for personal income and power. The Mafia in Italy, the United States, and elsewhere evolved from peasant organizations for revolt against exploitation by absentee landlords in Sicily, but they now use violence to corrupt unions, segments of political parties, businesses, and other organizations (Servadio, 1976). There are also many reports of guerrilla movements currently in Lebanon, Colombia, and other countries, initiated idealistically to combat tyrannically repressive governments, but eventually splintering into numerous small units, some of which became bandit gangs. This sequence in violence has been frequent throughout recorded history, according to Hobsbawm's (1959, 1981) classic accounts.

By far the most horrendous example in human history of the escalation of violence, and of its shifts from one target to another, is the record of Hitler's Nazis. Beginning as a small political party in the 1920s with beer hall and street roughness against their political opponents, their violence escalated and spread year by year, their brute force effective in expanding their power within Germany during the mid-1930s and in most of the European continent during the mid-1940s. Only a crushing counterforce, followed by a rule of law—of words—in Germany could reverse their escalation and spread of violence.

Nothing since the Holocaust compares to the Nazi outrages, but events in many countries have repeatedly demonstrated that habitually thinking of other people in a category, rather than as diverse individuals, can create indifference to extreme violence against those who are thus categorized. Making sweeping derogatory generalizations about all people in a particular racial, national, religious, political, or other group is a first step towards treating them inhumanly.

Any group that is treated violently as a whole tends to be unified thereby, and most groups then mobilize for counterviolence, either by themselves or by any force that they can mobilize on their behalf, such as the police. Any group that cannot argue peaceably about its complaints to lawful and responsive executive, legislative, or judicial bodies, or to the electorate, is likely to resort to recurrent and escalating intergroup violence. As with interpersonal violence, strife between organizations can only be resolved peacefully if there are appropriate agencies to facilitate free communication, and to enforce just laws.

Nations are but larger groups. Italy, Greece, Egypt, Israel, India, China, Latin America, and most other parts of the world have ruins of ancient civilizations, all destroyed, damaged, or plundered by wars. Technological advancement has only increased humanity's power to destroy cities and other human constructions, a power that has more than doubled every 20 years in this century. Wars today can produce more vast and devastated ruins. Each of the two major powers has tens of thousands of nuclear explosives, each of these separate explosives able to make a city uninhabitable, and the explosion of several hundred in a short war could create enough radioactive dust around the world to destroy most human and other life on the earth's surface.

The generalizations that were made at the beginning of this chapter on common features in all violence interrelate physical aggressions, whether they are between nations, smaller groups, or individuals. For example, the tendency for violence in one relationship to spread to others is shown by the eventual involvement of other countries in most wars that start between two countries, but also in the demonstration by Dane Archer and Rosemary Gartner (1976) that interpersonal violence increases during and after wars.

One highly pertinent fact in considering all types of violence is that *there has never been a war between two countries with elective governments* (Babst, 1964, 1972). This often overlooked fact seems to be applicable to all recorded history if one defines an elective government as one in which a majority of at least the adult male population can vote by secret ballot to select the nation's legislators from a slate of alternative candidates. Britain achieved elective government, so defined, only after its Great Reform Bill of 1832, and France during the periods when it was a republic. Britain fought France and the United States only before these dates. No international war has ever been waged between elective governments, although there have been civil wars and colonial independence wars in which one side was fighting such a government but claimed that it planned to establish its own elective regime if it won.

One can only speculate as to why elective governments have not warred against each other, but this author suspects it is because these nations make most of their major decisions only after relatively open and prolonged legislative debate that is fairly well reported and discussed in the mass media. In each country this process creates diverse alignments of opinion that cut across national boundaries, creating a high prospect of eventual negotiation and some compromise of their differences. As with interpersonal and intergroup strife of all types, open discussion reduces the risk that quarrels will escalate to the point where physical force is used to try to resolve them. Increasing the use of democratic procedures in all relationships, however, requires that more of the population be trained in and accustomed to their use.

## PERSONAL SKILLS AND VIOLENCE IN A SOCIETY

Thinking about what one should do or how one should act, like other thought, requires effort. People become tense and anxious if they are long in a situation in which they are uncertain about how they should behave. They struggle in deciding what would be an appropriate line of conduct, and in performing it. Once they make a decision about how to act, are absorbed in carrying it out, and encounter no difficulties in it, their tensions are relieved.

An emotional outburst is one way to get instant relief from thinking. Psychologist Patricia Brown (1983), of Australia's University of Melbourne and Melbourne Children's Court, finds that delinquents, when compared to nondelinquents, are generally deficient in verbal ability, thus deficient in capacity to think about their conduct. Consequently, most delinquents from an early age on find complex discussion frustrating and try to avoid it by acting impulsively. She finds that violent children tend to dislike language that is more complex than emotional expressions; therefore, they tend to adopt a "no-think" policy of immediate action in stressful circumstances. Their conduct is less well-planned than that of nondelinquents because planning is a verbal process which the delinquents are more likely to find stressful and thus to interrupt by emotional outbursts. Such youths, she suggests, "have a tendency to cut off from verbal material when under stress," and therefore, "verbally loaded interventions such as those normally used by probation officers and therapists would be contraindicated," but "techniques which are more action-oriented, like assertion training . . . need more consideration" (Brown, 1983, p. 106). Many people never fully outgrow their juvenile behavior patterns, especially in less formal situations like their homes, where society's controls are less constraining than elsewhere.

Linguistic disabilities may reflect either physiological handicaps or learning deficiencies, or both. Weak inhibition of emotional impulses has been linked by psychophysiological research to sluggish autonomic systems (as measured by the GSR), frontal lobe damage, slow alpha wave electroencephalographic frequencies, endocrine imbalances, and abnormal blood sugar levels (Moffitt & Mednick, 1984). All people, however, learn more or less successfully to control aggressive impulses. This learning is primarily a function of the reinforcements for different types of conduct that they experience, beginning in early childhood and continuing throughout life (Bandura, 1971, 1973).

Usually the most influential reinforcements, positive and negative, for learning how to express or to inhibit emotions, are the responses of others. However, people tend to seek the companions with whom they are most gratified. Violence-prone youths tend to "hang out" together partly because they share discomfort in formal situations, and partly because they are rejected by more conventional people of all ages.

The social separation of the most aggressive delinquents from the juveniles most conforming to school expectations becomes especially evident in junior high school, and intensifies in the school years thereafter, as students who are academically oriented and those who are not have different friends. Some youths respond negatively and some positively to the school's efforts to give all of them the types of skills and habits that are necessary for executive, administrative, and professional roles in the large formal organizations of today's society.

Schools, especially at the secondary level, prepare students for upward mobility in adult occupations by emphasizing punctuality, diligence, writing ability, public speaking, and the prerequisites, such as mathematics and the sciences, for college work. This training occurs not only in classes, but also in a variety of extracurricular organizations, such as school newspapers, drama groups, student government, and teacher-sponsored clubs. Follow-up studies show that the students who do well in school and those who are most active in school organizations other than athletic teams, are most likely to be upwardly mobile in status as adults. Conversely, those who do poorly in school by any indicator—i.e., low grades, disciplinary infractions, or truancy—have a high probability of involvement in delinquency of all types, including acts of violence (Hirschi, 1969; Jensen, 1976; Otto, 1976; Polk & Schafer, 1972; Spady, 1970).

There is a sharp contrast between the behavioral requirements of formal and informal youth groups, Rita Loeb (1973) and Reuven Kahane (1975) have pointed out. These become especially evident during adolescence. Informal groups, such as a clique of friends, are uninstitutionalized, in that they change or terminate readily, whereas formal groups, such as the Boy Scouts or a high school club, have continuity as organizations especially when adults are involved in them, despite turnover in membership. Informal groups are without clear purpose other than the attraction of the members to each other's company, whereas formal groups are organized for particular purposes, and engage in activities planned to serve those purposes. Informal groups have free-flowing, face-to-face conversation, usually without intermediaries, whereas formal groups have more deliberate and orderly communication, often through representatives, and much of it in writing of memos and minutes that are cited later. Informal groups do not assign very definite roles and offices to members, as is done in formal groups. Informal groups are governed by the members who happen to exert the most personal influence, sometimes achieved by verbal or physical aggression to which others defer; formal groups are governed by more deliberate procedures, rules, discussions, and voting.

The home, as a source of vocabularies and behavior models, may greatly aid or hinder schools and clubs in their unofficial but very important instruction in resolving differences nonviolently. Although there is by no means a perfect correlation between education or occupation and parental behavior at home, children from homes in which both parents are well educated and the children of white-collar workers generally have advantages in their schools and clubs over most children with less educated parents or with parents whose work does not require verbal skill.

For children in "culturally deprived" homes, Headstart programs that provide preschool reading and writing instruction, as well as more contact with verbally fluent adults than are available at home, plus nutritional supplements tend to offset the disadvantages of the home. A 20-year follow-up of children in such a program and of children from similar homes without this program, in Ypsilanti, Michigan, found that for the former Headstart children there was about a 50% higher rate of employment, less than half as large a percentage who at one time or another in school had been classified as mentally retarded, little more than half as large a percentage who had been on welfare, and only two-thirds as high a proportion who had ever been arrested; it was estimated that every dollar spent on Headstart saved the government seven dollars in subsequent outlays ("Preschool Pays Off," 1984).

## CONCLUSION

Violence in individuals is a function of how physiological arousal is shaped by learned ways of interpreting experience, and verbally justifying behavior. The prospects of acquiring norms and values that prevent violence, as well as skills and habits necessary to settle differences amicably, are greatly affected by a person's learning environment. This environment consists primarily of one's culture, which in the United States has included much endorsement of violence since its earliest days.

Segments of our nation, insofar as they are somewhat isolated from the rest of the population, develop subcultures which, in their support for violence, vary by region, social group, and neighborhood, as well as from one home to the next in today's predominantly mixed neighborhoods. The mass media, particularly television, is a part of the learning environment, and it is packed with violence, to which children are especially sensitive.

Classrooms and formal groups, aided or impeded by home experiences, prepare youths for participation in the large government and corporate organizations of today's advanced industrial society. When these organizations work as prescribed by law, nonviolent bureaucratic and legal procedures resolve differences, and physical aggression is not tolerated. Learning to fit in them and to make them capable of peaceful change is a matter of developing procedures in government and other organizations for making effective organizational decisions. Such decision making requires an ability to resolve differences nonviolently, even differences that arouse emotion; for groups to be peaceful, all members must become habituated to interacting nonviolently even when emotionally aroused.

Acquiring such skills and habits does not guarantee that adults who are orderly in their workplace will not become violent in their homes, but it increases their ability to resolve differences nonviolently if they feel that they should or must. Often formal controls are necessary to get people to use the nonviolent dispute resolution methods that they have mastered, and the controls of the work place may be absent in the home. Indeed, the government's ultimate monopoly of force and its power to arrest may be necessary to coerce the development and utilization of nonviolent methods of interaction among some persistently violent individuals and groups. This may become necessary in any setting, even in the home.

The increased organization of human activity in large corporations, many of them parts of international conglomerates, as well as the mobility of people through many communities in the course of their daily lives, increases the extent to which life in developed countries is highly formalized. The American society's tradition of violence, the subcultures of violence that still seem to characterize segments of it, and the models of physical aggression which clog our video screens clash with the behavioral requirements of life in today's work world. The school and the home are the major sources of preparation for adult employment and for other activities in formal organizations that are intolerant of violence. When these socializing agencies are inadequate for this task, special programs are needed to compensate for their deficiencies. Such programs more than repay their cost when operating effectively in reducing violence.

The tendency of violence to escalate and to spread is repeatedly evident in interpersonal, intergroup, and international relations. The accelerating rate of technological change makes it more urgent than ever that organizations as well as individuals be capable of rationally coping with new problems as they emerge, but this rationality requires the replacement of physical strife with nonviolent methods of dispute resolution. Now that nations are equipped with weapons that can exterminate most life on earth, the fate of the world depends on how well humans can develop verbal alternatives to violence.

## REFERENCES

Archer, D., & Gartner, R. (1976). Violent acts and violent times: A comparative approach to postwar homicide rates. *American Sociological Review, 41*, 937–963.

Babst, D. V. (1964). Elective governments: A force for peace. *Wisconsin Sociologist, 3*, 9–14.

Babst, D. V. (1972). A force for peace. *Industrial Research, 14*, 55–58.

Baldwin, J. D., & Baldwin, J. I. (1978). Behaviorism on verstehen and erklaren. *American Sociological Review, 43*, 335–347.

Ball-Rokeach, S. J. (1973). Values and violence: A test of the subculture of violence thesis. *American Sociological Review, 38*, 736–749.

Bandura, A. (1971). *Social learning theory*. New York: McCaleb-Seiler.

Bandura, A. (1973). *Aggression*. Englewood Cliffs, NJ: Prentice-Hall.

Benedict, R. (1934). *Patterns of culture*. Boston: Houghton Mifflin.

Berkowitz, L. (1962). *Aggression* (Ch. 9). NY: McGraw-Hill.

Blau, J. R., & Blau, P. M. (1982). The cost of inequality: Metropolitan structure and violent crime. *American Sociological Review, 47*, 114–129.

Blumer, H. (1969). *Symbolic interactionism*. Englewood Cliffs, NJ: Prentice-Hall.

Bohannon, P. (1960). *African homicide and suicide*. Princeton, NJ: Princeton University Press.

Brown, P. (1983). Delinquency, a failure in language coping? In D. Biles (Ed.), *Review of Australian criminological research*. Canberra: Australian Institute of Criminology.

Brown, R. M. (1969a). Historical patterns of violence in America. In H. D. Graham & T. R. Gurr (Eds.), *Violence in America* (National Commission on Causes & Prevention of Violence Report). New York: New American Library.

Brown, R. M. (1969b). The American vigilante tradition. In H. D. Graham & T. R. Gurr (Eds.), *Violence in America* (National Commission on Causes & Prevention of Violence Report). New York: New American Library.

Clinard, M. B., & Abbott, D. J. (1973). *Crime in developing countries*. New York: Wiley.

Clinard, M. B., & Abbott, D. J. (1976). Community organization and property crime. In J. F. Short, Jr. (Ed.), *Delinquency, crime and society*. Chicago: University of Chicago Press.

Curtis, L. A. (1974). *Criminal violence*. Lexington, MA: D.C. Heath.

Della Fave, L. R. (1974). The culture of poverty revisited: A strategy for research. *Social Problems, 21*, 609–621.

Doerner, W. G. (1978). The index of Southernness revisited: The influence of wherefrom upon whodunit (with comments by Loftin & Hill, and by Gastil). *Criminology, 16*, 47–66.

Durkheim, E. (1947). *The division of labor in society* (G. Simpson, Trans.). New York: Free Press. (Original work published 1893)

Durkheim, E. (1951). *Suicide* (J. A. Spaulding & G. Simpson, Trans.). New York: Free Press. (Original work published 1897)

Eberts, P., & Schwirian, K. P. (1968). Metropolitan crime rates and relative deprivation.

*Criminologica, 5,* 43–52. (Reprinted in D. Glaser (Ed.), *Crime in the city.* New York: Harper & Row, 1970.)

Erlanger, H. (1975). Is there a 'subculture of violence' in the South? *Journal of Criminal Law and Criminology, 66,* 483–490.

Federal Bureau of Investigation. (1935–1984). *Crime in the United States* (formerly *Uniform Crime Reports*) (Annual Report). Washington, DC: U.S. Government Printing Office.

Feshbach, S. (1961). The stimulating versus cathartic effects of a vicarious aggressive activity. *Journal of Abnormal and Social Psychology, 63,* 381–385.

Feshbach, S., & Singer, R. D. (1971). *Television and aggression.* San Francisco: Jossey-Bass.

Frantz, J. B. (1969). The frontier tradition: An invitation to violence. In H. D. Graham & T. R. Gurr (Eds.), *Violence in America* (Report of the National Commission on the Causes and Prevention of Violence). New York: New American Library.

Gastil, R. D. (1971). Homicide and a regional culture of violence. *American Sociological Review, 36,* 412–427.

Glaser, D. (1979). Capital punishment—Deterrent or stimulus to murder? Our unexamined deaths and penalties. *University of Toledo Law Review, 10,* 317–333.

Glaser, D., & Zeigler, M. S. (1974). Use of the death penalty v. outrage at murder. *Crime and Delinquency, 20,* 333–338.

Greenberg, B. S., & Dervin, B. (1970). *Use of the mass media by the urban poor.* New York: Praeger.

Hackney, S. (1969). Southern violence. In H. D. Graham & T. R. Gurr (Eds.), *Violence in America* (Report of the National Commission on the Causes and Prevention of Violence). New York: New American Library.

Hannerz, U. (1969). *Soulside.* New York: Columbia University Press.

Heller, C. S. (1966). *Mexican American Youth* (pp. 35–36). New York: Random House.

Himmelweit, H. T., Oppenheimer, A. N., & Vince, P. (1958). *Television and the child.* London: Oxford University Press.

Hirschi, T. (1969). *Causes of delinquency.* Berkeley: University of California Press.

Hobsbawm, E. J. (1959). *Primitive rebels: Studies in archaic forms of social movements in the 19th and 20th centuries.* New York: Norton.

Hobsbawm, E. J. (1981). *Bandits* (rev. ed.). New York: Pantheon Books.

Hochschild, A. R. (1979). Emotion work, feeling rules, and social structure. *American Journal of Sociology, 85,* 551–575.

Hofstadter, R., & Wallace, M. (Eds.). (1970). *American violence* (pp. 11–24). New York: Knopf.

Horowitz, R., & Schwartz, G. (1974). Honor, normative ambiguity, and gang violence. *American Sociological Review, 39,* 238–251.

Howitt, D., & Cumberbatch, G. (1975). *Mass media, violence and society.* New York: Wiley.

Jensen, G. F. (1976). Race, achievement and delinquency: A further look at delinquency in a birth cohort. *American Journal of Sociology, 82,* 379–387.

Kahane, R. (1975). Informal youth organizations: A general model. *Sociological Inquiry, 45*(4), 17–28.

Kennett, L., & Anderson, J. L. (1975). *The gun in America* (Chapters 1 & 2). Westport, CT: Greenwood Press.

Lane, R. (1976). Criminal violence in America: The first hundred years. *Annals of the American Academy of Political and Social Science, 423,* 1–13.

Lewis, O. (1966). *La vida: A Puerto Rican family in the culture of poverty.* New York: Random House.

Leyens, J. P., Camino, L., Parke, R. D., & Berkowitz, L. (1975). Effects of movie violence on aggression in a field experiment as a function of group dominance and cohesion. *Journal of Personal and Social Psychology, 32,* 346–360.

Liebert, R. M., Neale, J. M., & Davidson, E. S. (1975). *The early window: Effects of television on children and youth.* New York: Pergamon.

Liebow, E. (1967). *Tally's Corner: A study of Negro streetcorner men.* Boston: Little Brown.

Loeb, R. (1973). Adolescent groups. *Sociology and Social Research, 58,* 13–22.

Loftin, C., & Hill, R. H. (1974). Regional subculture and homicide: An examination of the Gastil-Hackney hypothesis. *American Sociological Review, 39,* 714–724.

Lundsgaarde, H. P. (1977). *Murder in Space City: Analysis of Houston homicide patterns.* New York: Oxford University Press.

McKeon, R. (Ed.). (1941). *The basic works of Aristotle.* New York: Random House.

Mead, G. H. (1934). *Mind, self and society.* Chicago: University of Chicago Press.

Mednick, S. (1977). A bio-social theory of the learning of law-abiding behavior. In K. O. Christiansen & S. Mednick, *Biosocial bases of criminal behavior.* New York: Gardner Press.

Merton, R. K. (1968). *Social theory and social structure* (3rd ed.). New York: Free Press.

Moffitt, T. E., & Mednick, S. A. (1984). Psychobiological relationships between crime and mental illness. In D. Weisstub (Ed.), *International yearbook on law and mental health.* New York: Pergamon Press.

National Commission on the Causes and Prevention of Violence (1969). *To establish justice, to insure domestic tranquility* (Final Report). Washington, DC: U.S. Government Printing Office.

Nighswander, J. K., & Mayer, G. R. (1969). Catharsis: A means of reducing elementary students' aggressive behaviors? *The Personnel and Guidance Journal, 47,* 461–466.

Otto, L. B. (1976). Social integration and the status-attainment process. *American Journal of Sociology, 81,* 1360–1383.

Pettigrew, T. F., & Spier, R. B. (1962). The ecological structure of Negro homicide. *American Journal of Sociology, 67,* 621–629.

Phillips, D. P. (1983). The impact of mass media violence on U.S. homicides. *American Sociological Review, 48,* 560–568.

Polk, K., & Schafer, W. E. (1972). *Schools and delinquency.* Englewood Cliffs, NJ: Prentice-Hall.

Preschool pays off for poor, study reveals. (1984, September 15). Los Angeles Times.

Rodman, H. (1963). The lower class value stretch. *Social Forces, 42,* 205–215.

Rusche, G., & Kirchheimer, O. (1939). *Punishment and social structure* (pp. 60–61). New York: Columbia University Press.

Servadio, G. (1976). *Mafioso: A history of the Mafia from its origins to the present.* New York: Stein & Day.

Sherman, L. W., & Berk, R. A. (1984). Deterrent effects of arrest for domestic assault. *American Sociological Review, 49,* 261–272.

Spady, W. G. (1970). Lament for the letterman: Effects of peer status and extra-curricular activities on goals and achievements. *American Journal of Sociology, 75,* 680–702.

Taft, P., & Ross, P. (1969). American labor violence: Its causes, character and outcome. In H. D. Graham & T. R. Gurr (Eds.), *Violence in America* (Report of the National Commission on Causes & Prevention of Violence, p. 270). New York: New American Library.

Thomas, M. H., & Drabman, R. S. (1975). Toleration of real life aggression as a function of exposure to televised violence and age of subject. *Merril-Palmer Quarterly, 21,* 227–232.

Valentine, C. A. (1968). *Culture and poverty.* Chicago: University of Chicago Press.

van der Voort, H., Vooijs, M. W., & Bekker, P. A. (1982). Kinderen en tv-geweld [Children and TV violence]. *Psycholoog, 17,* 370 (in *Psychological Abstracts, 70,* July–September 1983, #5403).

Voss, H. L., & Hepburn, J. R. (1968). Patterns in Criminal Homicide in Chicago. *Journal of Criminal Law, Criminology, and Police Science, 59,* 499–508.

Williams, K. R. (1984). Economic sources of homicide: Reestimating the effects of poverty and inequality. *American Sociological Review, 49,* 283–289.

Williams, P. A., Haertel, E. H., & Welberg, H. J. (1982). The impact of leisure-time television viewing on school learning: A research synthesis. *American Educational Research Journal, 19,* 19–50 (reprinted in Evaluation Studies Review Annual, Vol. 8, Beverly Hills, CA: Sage).

Wolfgang, M. E. (1958). *Patterns of criminal homicide.* Philadelphia: University of Pennsylvania Press.

Wolfgang, M. E., & Ferracuti, F. (1967). *The subculture of violence* (pp. 262–263, 279–280). London: Tavistock.

# 2

# The Changing Role of the Family

## Laura Lein

This chapter discusses major trends in family life in the United States and their implications for the well-being of families and the individuals in the family. A discussion of three important shifts in family demography begins the chapter, followed by a discussion of seminal perspectives from which the family has been studied. Current weaknesses in our study of the family are examined in the next section, and the chapter concludes with a number of proposals for research directions relevant to American families.

## INTRODUCTION AND OVERVIEW

The last two decades have been a period of rapid change for American families. At least three basic demographic shifts have occurred with a number of significant implications for the quality of family life and the role played by the family and family members in the society at large. First, and perhaps most dramatic in its implications for family life, women have steadily increased their participation in the paid labor force. That change has been most rapid among the mothers of very young children. Second, the divorce rate has increased. And third, the birth rate has generally declined. Together, these three trends have changed the profile of the American family.

### Women's Employment

In 1950 only 18% of wives with children under eighteen were employed. By 1980 that figure had risen to 54% (Lueck, Orr, & O'Connell, 1982). While our traditional stereotype of the American family has included an employed father and an unemployed mother at home caring for children, now only 12% of American households fit that model (Johnson &

Hayghe, 1977). This "normative" family described so often in literature, particularly literature for children, represents only a small minority of American households now. Furthermore, among married couples today, husbands do not bear the wage-earning responsibility alone. In nearly half of all married couples in the United States, husband and wife are both employed. In roughly 25% of married couples is the husband employed and the wife unemployed. In less than 25% both husband and wife are unemployed, due to time-out for schooling, retirement, or other unemployment (Hayghe, 1982).

Change in women's employment has occurred in a specific social and historical context. First, over the last two decades, feminism and the women's liberation movement have developed and strengthened as social movements. Although it remains the case that many women would not describe themselves as feminist and, in fact, believe that the women's movement has had little effect on their lives, a majority of women now appear to support the right to abortion, equal pay for equal work, and the need for child care (Lein & O'Donnell, 1984b). Women's needs and problems, their political perspectives, and their votes have become significant factors in the political life of our country (Klein, 1984).

Since the early 1970s, families have experienced an era of continuing inflation which is just beginning to subside. Families have found it increasingly necessary for two members to be employed in order to sustain what they consider an acceptable standard of living. More women have needed to earn in order to support their families. In fact, the Department of Labor asserts that two-thirds of employed American women are working out of clear economic need: They are either the sole earners in their household, or they are married to spouses earning less than $15,000 per year (U.S. Department of Labor, 1984).

During this same 20-year period, women have entered formal educational programs in such increasing numbers that they are now beginning to close what had been known as the "education gap," the gap between women and men in higher education that had remained substantial until the last decade. Thus, although the education differential continues for older women, younger women are rapidly closing it. Women now make up over half the student population in higher education. In the last several years women have earned almost half the bachelor's degrees awarded (U.S. Department of Commerce, 1979b).

As a result of their increased educational experience and expanding opportunities, women are entering occupations previously almost entirely dominated by men. These occupations range from the trained blue collar and construction trades to corporate management and the professions of law and medicine. Only in the last decade has the first wave of women since World War II been admitted to apprentice welding programs; they have become telephone line installers and machinists (O'Farrell & Harlan, in press). For instance, two and a half million women have entered management jobs as of 1979, compared to approximately 1,000,000 at the time of the passage of the 1964 Civil Rights Act (Wellesley College Center for Research on Women, 1982).

But in spite of all these changes—women's increasing labor force participation, their increased level of education and technical training, and their entry into previously male dominated occupations—women's opportunities in the paid labor force continue to be limited by a variety of barriers including job discrimination by sex, sexual stereotyping by supervisors, and sexual harassment. Furthermore, many women's opportunities in paid work are limited by the exigencies of life in a dual earner family or as a single head of household, often allowing them little time to devote to extra responsibilities on the job or to take advantage of opportunities for further training. Women still earn significantly less than men. Over the last two decades women have continued to earn roughly 60 cents for every dollar earned by men (U.S. Department of Labor, 1984). Thus, women are at a significant disadvantage in wage earning and in supporting a family. Hour for hour, they bring home less money, while carrying substantial responsibility for earning at least part of the family living.

Women's limited opportunities and income and the stress of combining work and family life affect the well-being of families, particularly in a time of inflation. In fact, families in which women are the wage earners tend to be poor. They are part of a recently documented trend termed the "feminization of poverty." Women, in general, and families headed by women, in particular, are more likely to be poor than men in general or families headed by men (Woody & Malson, 1984). Almost a quarter of employed women have incomes within a few percentage points of the government established parameters of poverty, and that figure is substantially higher for black women and other ethnic minority women (Malveaux, 1982). For women, employment is not necessarily the answer to their poverty.

All of the material presented thus far on women's wage-earning activities are aggregate data. Important though these data are for understanding employment trends for American women and the implications for their families, it is also possible for such aggregate material to mask the distinctively different experiences of minority women and their families. Black women have been employed at much higher rates than white women right through the 1950s and 1960s (Wallace, 1980). However, although more likely to be employed and to be continuously employed, black women and their families suffer a wider wage gap with white male employees than do white women and are more likely to be poor (Woody & Malson, 1984). Both black men and women are more likely to be poor than are their white counterparts. Other significant minorities in the United States also have employment patterns different from the aggregate, and women and families in these groups deal with starker realities of poverty, even if they are employed. Hispanic women are at least as likely as black women to be poor, and at least as likely to suffer poverty in spite of full time employment.

## Divorce

Changes in employment are not the only substantial demographic shifts in American family life. Single parent families have been part of the social scene since the early years of this country. However, until quite recently they were more likely to be a result of the death of one spouse or the other, rather than the result of separation or divorce (Bane, 1976). In fact, the number of family dissolutions due to the death of a spouse occurring during the family life cycle stage when there are dependent children at home has fallen dramatically, due primarily to decreases in the rate of maternal death in child-birth, other deaths related to acute illnesses such as pneumonia, and deaths due to industrial and other work-related accidents.

The rate of divorce has been rising steadily over the past several decades. Of the children born between 1941 and 1950, about 11% were involved in a period of family disruption due to the divorce of their parents. This compares to an estimate of at least 18% for children born around 1970. Census data indicate that in 1982 8.4 million women were in households with a child under 21 whose father was not in the household (U.S. Department of Commerce, 1983). The number of divorces and separations for families has overtaken the previously combined separation, divorce and death rate for younger married adults, so that the rate of family dissolution is now at its highest ever (Bane, 1976). Thus, more families with dependent children now undergo family dissolution than has been the case earlier this century, and, because such dissolution is more likely to be due to divorce or separation, it results in two separated households, rather than one remaining household.

The division into two households out of one household presents a number of problems to individual family members. In particular, aggregate data indicate that the household headed by the husband (usually without custody of children) maintains a standard of living similar to the original family. The standard of living of the household headed by the female (usually the household with responsibility for any dependent children) tends to plummet (U.S. Department of Labor, 1983).

In addition to the impact of women's decreased earning potential, families with children headed by women receive relatively little financial support from the ex-husband and father. Recent research indicates that the average child support award is $2,050 (U.S. Department of Commerce, 1983). Furthermore, in less than half of those cases where child support is awarded is it fully paid (Hunter, 1983). Overall, the partner with the more limited earning ability is left with the remaining major family responsibilities and relatively little financial support.

## Children

The third major demographic trend representing change in family life has been the number and timing of children born most recently to women of childbearing age. Over the last two decades the trend has been for women to bear fewer children. However, while many women are waiting longer than ever to have their first baby, another group of women are having children in their teen years. Thus, at the same time we are finding an increase in the proportion of children born to teenage mothers or "children having children," there is also an increase in the numbers of women in their thirties and even early forties having their first child (U.S. Department of Commerce, 1979a).

Both of these changes in women's childbearing appear to be related to changes in society-wide attitudes about having children and the relationship between responsibility for children and other aspects of women's lives. Many women are having fewer children and delaying their child rearing in order to get a job or career off the ground. These women feel the need to complete their education and launch their professional lives before assuming responsibility for children. The issues surrounding such delayed childbearing and child rearing are both medical and social. Studies and media reports indicate that while such women have somewhat increased medical risks both to themselves and their children, they are also among the women most likely to seek out and receive excellent pre- and postnatal medical care (Daniels & Weingarten, 1982). While such women are often well launched in respected professional careers, they also often report considerable anxiety and tension over the decision of when to return to the job after the birth of their young child. They do not anticipate the strength of the pull many of them feel to remain home longer than the maternity leave they have negotiated (Toman, 1983).

The phenomenon of an increasing proportion of children in the United States being born to very young mothers results from 1) the proportion of teenagers having children remaining steady with slight increases, and 2) the proportion of other women having children has decreased somewhat. Thus, an increasing percentage of America's children are being born to teenage mothers (Bane, 1976). These mothers and their children face a series of problems. Many teenage mothers find their schooling ended or dramatically slowed down following the birth of a child. The curtailing of their education has lifelong effects on the ability of young women to earn a living and, in particular, on their ability to support themselves and their child. Overall, very young mothers are ill-equipped for many of the activities associated with adequate parenting in today's society, ranging from the increasingly heavy financial demands put on parents to the continuing demands for patience, understanding, and emotional maturity.

Increasing rates of women's employment, particularly the employment of mothers of young children, increasing rates of marital dissolution, and new trends in birth patterns are all changing the stresses faced by American families today. Furthermore, these changes, in the context of continuing inflation, have often increased pressures without increasing the resources available to families. There is a continuing need for research that will delineate the results for family well-being and suggest services and supports to assist families in meeting the demands placed on them.

## RESEARCH PERSPECTIVES AND ANALYSIS OF FAMILY LIFE

Changing trends in family demography have an impact on family life as it is examined from a number of different research directions. Given the huge body of literature on family life, it is impossible to develop a description of all of the perspectives that have been used in the study of the family; however, three principle models provide settings for much of the more recent research on American families. The family has been examined as an economic unit, a political unit, and as a socioemotional system both within a wider social system and in isolation. Researchers drawing on each of these perspectives have explored issues related to employment, family dissolution, and the responsibilities for children, although work from each perspective has tended to concentrate on specific themes.

## *The Family as an Economic Unit*

The family is productive in at least three different ways: The family is the source of sustenance for paid laborers, where workers "go home" for food, sleep, warmth, and the other necessities of life. Thus, the family is also the setting for the unpaid labor of homemaking and community building; families fit into the socio-economic system because they require the financial returns of paid labor and then turn that money earned into the goods and services required for maintaining a labor force able to perform on the job. Also, families are responsible for rearing the next generation of society's workers.

There is now a considerable body of research illuminating the relationship between paid jobs and family life (Pleck, 1983). Originally, such research concentrated on the impact of earnings on family life and the significance of family and household to the well-being of the paid worker. Such work, often performed cross-culturally, indicated the importance of family life to the well-being of the individual (Szalai, 1972). Married men, perceived as the more-often employed members of the family, were in better health and expressed more personal well-being, in this country and in most other countries. Such research indicated that the work of the homemaker and the support of family life is indeed essential to the well-being of the national labor force. Furthermore, both women and men in the United States appear to recognize the significance of family life to their overall well-being. When asked about the relative importance of their life on the job compared to their experiences in the family, both women and men are more likely to name family life as the most important basis for their overall sense of life satisfaction (Pleck & Stains, 1981).

There is increasing concern that life on the job has an important influence on the quality of home life. More recent ethnographic studies provide powerful illustrations of the ways in which tensions on the job are fed back into the family, and the impact of these tensions as they play out in family life are borne by all family members. Men and women in demanding jobs bring the impact of these job-related stresses home with them.

In fact, men and women both are fully alert to the fact that their life on the job makes a substantial difference to the quality of home life (Piotrkowski, 1979). Both men and women realize the significance of their earnings in supporting the family. They also find it relatively easy to pinpoint those aspects of their jobs that put the heaviest burden on their families. Women, in particular, emphasize the difficulties created by the rigidity of work schedules when they also face responsibilities for family emergencies and the daily needs of children. Men are more likely to emphasize the strains on the job that leave them tired and irritable when they return home (Pleck, 1979).

The requirements of any one family member's job affects the family in large part because the characteristics of life in the paid labor force have a powerful impact on the mental and physical health of individual workers, which can, in turn, place additional burdens on the family. Research on the health risks of paid employment originally concentrated on heart disease and other disorders suffered more by men, and resulting from work in the upper levels of company management—work requiring rapid, high-risk decision making. Workers, almost overwhelmingly men, engaged in such occupations as high-level corporate management were considered at relatively high risk due to the tension of their jobs.

More recent research suggests that another group of workers, primarily women, are also at considerable risk of work-related, tension-produced disease. Women in traditional service occupations, such as social worker and nurse, often have to make frequent, fast, sometimes high-risk decisions, but, unlike corporate managers, they have little power or control over their own work environment or work schedules. The combination of the need for fast decisions and reactions with relatively little power or control over the work environment can be as detrimental to the health of workers as the fast-paced, high tension work of corporate management (Karasek, Schwartz, & Theorell, 1982).

Detailed studies of family life have also made clear the relationship between stress on the job and stress in the home. The pragmatics of family living, such as meal and housework schedules, children's bedtimes, and medical appointments are all clearly affected by the employment of either spouse, the tensions of their jobs, and the hours of their employment. The tensions of the job affect an individual's ability to parent, to be a loving husband or wife, and to be a good neighbor and member of the community.

The family is not only the "rest and recreation" site for society's paid workers; it is also the setting for the unpaid, but productive, labor of homemaking. The significance of homemaking as economic work has become increasingly visible in the last two decades. Studies have examined both the drop in standard of living that results when a family loses a homemaker and the financial worth, at current wages, of the work produced by homemakers (Howe, 1977). Thus, whether or not men and women are earning income for their work, they are likely both undertaking work that can have a dramatic effect on family standard of living, and work for which it is becoming increasingly possible to develop an economic evaluation. Housework and child care, as well as paid work, are productive in the economic sense and contribute directly to the family's standard of living.

The significance of homemaking to family well-being and the amount of work it entails has become more obvious and more studied with the entry of dual-earner families into the mainstream of American family life. With more women in the paid labor force, and particularly more women with young children, the occupation of homemaking and the resources required for homemaking have appeared simultaneously to become both more at risk and more important to the well-being of families. Furthermore, the accomplishment of the tasks demanded by homemaking has become a lively issue for negotiation between husbands and wives in families where both are employed.

Over the last 20 years, there have been several major studies of homemaking activities. According to an early study of time use in the home conducted in the 1960s, an unemployed wife in a two-parent, two-child household contributed an average of 58 hours a week in household labor, while her husband contributed an average of 11 hours a week (Walker & Woods, 1976). An employed wife in similar circumstances contributed 41 hours per week to the household in addition to her hours on the job. Although there have not been major changes in task allocation in the home, analysis of a more recent 1975–76 survey study (Pleck, 1983) indicated that the time devoted by employed wives to family work is dropping while the time devoted by husbands is increasing slightly.

One recent research study (Lein, 1984) indicates that men's and women's attitudes toward homemaking and their actual daily practices in the home are inextricably tied to their attitudes towards husbands' and wives' earned income. In families where there is recognition, as is the case in a growing number of families, that the wife's income is essential to maintaining the family's standard of living, husbands and wives are more likely to believe that the responsibility for the tasks of raising a family, including both homemaking and earning the family living, can no longer be strictly defined as either men's or women's work. If the family members perceive the wife's income as "extra," to be spent on luxuries but not on essential goods and services for the family, then husband and wife are also more likely to believe that it is the husband's job to earn the family living and the wife's job to perform the unpaid work of homemaking (Lein, 1984). Of course, there is a great deal of room for disagreement between husband and wife in this schema. Husbands and wives can disagree on the significance of the wife's earned income. Or the husband and wife may agree that the wife's income is essential to the family, but one or both of them may feel that such circumstances are detrimental to the family's well-being. In sum, while there is evidence that men's and women's relative contributions to the work of homemaking are changing, there is little evidence yet that the change is sufficient to ease the tensions around housework negotiations between husbands and wives.

Again, the results of aggregate data analysis can mask the sometimes very different experiences of minority families. Black dual earner families tend toward more of a partnership model for allocating household responsibilities. The recent tensions in white families over homemaking, related as they are to the swiftly changing demography in white women's employment, do not appear to be matched in black dual earner families, who have experienced a longer history with the dual-earner family structure (Peters, 1976).

The current paid workers are not the only workers for whom the family is considered primarily responsible. The family is also responsible for making a major investment in the next generation of society's workers. Thus, through their investment in children, families are investing in the well-being, education, and healthy development of the future labor force. Families hold much of the financial responsibility as well as other responsibilities for the caring and training of children. Over the last two decades there has been an increasingly close scrutiny of the average financial costs of raising a child, with estimates skyrocketing (Keniston & The Carnegie Council on Children, 1978).

Family responsibilities toward children are dependent not only on how many and how old their children are, but also on societal demands made on parents based on its standards of good parenting. Children create for their parents a network of social ties to other parents, to professionals who are involved with children, and to the institutions that serve children and families. While these networks can offer parents much support, the demands made on parents and their reactions to the pressures of parenting change with each generation and are often expressed through their social networks.

The definitions of what constitutes a good parent have changed dramatically. Parents are considered responsible for their children—their behavior, their healthy development, and their future. Furthermore, their behavior as parents is under an increasing amount of regulation and scrutiny. The growing recognition and reporting, and possibly the increased presence, of such social problems as child abuse have led to a continuing increase in the regulation of parenting. Essential though research and service programs are to prevention of and intervention in abuse, it is clear that the presence of such checks on parenting take their toll on all parents.

Intensive research with parents of young children indicates a growing concern among many parents that they might be considered abusive. There have been substantial attacks on American families, highly publicizing and presenting in the public media, descriptions of parents who are both abusive and too permissive, and thus are to blame for many of the ills of society today. There are, in fact, many troubled families today. However, generalized attacks on parents may undercut their ability to parent, rather than lead to improvement. And the ability of parents to rear their children is of urgent importance to our society.

Thus, families are key economic units. Families are the key social unit through which unpaid work is channeled to the benefit of paid workers and through which money and expensive services are made available to the children who will be the next generation of society's laborers.

## Family Life and Politics

Many men and women feel particularly vulnerable in their role as parents and as earners. And their increasing sense of vulnerability may well have contributed to what many perceive as the family's growing presence in the political arena. Families are increasingly becoming a focus of national politics. First, the increasing "gender gap," the difference between men's and women's voting patterns on issues and candidates, seems to reflect, at least in part, the commitment women feel to their homes, neighborhoods, and communities. Second, questions regarding the rights and responsibilities of families versus the rights and responsibilities of individuals in families have become part of an increasingly heated national debate.

During the suffrage movement women activists drew on their belief that women's votes might well transform American politics. However, right through the 1950s scholars found that women's enfranchisement did not lead to a significant change in the political scene, and politicians continued to assume that women would generally vote just as their husbands voted, and that, in fact, political opinions were held by families rather than by individuals. Only in the last 10 years, with the discovery of the now widely discussed gender gap, has there come the realization that members of families, women and men with their different perceptions of the role of family life, their different socialization and life experiences, and their different responsibilities, may well have different interests and perspectives, and vote from these divergent points of view (Smeal, 1984).

Accompanying the development of the gender gap in attitudes and voting behavior has come an increasing recognition that many of the tasks of parenting, the protection and nurture of children, require parental activity in the more public political sphere. Parents concerned with the education of their children find, for instance, that they cannot have impact on their children's education only through their influence at home. Children's education is too directly affected by the education systems controlled outside the home. There has been increasing research on the importance of parents' involvement in their children's school system for the children's own well-being and success in education (O'Donnell, 1984).

An increasing number of parents seem to be recognizing the significance of many public policy issues for their children's future. Being a parent means taking a stand on issues from the nuclear freeze and national security to toxic waste and the economic health of the country, at least in part, because these issues affect one's children in ways sufficiently direct to demand the involvement of a responsible parent. Furthermore, as children themselves become cognizant of these issues, parents wishing to reassure and empower their children feel the need to demonstrate to them through their political action the fact that as parents, they care and that they can continue to work for their children's welfare, even if outside the family (Lein & O'Donnell, 1984a).

But the family and family members are not simply finding their political voice. The family is also becoming a focus of political debate. Issues connected with family life and with the power and control of husbands over wives and parents over children have become an important and visible issue in national and state politics (Klein, 1984). A political "woman's agenda" has developed including such issues as national child care, affirmative action, the right to abortion and the need for a nuclear freeze (Lein & O'Donnell, 1984b). Furthermore, struggles over control in the family deal with issues ranging from the identification and intervention in cases of child abuse and wife beating to the development of mechanisms for determining when to use heroic medical measures in treating newborns and the elderly (Lein & O'Donnell, 1984c). Struggles over all these issues are related to the impact of these issues on family life and to questions about the rights of the family versus the rights of individual family members and the responsibility of the society at large to protect the individual.

## Social and Emotional Life

The family is an important context for both the creation and resolution of socioemotional conflicts. Material on managing interfamilial relationships—parents with children, spouse with spouse, sibling with sibling—is extensive. For instance, there has been a surge in the research undertaken on childhood development and education and on writing pertaining to the requirements for good parenting. Literature on the nature of parenting, including advice to parents, can make extraordinary demands on them.

During this country's early years and various other periods including the Depression (Working Family Project, 1974), demands on parents, although strenuous, were relatively straightforward and easy to encapsulate. For many parents it had taken and continues to take enormous effort to ensure that their children are adequately clothed, cleaned, fed and formally educated. During the Depression, for instance, parents tended to perceive that success in these areas meant that they were good parents. Simply giving their children a chance at a good life was very hard work. Certainly, parents were responsible for the behavior of their children, but it was also widely accepted that some children were harder to raise than other children. Parents were not necessarily to blame if things did not work out well for their children.

No longer do we have such relatively clear social expectations for the role of parents. Current advice instructs parents in the language to use with their children, the kinds of games to play with them, and the exact wording to use in discipline. Furthermore, theories of the role of parenting place considerable responsibility on parents. Some experts explain to parents that the first three years of a child's life determine his or her future, and those three years are in the hands of parents.

Accompanying the growth of literature on the child-parent bond, there has been significant work on other family bonds, including husband-wife and sibling relationships, and the role of grandparents, aunts, uncles, and other relatives (Lein & Sussman, 1982). All of these relationships are complex, sometimes tenuous, and accompanied by heavy responsibilities: The implicit demands made on parents, brothers and sisters, and other relatives are great and the concrete and pragmatic demands made on many of these relationships have intensified.

## GAPS IN RESEARCH ON THE CHANGING AMERICAN FAMILY

The family is a focus of policy and research, but the direction of that policy development and the kinds of questions asked by researchers are clearly influenced by current attitudes about family life, the current expectations of how families should meet their responsibilities, and current assessments of the health and well-being of American families in general. Therefore, while research on family life has accomplished a great deal, there has also been only limited consideration of some significant issues. Today, both control over what happens in families and expectations of what families should accomplish are heated political and research questions. As a result, over the last several decades, research on families has tended to put families on the defensive.

For example, the largest body of research on women's employment and family life has been in response to concern over the impact of mother's employment on their young children (Howrigan, 1973). Certainly, this is an important and significant problem, but research consideration of this issue has overshadowed the development of research, for instance, on the impact of responsibility for children on adults' lives. In spite of continued national concern about who is having children, how many and when they are being born in the adult life span, there are still relatively few resources determining what it means to adults—to their personal development, jobs, and career development, integration into different social communities, and quality of life—to have responsibility for young children (Lein & O'Donnell, 1984a).

The impact of responsibility for dependent children on adults is evident when the family is examined in terms of each of the perspectives we began with. First, responsibility for children colors the commitment to the paid labor force of mothers and fathers, and parental images of children's possible futures influence patterns of family spending. Second, responsibility for children both motivates parents in their political activity and motivates much of the public examination of family life. Third, the arrival of children into the family makes a significant difference in the management of family responsibilities and in the nature of negotiations between adults in the family.

In 1974, Kanter called for research on the mutual impact of employment and home life for families. In her analysis of the studies on work and family life up to that time, she discovered gaps in research on the interrelationship between these spheres of life. Such a lack is symptomatic of overall weaknesses in research on families. There needs to be continued study of these and other spheres of family life and paid work and the different functions fulfilled by families in the society at large as they have an impact on each other. Thus, in the same way that a decade ago there was relatively little study of the relationship between life on the job and life in the home, there continues to be little exploration of the relationship between life on the job and family politics and between family political life (both inside the family and in national politics) and the socioemotional life played out in the internal dynamics of daily family life.

Our vision of family life has been limited because relatively little research has been designed from the point of view of the family as, simultaneously, an economic, political and social institution in the larger social world it inhabits. Because any given study has tended to examine families from one perspective and with a concentration on one mode of functioning, it has been relatively easy to underestimate the pressures on today's families. And it has been relatively easy to blame families, and, even more importantly, the individuals in families, for any inability on the part of families to meet societal expectations of what family life should entail.

Researchers, as well as those in policy and political arenas, often question the current quality of family life. For example, as women have entered the paid labor force, there has been public concern that, as a result, they will abdicate responsibility for the work of the home—child care, housework, and the work of maintaining a marriage. One of the most frequently asked questions in the media and elsewhere in connection with women's paid jobs has been, "Who will care for the children?" However, the questions suggesting a vision of women's paid work as a relinquishing of responsibility for home and family fail to recognize the realities of economic life for many women and families. First, we need to recognize the economic need of many women to work to help support their families, and the particularly stringent conditions experienced by single heads of household, the large majority of whom are women.

Second, as mentioned earlier, the aggregate statistics have masked the fact that black and other ethnic minority women have been and continue to be represented in the paid labor force at a level significantly higher than the national average. For many women with limited economic resources, earning a living is not an abdication of responsibility to the family; rather, it is an essential part of being a responsible wife and mother. Family roles are particularly demanding in single-parent families and in families with very restricted economic resources. Research on changes in family life in the United States continually needs to recognize the diversity of kinds of families and the constraints under which they live.

Analysis of the responsibilities and experiences of women in families has tended to concentrate on housework and child care to the exclusion of several other significant tasks involved in maintaining a family and household. Maintaining a marriage—apart from the tasks of homemaking and child care—requires significant work. In many households, most of the complications of scheduling and the negotiations over family activity, expenditure and location occur between husband and wife. One outcome of initial research on divorce (Weiss, 1975) is the recognition of the work entailed to maintain a marriage. Even in the midst of the upheaval of marital dissolution, wives and husbands recognize that part of the workload of family life disappears with the absence of the spouse.

An additional set of tasks is just beginning to receive formal recognition as part of the unpaid work traditionally undertaken by women. Women have held the primary responsibility for work in the community. They have managed the exchanges with neighbors and friends, communicated on a regular basis with relatives, and participated as volunteers in the school, church, and other community and neighborhood organizations. This work has a substantial impact on the quality of living in families, neighborhoods, and communities.

As part of their unpaid service to the neighborhood and community, women assume more of the daily activities of caring for elderly members of the family in need of regular assistance. While men are more likely to assume responsibility for such tasks as managing the income and finances of an elderly relative, women are more likely to assist others by writing and phoning regularly, visiting, and undertaking the chores of daily household maintenance (Bahr & Nye, 1974).

Furthermore, this work on behalf of the older generation has assumed a dramatically increased level in the last two generations. Families have become smaller with more single-child and two-child families. Therefore, as each child becomes an adult, he or she is more likely to be called on to assume responsibility for parental needs. In particular, the odds of being the only surviving daughter are on the rise. And of course, at the same time, all of us are living longer, and the causes of death have changed from the acute (pneumonia, accident) to the chronic (cancer, heart disease), so that more sons and daughters will be called on to offer support to their parents and other elderly family members over a longer period of time.

Research on families undertaken in the light of women's increasing labor force participation has tended to neglect the implications of the necessity for women's earnings in family life. It has also neglected the wealth of unpaid work essential to maintaining family standards of living as we now know them. This has resulted in a tendency to blame women for their paid work and for the accompanying changes in family life, rather than acknowledge the commitment to family and community represented by women's ability to face pressures on the family by assuming additional tasks.

A more recent question in contrast to that outlined above asks in what ways men are to blame for their relatively low time and energy commitment to the daily pragmatic and emotional life of the family. However, this line of research questions and the resulting analyses of the interior of family life rest on the assumption that the pressures under which families continue to exist and the actions they take to meet these pressures do not explain the tensions and difficulties faced by families: Someone in the family must be to blame. The recognition that families are taking on more work in response to greater pressures may be a significant part of the explanation of why some families fail to assume all of their responsibilities.

Not only do families fall under censure for their failures, but increased blame for family disorders has been put on professionals offering direct services to families—and of course, most of these are women. This concentration on the failings of teachers, social workers, and child-care workers to help families again entails a lack of recognition of the pressures under which families labor and the tensions of women in the typically female-dominated serving professions. It is important to understand that there may be all too many situations where low income, heavy responsibility and lack of expertise may make it difficult, if not impossible, for families to meet all of their responsibilities.

## NEW RESEARCH DIRECTIONS

Our approach to families, then, has limited research horizons in a number of ways. In particular, if we are to reach out appropriately to families under stress, we need to learn more about families in a variety of domains, and to use new knowledge and information to frame theories that allow for more concrete understanding of the ills that can occur in family life, rather than simply blame families, individual family members, or family service workers. Such a need requires continuing work on a number of research questions:

- How does changing family demography affect both the impact of public policies on families and the ways in which family members are motivated to become politically active?
- What are the distinctive family strategies in those communities of families where women's labor force participation has been a long-established pattern? We need to examine the constructive patterns for undertaking family responsibility that emerge with long-term responsibility for multiple roles. New research on women's lives suggests that multiple roles and responsibilities may well be an asset to women's mental health: The problem for families is not that women are taking on multiple roles; the problem is that the pressures on families are becoming more than they can support.
- How can we delineate and define the responsibilities of families today in all three domains: labor force (paid and unpaid), political and socio-emotional? What are the responsibilities in each domain that families are currently expected to meet, and what demands

do these responsibilities entail? In other words, how much are we demanding from families?

- What are the implications of changing role definitions for children, women and men in families? What new demands are being placed on members of families, and what resources are available to them in meeting their new responsibilities? Furthermore, what are the implications of these responsibilities for adults as well as children: How do changes in adult lives affect healthy adult development?

## REFERENCES

Bahr, H. M., & Nye, F. I. (1974). The kinship role in a contemporary community: Perceptions of obligations and sanctions. *Journal of Comparative Family Studies, 5,* 17–25.

Bane, M. J. (1976). *Here to stay: American families in the twentieth century.* New York: Basic Books.

Daniels, P., & Weingarten, K. (1982). *Sooner or later: The timing of parenthood in adult lives.* New York: W. W. Norton.

Hayghe, H. (1982). Marital and family patterns of workers: An update. *Monthly Labor Review,* May, 53–56.

Howe, L. K. (1977). *Pink collar workers.* New York: Avon Books.

Howrigan, G. (1973). *The effects of working mothers on children.* Reprint. Cambridge, MA: Center for the Study of Public Policy.

Hunter, N. (1983). Child support law and policy: The systematic imposition of costs on women. In I. Diamond (Ed.), *Families, politics and public policy: A feminist dialogue on women and the state.* New York: Longman.

Johnson, B. L., & Hayghe, H. (1977). Labor force participation of married women, March, 1976. *Monthly Labor Review,* June, 32–36.

Kanter, R. (1974). *Work and family life.* New York: The Russell Sage Foundation.

Karasek, R. W., Schwartz, J., & Theorell, T. (1982). *Job characteristics, occupation and coronary heart disease.* Final Report, National Institute of Occupational Safety and Health, Contract No. R-01-0H00906. New York, Columbia University.

Keniston, K., & The Carnegie Council on Children. (1978). *All our children: The American family under pressure.* New York: Harcourt Brace Jovanovich.

Klein, E. (1984). *Gender politics: From consciousness to mass politics.* Cambridge, MA: Harvard University Press.

Lein, L. (1984). *Families without villains.* Lexington, MA: Lexington Books.

Lein, L., & O'Donnell, L. (1984a). *Children.* Philadelphia, PA: Westminster Press.

Lein, L., & O'Donnell, L. (1984b). The mainstream woman: A new voice in American politics (Working Paper No. 142, Fall). Wellesley College Center for Research on Women, Wellesley, MA.

Lein, L., & O'Donnell, L. (1984c). A Woman's Influence. Press kit, *Woman's Day,* April.

Lein, L., & Sussman, M. (Eds.). (1982). *The ties that bind: Men's and women's social networks. Marriage and Family Review, 5*(4). New York: Haworth Press.

Lueck, M., Orr, A. C., & O'Connell, M. (1982). Trends in child care arrangements of working mothers. *Current Population Reports,* Special Studies P-23, No. 117, U.S. Department of Commerce, Bureau of the Census, June.

Malveaux, J. (1982). Recent trends in occupational segregation by race and sex. Unpublished paper, presented at the Committee on Women's Employment and Related Social Issues: National Academy of Sciences, Washington, DC, May.

O'Donnell, L. (1984). *The unheralded majority: Contemporary women as mothers*. Lexington, MA: Lexington Books.

O'Farrell, B., & Harlan, S. (in press). Job integration strategies: Today's programs and tomorrow's needs. In B. F. Resking (Ed.), *Sex segregation in the workplace: Trends, explanations, remedies*. Washington, D.C.: National Academy Press.

Peters, M. (1976). A study of household management and child-rearing in black families with working mothers. Unpublished dissertation, Harvard University.

Piotrkowski, C. (1979). *Work and the family system*. New York: The Free Press.

Pleck, J. (1979). Men's family work: Three perspectives and some new data. *The Family Coordinator, 26*, 481–488.

Pleck, J. H. (1983). Husbands' paid work and family roles: Current research issues. In H. Z. Lopata & J. H. Pleck (Eds.), *Research in the interweave of social roles, families and jobs*. Greenwich, CT: JAI Press.

Pleck, J. H., & Stains, G. L. (1981). Work schedules and work-family conflict in two earner couples. In B. Forisha & B. Goldman (Eds.), *Outsiders on the insider: Women in organizations*. Englewood Cliffs, NJ: Prentice-Hall.

Smeal, E. (1984). *Why and how women will elect the next president*. New York: Harper & Row.

Szalai, A. (Ed.). (1972). *The use of time: Daily activities of urban and suburban populations in twelve countries*. The Hague: Mouton.

Toman, B. (1983, September 7). Maternity costs, parenthood and career overtax some women despite best intentions. *The Wall Street Journal*, p. 1.

U.S. Department of Commerce. (1979a). *Households and families by type: March 1979*. Current Population Reports, Series P-20, No. 345.

U.S. Department of Commerce, Bureau of the Census. (1979b). School enrollment—Social and economic characteristics of students: October, 1978. *Current Population Reports*, Series P-20, No. 335.

U.S. Department of Commerce. (1983). *Child support and alimony: 1981*. Current Population Series D-23, No. 124.

U.S. Department of Labor. (1983). *Handbook of labor statistics*. Bulletin 2175, December.

U.S. Department of Labor. (1984). *20 facts about women workers*.

Walker, K. E., & Woods, M. E. (1976). *Time use: A measure of household production of family goods and services*. Washington, D.C.: American Home Economics Association.

Wallace, P. (1980). *Black women in the labor force*. Cambridge, Massachusetts: MIT Press.

Weiss, R. (1975). *Marital separation*. New York: Basic Books.

Wellesley College Center for Research on Women. (1982). *Summary description of the "Women in Management" Project*. (research report) Wellesley College Center for Research on Women.

Woody, B., & Malson, M. (1984). In crisis: Low income black employed women in the U.S. workplace. Wellesley College Center for Research on Women Working Paper No. 131, Fall.

Working Family Project (Laura Lein, Principal Investigator). (1974). Work and Family Life. Unpublished Preliminary Report to The National Institute of Education, Grant No. 3094, Cambridge, MA: Center for the Study of Public Policy.

# 3

# *The Violent Family*

## Suzanne K. Steinmetz

During the last decade tremendous activity has occurred in the field of family violence. While participating in television interviews conducted during 1974–75 in conjunction with the publication of *Violence in the Family* (Steinmetz & Straus, 1974), this author often had to reaffirm, off camera, the existence of the problem. One decade later we have nationwide task forces on domestic violence, over 700 shelters for abused women, legislation protecting abused children, battered spouses and vulnerable adults and, in a growing number of states, marital rape, elder abuse, and warrantless arrest laws.

This essay, which provides an overview of over a decade of research, is arranged around the most commonly asked questions regarding family violence.

1) What is family violence?
2) Is family violence a new phenomenon? Are we more violent today? Is it the result of our fast-paced technology-oriented society which ignores traditional family values?
3) Is family violence widespread? Who are the victims? We hear about child abuse, what about parent abuse? We hear about wife abuse, what about wives who abuse their husbands?
4) Are there characteristics such as social class, alcoholism, mental illness, unemployment which distinguish violent families?
5) Can we stop family violence, predict family violence, prevent family violence?

I gratefully acknowledge Cathy Sullivan for technical editing and manuscript preparation.

51

## WHAT IS FAMILY VIOLENCE?

For the purpose of this paper, violence is defined as an act carried out with the intention of, or perceived as having the intention of, physically hurting another person. This physical hurt can range from slight pain, as in a slap, to murder. In addition to this definition of violence, other characteristics of these violent acts must be considered. For example, is the act instrumental to some other purpose, such as disciplining a child for a specific wrongdoing, or expressive, i.e., an end in itself? Is this act culturally permitted (or required), such as spanking a disobedient child, i.e., is it a legitimate act versus one which runs counter to cultural norms such as murder, which is illegitimate violence? Thus, the basis for the "intent to hurt" may range from a concern for a child's safety (as when a child is spanked for going into the street) to hostility so intense that the death of the other is desired. The former would be an example of *legitimate instrumental violence* and the latter of *illegitimate expressive violence*.

Our knowledge about family violence is influenced by methodological limitation in research. Social desirability, for example, can result in the reporting of a behavior in more acceptable terms, i.e., a punch with a closed fist is reported by the interviewee as a slap. The retrospective nature of survey research data allows the participants to "forget" or redefine the behaviors in accordance with the current state of their relationship. Since there is the tendency for the data on spouse and child abuse to be from the perspective of one spouse, usually the wife, our view of family violence may be skewed.

## IS FAMILY VIOLENCE A NEW PHENOMENON: ARE WE MORE VIOLENT TODAY?

As an academic topic of research, family violence is a new phenomenon. A special issue of *Journal of Marriage and the Family* in 1971 devoted to family violence represented the first research effort not limited to child abuse or a few psychiatric studies of abused wives.

The fact that this had not been a topic of research should not be construed as indicating the absence of violent family interaction. For example, a Massachusetts law during the colonial period required that cohabitation be peaceful, and yet there were numerous examples that this requirement was not met and that not all citizens upheld the law. The First Church of Boston excommunicated Mary Whorten for "reviling of her husband and sticking of him in other vile and wicked courses" (Morgan, 1966, p.

141). One man in Plymouth Colony was punished for abusing his wife by "kicking her off from a stoole into the fier," and another for "drawing his wife in an unciviel manner on the snow." Joan Miller was charged with "beating and reviling her husband and egging her children to healpe, her bidding them to knock him in the head and whishing his vitals mights chock himme" (Demos, 1970, p. 93). The husband's right to chastise his wife with a whip or rattan no bigger than his thumb, a remnant of ancient law, was upheld by a Mississippi court in 1928. This law, which prevailed for nearly a half century, limited the husband's use of corporal punishment to those "in great cases of emergency" and with "salutatory re-straints" (Bradley v. State, Walker, 158, Miss. 1824).

A North Carolina court, in 1874, ruled that the husband has no right "to chastise his wife under any circumstances." This ruling did note, however, that if "no permanent injury has been inflicted, nor malice, cruelty, or dangerous violence shown by the husband, it is better to draw the curtains, shut out the public gaze, and leave the parties to forget and forgive" (State v. Oliver, 70, N.C., 60, 61, 1874).

In 1885 a member of the Pennsylvania legislature expressed concern about the economic cost to society for providing for the imprisoned wife beater and his family. Following the lead set by the state of Maryland, this state governing body suggested that public whippings be used as an alternative punishment (Steinmetz & Straus, 1974).

The phenomenon of the battered husband has also been documented (Steinmetz, 1977–78). The charivari, a post-Renaissance custom, attempted to shame and humiliate wayward individuals who were considered to be a threat to the social order of the patriarchal community. For example, in France, the battered husband was forced to wear outlandish outfits, and ride backwards around the village on a donkey while holding on to the tail. The Brittons treated the beaten husband by strapping him into a cart and parading him through the booing crowds, while the assaultive wife was forced to ride backwards on a donkey, drink wine, and wipe her mouth with the animal's tail (Shorter, 1975).

Children were also not immune from abuse. The Hammurabi code of 2100 B.C. and the Hebrew code of 800 B.C. considered infanticide to be an acceptable practice (Bates, 1977). The Bible provided parents with specific guidelines on education: "He who spares his rod hates his son, but he who loves him disciplines him diligently" (Proverbs 13:24).

The practice of burying children in the foundations of buildings existed throughout history and as recently as the sixteenth century German children were buried alive beneath the steps of public buildings (Bates, 1977).

In 1646, a law attempted to help parents control their rebellious children. This law noted that "unless the parents have been very unchristianly negligent in the education of such children or have so provoked them by extreme and cruel correction any child over 16 years of age and of sufficient understanding who cursed, smitted and would not obey his natural mother or father, then would be put to death" (Bremner, 1970, p. 37).

During the Industrial Revolution children endured long hours of labor, extreme physical hardship and numerous beatings to ensure that they would exhibit no laziness. In 1874, the New York courts were forced to label Mary Ellen, a nine-year-old battered child, a member of the animal kingdom in order to protect her. The need to use laws enacted by the Society for the Prevention of Cruelty to Animals to protect children was instrumental in the founding of the Society for Prevention of Cruelty to Children. However, it was nearly a century later before all states had laws mandating the reporting of child abuse, requiring the investigation of reported cases, and providing services to these children and their families.

In the early 1980s abuse of elders was considered to be the new domestic violence problem and social critics mused over this latest indication of the breakdown of the American family. However, historical analysis of the treatment of and role performed by adults in earlier periods in the United States suggest that contemporary United States represents a considerably more humane period (Steinmetz, 1981, 1984). This stance has also been supported by Radbill (1968) and de Mause (1974) who suggest that children today are exposed to less neglect, mistreatment, and violence than at any other time in history.

To examine violence levels in the recent past, Straus, Gelles, and Steinmetz (1980) compared parent-child violence used by 306 couples with teenage children between 13 and 17 and the violence these parents experienced when they were teens. Over one-third of these parents had used physical punishment during the year of the survey. Results indicated an "almost" identical rate of hitting teenagers by the grandparent generation: 37.3%. Thus parents were physically punished as teenagers in about the same numbers as they are currently punishing their own teenage children. Straus et al. (1980) suggest that the seeming increase in child abuse is probably the result of greater public awareness, less public toleration of cruelty to children, and the uncovering of cases through new laws that require doctors and others to report cases of child abuse.

## IS VIOLENCE WIDESPREAD?

Domestic quarrels were a factor in 31% of homicides in Georgia during 1972 (Boston Globe, 1973); 13% of nationwide homicide in 1969 (Truninger, 1971); 23% in a Detroit study (Wilt & Bannon, 1976); and

24.7% of Philadelphia homicides between 1948 and 1952 (Wolfgang, 1958).

Besharov (1975) estimated that 2,000 children were the victims of homicides at the hands of their parents that year. Nationally, sibling homicides in 1983 constituted nearly 2% of all homicides (U.S. Department of Justice, 1985); over 3% of the homicides between 1948 and 1952 that occurred in Philadelphia (Wolfgang, 1958) and 3% of the homicides in New York City in 1965 (Bard, 1971) were sibling homicides.

Numerous studies document that between one-half and three-fourths of all women have probably experienced physical violence from their partners at some time (Gelles, 1974; Steinmetz, 1977a; Straus et al., 1980). However, since most of these studies surveyed intact couples and confined their questions to interaction with the current mate, these findings are probably underestimates. For a large number of women, about one out of five, the abuse is not an isolated incident, but occurs repeatedly (Straus et al., 1980; Walker, 1979); for one out of 15 to 20 women severe physical battering occurs (Gelles, 1974; Kentucky Commission on Women, 1979; Steinmetz, 1977b); and for about 1,700 women each year, the violence results in death (Steinmetz, 1978b).

A national survey of 2,143 intact families (Straus et al., 1980) revealed that almost seven out of every 100 couples had thrown something at a spouse in the previous year; 7% had slapped; 13% had pushed, shoved or grabbed; 1.5% had experienced a "beating up"; and one out of every 200 couples used a gun or knife on a spouse. When respondents reported on behaviors over the entire marriage the ratio was considerably higher: 16% threw something; 18% slapped, almost one out of four pushed, shoved or grabbed; 5% beat up; and about 3% used a gun or knife on a spouse.

Although husbands and wives appear to be equal as victims and perpetrators of homicide (Wolfgang, 1958) and the less extreme forms of spouse violence (Steinmetz, 1977–78, 1980a; Straus et al., 1980), husbands as victims constitute an extremely small amount of incidents resulting in serious (but not fatal) injury. While the Straus et al. (1980) study found that one-fourth of wives perpetrated violence that was not retaliated by husbands or in response to that of the husband, clinicians and police document that much of the violence that wives perpetrate is in self-defense. Furthermore, these data do not reveal the actual frequency with which these acts occur, the duration of the act, the intensity or severity of the violence, or the degree of injury. Clinical data suggest that when these factors are considered, women are more frequently victims of severe abuse.

Based on police records and a random sample of families, it was estimated that 7% of the wives and just over a half of a percent (.6) of the husbands would be victims of severe physical abuse by their spouse (Steinmetz, 1977b). This ratio of 1 : 13 was found in a recent update although the numbers of abuse incidents increased dramatically (Steinmetz, in press). Ian Oswald (1980) examined the histories of patients admitted to the Royal Infirmary of Edinburgh because of parasuicide. During 1977 and 1978, 592 admissions of women who were married (or living with a man) and between 20 and 40 years of age, answered 30 items which contained questions on victim and perpetrator of violence. Oswald found 299 reported domestic violence; and 263 were victims of violence. Of this number 124 (46%) reported that they were excessively violent and 36 (12%) had been perpetrators of violence but were not the victim of violence.

Spanking, the most prevalent form of family violence, has been reported to occur in between 84% and 97% of all families (Blumberg, 1964–65; Erlanger, 1974; Stark & McEvoy, 1970). A high percentage of these families continue to use corporal punishment for disciplining their children until tenth grade (Bachman, 1967) and twelfth grade (Steinmetz, 1971, 1974; Straus, 1971).

The American Humane Association (1978) found that 36% of reported abuse cases involved children between 10 and 18; Gil (1970) found nearly 17% of abused youth were over 12. Straus et al. (1980) reported 66% of youths 10–14 were struck; 34% of those 15–17 had been hit. In fact, the abuse had two peaks: 3–4-year-olds and 15–17-year-olds. A nationwide study of adolescent girls revealed that 12% had been beaten and 9% had been raped (Knopoka, 1975).

Physical punishment is also used on the very young. Korsch, Christian, Gozzi, & Carlson (1965) interviewed 100 mothers of infants who were outpatients in Los Angeles clinics and found almost half spanked infants under 12 months of age and one-fourth started spanking before the infants had reached six months of age. Wittenberg (1971) found no social class differences in methods used to discipline children, but 41% of his sample used some form of physical punishment for babies under 6 months of age; 87% had used physical force before their children were two.

A national study of 2,143 intact families with children aged 3–17 found that each year 3% were kicked, bitten, or punched and more than 1% are beaten each year; 1 child in 1,000 has been attacked with a gun or knife each year (Straus et al., 1980). When the data-recording period extended beyond the "previous year" to include "ever happened," 8% were kicked, bitten, or punched, about nine times per year; 4% were beaten and this occurred about six times per year; and 3% had a gun or knife used on them.

Parent-child violence is not unidirectional. Children perpetrated acts of violence on their parents: 18% or one out of five American children engage in one or more acts (Straus et al., 1980).

Sibling violence, considered by most to be normal interaction, had rates ranging from 63% to 73% (Steinmetz, 1977a, 1977b). The Straus et al. (1980) study which contained 733 families with two or more children ages 3–17, reported that 75% used physical violence and averaged 21 acts per year. Thirty-eight percent of siblings kicked or hit, 14% "beat-up," 0.8% threatened to use a gun or knife, and 0.3% used a gun or knife. When these percentages are extrapolated to the 36.3 million children between ages 3 and 17 who have siblings, we find that 6.5 million children have been beaten up by a sibling and that nearly 2 million children at some time during their childhood have faced a gun or knife.

As life expectancy increases and the cost and availability of nursing care limits the accessibility, one can expect more families to provide care for their elderly kin. Preparation for this caregiving role is not usually provided in a formal setting and informal role models are rare. This lack of knowledge, combined with limited support services, assures difficulties when competing demands for financial, emotional and physical resources arise.

During a 12-month period, Family Service Association of Greater Lawrence, Massachusetts investigated 82 referrals, of which one-fourth were elders living with their family who experienced abuse or neglect (Langdon, 1980). Baltimore police in a single year reported 149 assaults against individuals 60 years old or older. They noted that nearly two-thirds of these assaults (62.7%) were committed by a relative other than the spouse (Block & Sinnott, 1980).

The above data reflect primarily physical abuse. Sexual abuse of children and marital rape are also part of family violence. Sexual abuse of children is greatly underestimated and underresearched (Tierney & Corwin, 1983). DeFrancis (1969) estimated 40 cases per million population or about 8,000 cases based on our current population. The National Center on Child Abuse and Neglect (1978) estimated between 60,000 and 100,000 cases each year. In an extrapolation from reported incidents of sexual offenses against children, Sarafino (1979) projected about 336,000 incidents per year. Finkelhor (1979) reported that about 20% of college women were victimized, about half the amount of men were victimized, and family members were the perpetrators in about half the cases.

Marital rape—sexual assault on women by their husbands—appears to be quite prevalent. In a review of the research in this area, Finkelhor and Yllo (1983) report the following: 36% of 304 battered women in 10 shelters had been raped by their husbands or cohabiting partner (Spektor, 1980); a similar rate was found by Giles-Sims (1983); 37% of a sample of 119 women in California experienced marital rape (Pagelow, 1980); and 14% of a sample of 930 women reported an "unwanted" sexual experience with husband or ex-husband (Russell, 1980). Finkelhor and Yllo surveyed 326 women in a childhood sexual abuse study and reported that the use or threat of physical force by the partner in order to have sex was experienced by 10% of the women; however, 3% of the women had this experience with a stranger. Although forced sex in marriage is probably the most frequent type of sexual assault, women who have been sexually assaulted by their husbands or partners avoid defining themselves as raped (Gelles, 1979).

## WHAT ARE THE CHARACTERISTICS OF FAMILIES EXPERIENCING FAMILY VIOLENCE?

In this section, five characteristics will be examined. These have been selected because they are consistently linked in the literature to family violence. These include: mental illness and psychiatric disorders; income; education; employment status (the components of social class); and substance abuse.

### *Mental Illness and Psychiatric Disorders*

It is easy to understand why child abusers or wife batterers are labeled as mentally ill—obviously normal people would not behave this way. Likewise, a battered wife is described as having psychiatric defects—why else would she allow herself to become a victim?

Although early studies of child abuse tended to attribute numerous psychiatric defects, such as depression, immaturity, impulsiveness, and dependency, to abusing parents (Elmer, 1971; Holter & Friedman, 1968; Steel & Pollock, 1974; Kempe & Helfer, 1972), evidence to the contrary is overwhelming. For example, Steel and Pollock (1974) showed that abusive parents did not exhibit characteristics different from a cross section of the general population; in Kempe and Helfer's (1972) study less than 10% of the abusers were seriously mentally ill; and 8 out of 35 batterers, about 13% more than expected in a normal population, evidenced organic dysfunctions in encephalographic examinations (Smith, Honigsberger, & Smith, 1973). In one study of 60 battered women, almost the entire sample had sought medical help for stress-related complaints and many evidenced symptoms commonly associated with the rape-trauma syndrome; more than half had evidence of prior psychological dysfunction; and 13 had been hospitalized with violent psychotic behavior. In fact, many of the characteristics attributed to victims of abuse appear to be the result of the battering rather than personalities that allow or encourage abuse (Steinmetz, 1979; see Steinmetz, in press for a review of this research).

The mental illness of elders has been reported as contributing to their abuse by caregiving kin (Steinmetz, 1981, 1984); and mental illness of caregivers a factor in the abuse of elders (Bergman, O'Malley, & Segars, 1980). In a study of caregivers who battered an elderly relative it was found that 14% of abusers were reported to be suffering from mental illness and 21% had a past suicide attempt (Bergman et al., 1980).

Earlier studies reported a negative relationship between social class and family violence (Blumberg, 1964–65; Elmer, 1971; Gil, 1970; Holter & Friedman, 1968) which was questioned by Erlanger (1974) and Steinmetz & Straus, (1974). It was noted that the use of public agency files may produce a bias towards the lower class.

## Income

Greater financial resources enable parents to procure stress-reducing mechanisms, such as baby-sitters, vacations, nursery schools, and camps which provide them with "time-out" from child rearing/homemaking responsibilities. The interactions between stress and income and the effect on family violence is critical. The national survey (Straus et al., 1980) found that increased stress, as rated by 18 items, had no effect on the very poor (family income below $6,000) or on those with family incomes above $20,000 (where income provides a cushion) but did increase the likelihood of child abuse of the middle-income group. Furthermore, a higher income enables one to secure medical and psychological help from a private physician (Prescott & Letko, 1977), thus reducing the potential for violence. Socioeconomic stress and inadequate resources accounted for 36% of the variance in rates of child abuse in another study (Garbarino, 1976). Finally, mothers in higher income families have had greater access to contraception and abortion, thus enabling them to have greater control over family size and spacing, a factor related to family conflict and violence (Farrington, 1977; Gil, 1970; Johnson & Morse, 1968; Straus, 1976; Young, 1964).

In general there is a consistent decrease in violence as income levels go up. Fifty-three percent of families with incomes under $6,000 reported abuse between siblings, 22% reported child abuse, 11% reported spouse abuse. In contrast, reported abuse for families with incomes of $20,000 and over were sibling abuse, 41%; child abuse, 11% and spouse abuse, 2% (Straus et al., 1980).

Income is also related to incidents of elder abuse. Twenty-three percent of caregivers in one study of elder abuse reported that they had financial problems; 16% were listed as long-term problems (Bergman et al., 1980). Twenty-seven percent earned less than $5,200; 23% earned between $5,200 and $9,000; thus 50% were extremely low income.

## Education

Levels of education have also been linked to family violence. Some studies show a negative relationship between the husband's education and spouse and child abuse and between the wife's education and spouse violence (Steinmetz, 1977a). Similar findings were reported by Gelles (1974) with the exception of high levels of violence for women college graduates. A curvilinear relationship was found when education was categorized into four levels: eighth grade or below, some high school, high school graduate, and college. For both men and women there was a positive relationship between the first three levels of education and child abuse (11, 15, and 18% for men; 12, 14, and 17% for women). It was among those parents who had been exposed to college that a decrease in child-abuse rates occurred—11% for both men and women.

A similar relationship was found between spouse abuse and education. High school dropouts had the highest abuse rates, 6% each, as well as the highest victimization rates, 7% each. A college education reduced the likelihood of a woman being victimized (2%), but increased the likelihood of victimization for men (5%).

## Unemployment

Unemployment, because it often represents personal (rather than societal) failure, has led to the use of violence as a controlling mechanism. In one study 48% of a sample of abusers had experienced unemployment during the year preceding the abuse (Gil, 1970). Families in which the father was employed full-time, consistently had lower levels of child and spouse abuse (Straus et al., 1980). Furthermore, part-time employment was more likely to predict family violence than was unemployment (Prescott & Letko, 1977).

## Substance Abuse

The actual relationship between alcohol and violence appears to be controversial. Do individuals drink, lose control, and then beat their spouses or children, or do they wish to vent their anger on their spouse and/or children and drink in order to gain the courage to do so and to provide an excuse for their action? Numerous studies have documented the relationship between alcohol use and child abuse (Bayles, 1978; Gil, 1970; Wertham, 1972; Young, 1964); and alcohol use and spouse abuse (Bayles, 1978; Gelles, 1974; Prescott & Letko, 1977; Roy, 1977). Twenty-eight percent of a sample of abusers of elderly (Bergman et al., 1980) were reported to be alcohol or drug abusers. MacAndrew and Edgerton (1969) suggest that the effects of alcohol on a social behavior is influenced by cultural expectation and socialization. Thus, in some societies the use of alcohol is associated with considerable violence; in some, no relationship exists; in others, violence is associated with alcohol, but only under certain conditions.

Unfortunately, much of the research on this topic is subjectively based on victims or third-party responses rather than chemical analysis of blood alcohol levels and an in-depth investigation of the abusers' total drinking behavior. Furthermore, a definition of alcoholism or accurate operational measure of the levels of intoxication is lacking.

In a comprehensive review of the research on the relationship between alcohol use and incidence of child abuse, Orme and Rimmer (1981) report the lack of empirical data to support the association between alcoholism and child abuse and conclude that estimates of alcoholism and alcohol problems in the general population appear to be identical as that in the child abusing population.

## IS THERE A CYCLE OF VIOLENCE?

The data supporting the cycle of violence theory are substantial. Although the statement "abused children grow up to be abusing adults" (Bryant, 1963; Craft, 1969; Oliver & Taylor, 1971; Silver, Dublin & Lourie, 1969; Wasserman, 1967; Zalba, 1966) needs qualification because we haven't studied abused children who grow up to be warm, loving adults, support for the influence of growing up in a violent home on later victimization and abuse are striking.

Relentless brutality, which was often condoned by other family members, characterized the backgrounds of children who committed murder

(Bender, 1959; Sargent, 1962). Studies of adolescents who committed parricide (Sadoff, 1971; Tanay, 1975) reveal that the adolescents' parents were cruel and frequently beat other members of the family, especially the children's mothers. Climent and Ervin (1972) found that 75% of a sample composed of 30 individuals admitted to the emergency room as a result of violent behavior had been assaulted by their fathers, and 14% had been assaulted by their mothers, while only 16% of the control group experienced assault by father and only 3% (one individual) was assaulted by the mother.

Brutalizing childhood was found to be characteristic of rapists (Brownmiller, 1975; Hartogs, 1951), split personalities (Schreiber, 1973), and suicides (Bender & Curran, 1940; Gayford, 1975; MacDonald, 1967). A study of the childhood environment of 14 political assassins revealed disorganized, broken families, parental abuse and rejection, and marginal integration into society (Steinmetz, 1977a).

Gayford (1975), in a study of 100 battered wives, discovered that 51 of the batterers and 23 of the victims had a violent childhood. Furthermore, 37% of abused wives and 54% of abusive husbands had abused their children. In a sample of battered women, Roy (1977) reported violence in the families of origin of 81% of abusive husbands and 33% of abused wives. Parker and Schumacher (1977) reported that about 68% of the abused wives in their sample had mothers who had been abused compared with 25% of nonabused wives who had witnessed their mothers being abused.

The effects of witnessing violence on later violent behavior is especially potent for boys. In a study of marital violence, Rosenbaum and O'Leary (1981) found that although abused wives were no more likely to have witnessed parental abuse than nonabused wives, a strong and significant relationship existed between the husband's witnessing parents abusing each other and using physical violence on his wife. These researchers also found that nearly 82% of husbands who witnessed marital violence as children were also victims of child abuse by their parents. Rosenbaum and O'Leary note that male children of couples in which there is wife abuse are clearly at high risk for development into the next generation of abusive households.

This is consistent with Feshbach's (1970) review of the aggression literature which showed that boys respond to severe punishment by exhibiting overt aggression, girls with inhibited passive behavior and conflict and anxiety about aggression.

Kinard (1979) found that abused children were more likely than nonabused children to use aggression as a response to frustration with peers.

The double whammy described by Straus et al. (1980) illustrates how the combined effect on the child of both witnessing violence and experiencing violence increases (about double) the acceptability of using violence to solve problems as well as actual use of violence years later as an adult. Furthermore, while the probability of nonviolent parents being violently attacked by their children is about one out of 400, the probability of parents who use severe violence on their children being attacked is 200 out of 400 (Steinmetz, 1980b).

## WHAT ARE SOME NEW AREAS FOR RESEARCH IN FAMILY VIOLENCE?

Two major needs must be addressed in order to improve research on family violence. The first is the need for longitudinal research designs allowing in-depth studies of families during different stages of the life cycles. The second is the need for multidisciplinary approaches. For example, genetic and hormonal influences on family violence need to be explored. The effect of the extra X chromosome on male violence has been demonstrated; more recently, the pre-menstrual syndrome (PMS) effect on women's violence is being explored. What effect might PMS have on child abuse?

Neurological data on organic brain syndrome and abuse are other rich avenues of exploration. Early research found that certain families over several generations that were predisposed to episodic violence displayed particular brain wave patterns. This raises the question of genetic transmission and represents a new dimension in the understanding of the cycle of violence.

How does alcohol contribute to violence? Without the benefit of scientific research, our own personal observations reveal that some people become the uninhibited life of the party when drunk, while others fall asleep, and still others become nasty and aggressive. We also know that there is a tendency in certain families for the members to become alcoholic. Therefore, the genetic variable of alcoholism and this effect on the cycle of violence between generations must be considered, as well as the social-learning role model from an intergenerational perspective.

The link between nutrition and abuse needs further research. The Feingold diet (1975), which posits a relationship between food additives and hyperactivity, while "disproven" in some research studies is clearly supported by clinical observations over time by families and institutional staff who have replaced candy, soft drinks, and cookie-type sweets with fruit and vegetables. Since much of the research on the Feingold diet is considerably flawed—extremely small samples, no control groups, no controls or adaptation of treatment diet for sex of children, age or weight, and limited observation after the ingestion of the "treatment" food (usually 30 minutes to two hours)—additional methodologically sound research on the relationship between diet and violence is needed (Adams, 1981; Prinz, Roberts, & Hantman, 1980; Stare, Whelan, & Sheridan, 1980).

Family violence affects all members: the victims, the abusers, and the witnesses. It has been demonstrated that the effect of this violence goes beyond the interactions of the family and pervade all aspects of our environment. Thus, even if we don't experience family violence directly, we all experience indirectly, the fallout resulting from family violence: higher insurance rates, higher taxes to support needed social services to victims and their families, as well as the legal cost of prosecuting and punishing offenders, and the social and emotional stress of living in an environment characterized by violence. It is in our best interest to direct financial and intellectual resources toward eliminating family violence.

## REFERENCES

Adams, W. (1981). Lack of behavioral effects from Feingold diet violations. *Perceptual and Math Skills, 52*(1), 307–313.

American Humane Association (1978). National analysis of official child neglect and abuse reporting. Denver, American Humane Association.

Bachman, J. G. (1967). *Youth in transition*. Ann Arbor, Michigan: University of Michigan, Institute for Social Research.

Bard, M. (1971). The study and modification of intrafamilial violence. In J. L. Singer (Ed.), *The control of aggression and violence*, pp. 149–64. New York: Academic Press.

Bates, R. P. (1977). Child abuse—The problem. Paper presented at the 2nd World Conference of the International Society on Family Law, June, Montreal, Canada.

Bayles, J. A. (1978). Violence, alcohol problems and other problems in disintegrating families. *Journal of Studies on Alcohol, 39*(3), 551–563.

Bender, L. (1959). Children and adolescents who have killed. *American Journal of Psychiatry, 116*, 510–513.

Bender, L., & Curran, F. J. (1940). Children and adolescents who kill. *Criminal Psychopathology, 1*, 297–322.

Bergman, J. A., O'Malley, H., & Segars, H. (1980). Legal research and services for the elderly. Elder abuse in Massachusetts: A survey of professional and paraprofessionals. *Elder abuse: The hidden problem*. (A Briefing) Select Committee on Aging, U.S. House of Representatives, 96th Congress (Boston, Massachusetts, June 23, 1979). Washington, D.C.: U.S. Government Printing Office.

Besharov, J. D. (1975). Building a community response to child abuse and maltreatment. *Children Today, 4*(5), 2.

Block, M., & Sinnott, J. P. (1980). Prepared Statement *Elder Abuse: The Hidden Problem*. Briefing by the Select Committee on Aging. U.S. House of Representatives: 96 June 23, 1979. Boston, Massachusetts pp. 10–12, Washington, D.C.

Blumberg, M. (1964–65). When parents hit out. *Twentieth Century, 173*, 39–44.

*Boston Globe* (1973). Home strife number one cause of murders in Atlanta. (Feb. 6), 12.

Bradley v. State, Walker, 158, Miss. 1824.

Bremner, R. H. (1970). *Children and youth in America: A documentary history* Vol. 1 (p. 37). Boston, MA: Harvard University Press.

Brownmiller, S. (1975). *Against our will: Men, women and rape*. New York: Simon & Schuster.

Bryant, H. D. (1963). Physical Abuse of Children: An Agency Study. *Child Welfare, 42*, 125–30.

Climent, C. F., & Ervin, F. R. (1972). Historical data in the evaluation of violent subjects. *Archives of General Psychiatry, 27*, 621–24.

Craft, M. (1969). The natural history of psychopathic disorder. *British Journal of Psychiatry, 115*, 39–44.

DeFrancis, F. (1969). *Protecting the child victim of sex crimes committed by adults*. Denver: American Humane Association.

de Mause, L. (1974). *A history of childhood*. New York: The Psycho-History Press.

Demos, J. (1970). *A little commonwealth*. New York: Oxford University Press.

Elmer, E. (1971). Studies of Child Abuse and Infant Accidents. In *The Mental Health of the Child*, U.S. National Institute of Mental Health, Washington, DC: U.S. Government Printing Office.

Erlanger, H. R. (1974). Social class and corporal punishment: A reassessment. *American Sociological Review, 39* (Feb), 68–85.

Farrington, K. (1977). Family violence and household density: Does the crowded home breed aggression? Paper presented at the Annual Meeting of the Society for the Study of Social Problems, September 5–9, Chicago, IL.

Feingold, B. F. (1975). *Why your child is hyperactive*. New York: Random House.

Feshbach, S. (1970). Aggression. In P. H. Mussen (Ed.), *Carmichael's manual of child psychology, Vol. 2*. New York: John Wiley.

Finkelhor, D. (1979). *Sexually victimized children*. New York: Free Press.

Finkelhor, D., & Yllo, K. (1983). Rape in marriage: A sociological view. In D. Finkelhor, R. Gelles, G. Hotaling, & H. Straus. *The dark side of families*. Beverly Hills, CA: Sage.

Garbarino, J. A. (1976). A preliminary study of some ecological correlates of child abuse: The impact of socioeconomic stress on mothers. *Child Development, 47*, 178–185.

Gayford, J. (1975). Wife battering: A preliminary survey of 100 cases. *British Medical Journal, 1*, 195–197.

Gelles, R. J. (1974). *The violent home*. Beverly Hills, CA: Sage.

Gelles, R. J. (1979). *Family violence*. Beverly Hills, CA: Sage.

Gil, D. (1970). *Violence against children: Physical child abuse in the United States*. Cambridge, MA: Harvard University Press.

Giles-Sims, J. (1983). *Wife beating: A systems theory approach*. New York: Guilford Press.

Hartogs, R. (1951). Discipline in the early life of sex delinquents and sex criminals. *Nervous Child, 9*, (March), 167–73.

Holter, J. C., & Friedman, S. B. (1968). Principals of management in child abuse cases. *American Journal of Orthopsychiatry, 38*(1), 127–138.

Johnson, B., & Morse, H. A. (1968). Injured children and their parents. *Children, 15*, 147–152.

Kempe, C. H., & Helfer, R. E. (Eds.) (1972). *Helping the battered child and his family*. Philadelphia: J. P. Lippincott.

Kentucky Commission on Women (1979). *A survey of spousal violence against women*. Frankfort, Kentucky.

Kinard, E. M. (1979). The psychological consequences of abuse for the child. *Journal of Social Issues, 35*(2), 82–100.

Knopoka, G. (1975). *Young girls: A portrait of adolescence*. Englewood Cliffs, NJ: Prentice-Hall.

Korsch, B. M., Christian, J. B., Gozzi, E. K., & Carlson, P. V. (1965). Infant care and punishment: A pilot study. *American Journal of Public Health, 55*, 1880–1888.

Langdon, G. (1980). Statement presented at the House of Representatives Select Committee on Aging (96), June 23, 1979: Boston, MA, pp. 16–21, Washington, DC: U.S. Government Printing Office.

MacAndrew, C., & Edgerton, R. B. (1969). *Drunken comportment: A social explanation.* Chicago: Aldine Press.

MacDonald, J. M. (1967). Homicidal threats. *American Journal of Psychiatry, 124*, 475–82.

Morgan, E. S. (1966). *The Puritan family.* New York: Harper & Row.

National Center on Child Abuse and Neglect. (1978). *Child sexual abuse: Incest, assault and sexual exploitation* Pub. No. (OHDS) 79-30166. Washington, DC: U.S. Department of Health, Education and Welfare.

Oliver, J. E., & Taylor, A. (1971). Five generations of ill-treated children in one family pedigree. *British Journal of Psychiatry, 119*(552), 473–80.

Orme, T. C., & Rimmer, J. (1981). Alcoholism and child abuse. *Journal of Studies on Alcohol, 42*(3), 273–287.

Oswald, I. (1980). Domestic violence by women. *The Lancet*, Dec. 6, p. 1253.

Pagelow, M. D. (1980). Does the law help battered wives? Some research notes. Madison, WI: Law and Society Association.

Parker, B., & Schumacher, D. (1977). The battered wife syndrome and violence in the nuclear family of origin: A controlled pilot study. *American Journal of Public Health, 67*, 760–761.

Prescott, S., & Letko, C. (1977). Battered: A social psychological perspective. In M. M. Roy (Ed.), *Battered women: A psychosociological study of domestic violence* (pp. 72–96). New York: Van Nostrand Reinhold.

Prinz, R. J., Roberts, W. A. & Hantman, E. (1980). Dietary correlates of hyperactive behavior in children. *Consulting and Clinical Psychology, 48*(6), 760–769.

Radbill, S. X. (1968). A history of child abuse and infanticide. In R. E. Helfer & C. H. Kempe (Eds.), *The battered child.* Chicago, IL: University of Chicago Press.

Rosenbaum, A., & O'Leary, D. (1981). Children: The unintended victims of marital violence. *American Journal of Orthopsychiatry, 51*(4), 692–699.

Roy, M. (1977). A current survey of 150 cases. In M. Roy (Ed.), *Battered women: A psychosociological study of domestic violence.* New York: Van Nostrand Reinhold.

Russell, D. (1980). The prevalence and impact of marital rape in San Francisco. Paper presented at the annual meetings of the American Sociological Association, New York.

Sadoff, R. L. (1971). Clinical observations on parricide. *Psychiatric Quarterly, 45*, 165–69.

Sarafino, E. (1979). An estimate of the nation-wide incidence of sexual offenses against children. *Child Welfare, 58*, 127–134.

Sargent, D. (1962). Children who kill: A family conspiracy. *Social Work, 7*, 35–42.

Schreiber, F. (1973). *Sybil.* New York: Warner Books.

Shorter, E. (1975). *The making of the modern family.* New York: Basic Books.

Silver, L. B., Dublin, C. C., & Lourie, R. S. (1969). Child abuse syndrome: The "gray areas" in establishing a diagnosis. *Pediatrics*, 44, 594–600.

Smith, S. M., Honigsberger, L., & Smith, C. A. (1973). EEG and personality factors in baby beaters. *British Medical Journal, 870*(3), 20–22.

Spektor, P. (1980). Testimony delivered to the Law Enforcement Subcommittee of the Minnesota House of Representatives, February 29.

Stare, F. J., Whelan, E. & Sheridan, M. (1980). Diet and hyperactivity: Is there a relationship? *Pediatrics, 66*(4), 521–525.

Stark, R., & McEvoy, J., III (1970). Middle class violence. *Psychology Today*, 4 November, 52–65.

State v. Oliver, 70, N.C., 60, 61, 1874.

Steel, B. F., & Pollock, D. A. (1974). A psychiatric study of parents who abuse infants and small children. In R. E. Helfer & C. H. Kempe (Eds.), *The battered child* (pp. 89–134). Chicago, IL: University of Chicago Press.

Steinmetz, S. K. (1971). Occupation and physical punishment: A response to stress. *Journal of Marriage and the Family, 33*, 664–666.

Steinmetz, S. K. (1974). Occupational environment to physical punishment and dogmatism. In S. K. Steinmetz & M. A. Straus (Eds.), *Violence in the Family.* New York: Harper & Row.

Steinmetz, S. K. (1977a). *The cycle of violence: Assertive, aggressive, and abusive family interaction.* New York: Praeger.

Steinmetz, S. K. (1977b). Wifebeating-husbandbeating—A comparison of the use of physical violence between spouses to resolve marital fights. In M. M. Ray (Ed.), *Women: A psychosociological study of domestic violence* (pp. 63–72). New York: Van Nostrand Reinhold.

Steinmetz, S. K. (1977–78). The Battered Husband Syndrome. *Victimology, 2,* 499–509.

Steinmetz, S. K. (1978a). Battered parents. *Society, 15,* 54.

Steinmetz, S. K. (1978b). Violence between family members. *Marriage and Family Review, 1,* 1–16.

Steinmetz, S. K. (1979). Wife beating: A critique and reformation of existing theory. *The Bulletin of the American Academy of Psychiatry and the Law, 6*(3), 322–334.

Steinmetz, S. K. (1980a). Women and violence: Victims and perpetrators. *American Journal of Psychotherapy, 34*(3), 334–350.

Steinmetz, S. K. (1980b). Violence-prone families. *Annals of New York Academy of Sciences, 347,* 251–265.

Steinmetz, S. K. (1981). Elder abuse. *Aging* (Jan/Feb), 6–10.

Steinmetz, S. K. (1984). Family violence towards elders. In S. Saunders, A. Anderson, C. Hart, & G. Rubenstein (Eds.), *Violent individuals and families. A handbook for practitioners*. Springfield, IL: Charles C Thomas.

Steinmetz, S. K. (in press). Family violence. In M. Sussman & S. Steinmetz (Eds.), *Handbook of marriage and family*. New York: Plenum Press.

Steinmetz, S. K., & Amsden, D. J. (1983). Dependent elders, family stress and abuse. In Th. H. Brubaker (Ed.), *Family relationships in later life*. Beverly Hills: Sage.

Steinmetz, S. K., & Straus, M. A. (Eds.). (1974). *Violence in the family*. New York: Harper & Row.

Straus, M. A. (1971). Some social antecedents of physical punishment: A linkage theory interpretation. *Journal of Marriage and the Family, 33,* 658–663.

Straus, M. A. (1976). Sexual inequality, cultural norms and wife beating. *Victimology, 1*(1), 54–76.

Straus, M. A., Gelles, R. J., & Steinmetz, S. K. (1980). *Behind closed doors: Violence in American families*. New York: Doubleday.

Tanay, E. (1975). Reactive parricide. *Journal of Forensic Sciences, 21*(1), 76–82.

Tierney, N. S., & Corwin, D. L. (1983). Exploring intrafamilial child sexual abuse: A systems approach. In D. Finkelhor, R. Gelles, G. Hotaling, & M. Straus (Eds.), *The dark side of families*. Beverly Hills, CA: Sage.

Truninger, E. (1971). Marital violence, the legal solution. *Hastings Law Journal, 23* (Nov.), 259–276.

U.S. Department of Justice (1985). *FBI uniformed crime report*. Washington, DC: U.S. Government Printing Office.

Walker, L. E. (1979). Social consequences of feminism: The battered women's movement. Paper presented at the Annual Meeting of the American Psychological Association, New York.

Wasserman, S. (1967). The abused parent of the abused child. *Children, 14,* 175–179.

Wertham, F. (1972). Battered children and baffled adults. *Bulletin of the New York Academy of Medicine, 48,* 887–898.

Wilt, G. M., & Bannon, J. D. (1976). *Violence and the police: Homicides, assaults and disturbances*. Washington, DC, The Police Foundation.

Wittenberg, C. (1971). Studies of child abuse and infant accidents. In J. Segal (Ed.), *The mental health of the child: Program reports of the National Institute of Mental Health*. Washington, DC: U.S. Government Printing Office.

Wolfgang, M. E. (1958). *Patterns in criminal homicide*. Philadelphia: University of Pennsylvania Press.

Young, L. R. (1964). *Wednesday's children: A study of child neglect and abuse*. New York: McGraw-Hill.

Zalba, S. R. (1966). The abused child: I. A survey of the problems. *Social Work, 11*(4), 3–16.

# Part II

# CAUSES OF FAMILY VIOLENCE

# 4

# *Psychological Causes of Family Violence*

## Lenore E. A. Walker

Prior to the early 1970s, the family was thought to be the peaceful, calm, tranquil refuge we all seek from the hectic and sometimes violent outside world. Locking doors at night supposedly kept most crime out of our homes. Although it was known that some families were troubled, it was thought to be only a small percentage. Physical, sexual, and psychological abuse of family members was something that happened to others. Imagine the surprise when it was learned that women and children were more likely to be hurt at home by the same men who loved them.

It is estimated that such criminal acts are taking place in nearly half of all families. Straus, Gelles, and Steinmetz (1980) conducted an epidemiological survey of 2,000 families and found that 28% of the adults engaged in at least one physically abusive act during the year about which they inquired. Children abused each other as well as parents and grandparents, also in unexpectedly high frequency. In research conducted with already identified battered women, it was found that the rate of child abuse and threatened or actual violence against family, friends, pets, and treasured objects frequently occurred (Walker, 1984a). The old adage that violence begets more violence is nowhere more true than inside the family. Yet, for so long the violence was not acknowledged and even hidden from the view of others.

History tells us that there always have been men who commit violence against women. For thousands of years, however, it was considered to be women's lot. Wives who were not beaten were considered lucky. Most simply hoped they could be good enough to minimize the danger. Susan Brownmiller (1975) suggests that in the early days a woman married a man in order to protect herself from the danger of being raped by other men. She calls rapists the *shock troops* who frighten unmarried women into

71

monogamous relationships. Ann Jones (1980) suggests that batterers are the *home guard*; the knowledge that they could be beaten like other women was said to keep all wives in their place.

Women were taught, then, how to behave so as to avoid being beaten. The Bible and other writings throughout the ages suggested ways for women to develop a better character. Subsequently, it became appropriate to assume that a man had the right to beat a woman who misbehaved. Children, too, were considered an extension of men's property and discipline was seen as necessary to develop their good character as well. Beatings, often administered with objects and weapons, were allowed for their own good.

Today's message to women and children is not all that different. Women's advocates teach women to be independent and of strong character so that they do not have to rely on or need men who could hurt them. Much attention is focused on helping a battered woman heal with a minimum of scars so she can get on with her life. Often, a systems approach is utilized, suggesting each family member change and become stronger, as though that would cause the violence to stop. Many of the newer teachings of the church suggest that parents return to using weapons (often recommended is a wooden spoon) to discipline children because they say, *hands are for loving not hitting.* No-hitting rules, the obvious answer, is seen as abdicating from the parental responsibility to discipline children. Rarely is it stressed that stopping the violence is the man's responsibility, that he must learn to keep his temper under control, and use other conflict resolution strategies without the assistance of other family members. Rarely is it considered reasonable to expect the abusive men to stop their battering behavior no matter what the women's character.

The long tradition of spouse abuse has been linked with the religious and legal rights giving men the responsibility for deeds of their wives and children, thus necessitating their right to discipline those who were disobedient (Martin, 1982). The *rule of thumb* expression comes from old common-law statutes limiting men's discipline to hitting women with a stick no wider than their thumb. Today, most police and sheriff departments have a *stitch rule* which regulates the amount of injury required before criminal charges are filed against a wife beater. It is not surprising, given this long tradition of male supremacy, to expect that family violence is so closely linked with discrimination against women.

A political perspective is critical to the understanding of family violence. If the traditional views prevail, then violence in the family is seen as occurring because of character flaws in the woman or the man or the children. An analysis of psychological causation of family violence must acknowledge this long history and the lack of societal intervention.

This chapter is written from the knowledge of the long and unfair history of men's violence towards women. It is assumed that the underpinnings of all violence in society is rooted in the violence that begins at home, most of which is directed by men towards women although, certainly, women behave in violent ways towards men and children, too. However, the most serious violence and the greatest injuries are caused by men (Straus et al., 1980). The battered women studied indicate that their violent behavior is most likely reactive to being abused by men who love them (Frieze, 1980; Straus et al., 1980; Walker, 1984a). Women are most likely to use "biting," "scratching," and other close contact violent acts while men were most likely to use more serious assaultive tactics. In any case, all available empirical analyses of family violence begin with acknowledging the likelihood that the man is the batterer and the women and children the most likely victims.

## THEORETICAL BASES FOR UNDERSTANDING FAMILY VIOLENCE

The major theories that explain spouse abuse can be classified in three major categories: feminist-political, sociocultural, and psychological. The differences between these three major ideologies have been detailed elsewhere (Walker, 1981) but a brief explanation is necessary.

*The feminist-political* theories suggest that men beat women to gain the power to which they feel entitled because of the structure of a patriarchal society which teaches men to expect to be dominant. Religious teachings reinforce the male-supremacy viewpoint and encourage battered women to endure and pray for their mates' salvation (Davidson, 1978). Patriarchy is shown to foster wife abuse in the research by Dobash and Dobash (1981), who further suggest that the American economic structure cannot tolerate a nonsexist, pluralistic society and suggest that a restructuring of the capitalistic system is necessary before women will cease being battered. Clinicalization of family members in the battering of women is frowned upon by those applying the feminist-political analysis and theorists such as Wardell, Gillespie, and Leffler (1983) caution against errors in understanding which will result from continuing to use an individual psychopathology model. It is suggested that rigid sex-role socialization patterns result in the stereotyped male aggression and female passivity which is often found in battering relationships (Walker, 1979). Little boys are taught to turn all their unpleasant feelings into anger and strike out, while little girls are expected not to show their angry feelings while they nurture and care for others. Any deviation from these stereotypical standards is seen as a breach of the norm and is not acceptable behavior. Such unacceptable behavior is punishable by men, the dominant class. Women, as members of the oppressed class, must learn to accept punishment when they are wrong.

There has been an ongoing debate between those who favor the feminist-political ideology and those empirical sociologists, such as Gelles (1981), who believe ideology negatively influences data collection and analysis. Dobash and Dobash (1983) and Wardell et al. (1983) believe that scientific empiricism is so fraught with sexist bias that it cannot offer sufficient understanding of the causes of domestic violence to make it worthwhile to use its methodology to study the problem. Further discussion into this highly emotionally charged debate can be found in Gondolf (1984), Schechter (1982), and Walker (1984a). For the purposes of this chapter, a dichotomy between feminist ideology and empiricism will not be assumed. All research has ideological values which influence questions to be answered whether or not they are specified. Feminist empiricists call for explicit assumptions and careful scrutiny of potential sources of bias. An example of such scrutiny can be found in Bograd's (1984) feminist critique of a family systems analysis of battering relationships. Much of the empirical research cited herein has met such scrutiny, though admittedly to varying degrees which have been reported along with research results.

*Sociocultural theorists* attempt to define the norms for our society by analyzing group behavior. There certainly is overlap with some of the feminist-political and psychological theories. However, an analysis of the dominant cultural values, especially those which tolerate expression of aggression, is included. Sociological theory suggests that we are a society that tolerates a great deal of violence, especially directed towards women and children. Most people whose attitudes are surveyed believe that physical punishment is justified in some circumstances other than self-defense (Gelles, 1972). Few parents believe that children shouldn't be spanked (Herzberger, 1984), and there are even professionals who believe that incest may facilitate some girls' sexual growth (Constantine, 1981; Helfer & Kempe, 1974). Violence is prevalent on television and on the street. The culture in which we live, then, is seen to encourage abuse.

One extreme example of so-called cultural relativity still occurs in some Third World cultures which practice the ancient rite of passage into womanhood with female clitoridectomies and male circumcisions. The woman, unlike the man, loses her ability to reach orgasm and derive physiological pleasure from sex following this procedure. Men, of course, do not. There are those who draw parallels between this practice and the extreme sexual jealousy often seen in batterers (Walker, 1983). Thus, it simply may be one more way to keep women in their place and may not have the cultural significance male anthropologists have attributed to it.

Other sociocultural theories that stress an environmental analysis have been raised by sociologists. Gelles (1983) proposes application of the resource-exchange theory which adds violence to a list of strategies family members use to control one another. The theory proposes that some men learn to use violence when other resources fail. This learning is said to take place in childhood after witnessing the successful use of violence to get needs met. It does not explain why some men who grew up with violence in their childhood homes do not use violent behavior as a resource in their own homes. Burgess (1984) has attempted to analyze development of social competence skills to explain these differences using a social-learning theoretical approach.

The *psychological* theories have not been much more illuminating about the causation of domestic violence. Early theories postulated that women were masochistic and somehow provoked their own abuse (Snell, Rosenwald & Robey, 1964). Psychological counseling was seen as a necessity to get women to stop behaving in ways that justified their being battered. Such victim precipitation theories still exist among some psychoanalysts (Blum, 1982), and despite the absence of empirical data, battered women are still being labeled masochists (Shainess, 1979). Dynamic psychology theories have not provided useful analyses to explain how domestic violence occurs or is perpetuated. Further, its emphasis on interpretations of observed phenomena renders much of the clinical anecdotal material invalid now that empirical research has challenged those interpretations. Conte (1984) provides a more complete discussion of how this has occurred in the child sexual assault literature with the growth of more sophisticated empirical analysis. The impact on the understanding of spouse abuse is less obvious due to fewer early publications by psychoanalysts who may not have isolated battering as a specific problem and therefore did not offer a treatment philosophy. The insidiousness of its effect, however, is seen in the tenacity with which clinicians continue to blame the victim for part if not all of their victimization.

Social psychology has offered insight into the impact of social conditions on battered women in general. Attribution theory analyzes people's beliefs in the causes of what happens to them. Battered women would be expected to have an external belief system; they would be more likely to attribute the causation of events to powerful others and uncontrollable forces (Frieze, 1980). In fact, battered women completing locus of control scales did demonstrate high scores on the external side of the continuum. However, on the Levinson Locus of Control Scale, three separate measures are given: one for internal locus of control and two for external locus of control measuring powerful others and chance beliefs. The battered women who completed that scale were found to have high scores on all three indices, consistent with clinical findings that they believe both that they control what happens as well as being controlled by outside influences (Walker, 1984a). Douglas and Der Ovanesian (1984) also found contradictory results, and more study is needed before we really understand battered women's attributions and its impact on acceptance of violence.

Another theory, that of cognitive dissonance, has also been applied to battered women. In an attempt to understand how women who are abused are able to remain with the abusers, Stahley (1978) postulated that the women begin to doubt their own reality and then substitute their men's world view in an attempt to reduce the conflict between the two opposing views. This theory also has theoretical logic, much like attribution theory, but still has not been empirically tested. Greenblatt (1984) has developed a simulation model designed to measure normative attitudes toward battering which should shed some light on this question.

Aggression theorists have begun to examine whether general interpersonal aggression theories fit the unique case of chronic, repeated family violence. Berkowitz (1983), for example, has developed a model which suggests that the interaction of victims with the aggressor can influence further aggressive behavior. His model includes understanding motive or intent of the violent behavior and he classifies aggressive acts as being *instrumental violence* designed to get what the aggressor wants from a victim or *expressive violence* designed to inflict pain on the victim. The battered woman's responses are seen to stimulate or reinforce the batterer who then continues his violent behavior. Browne (in press a) points out the difficulties of the application of this theory in relation to battered women. Too many reported battering incidents are known to occur solely because of the man's internally or externally influenced state of mind. Rarely are instrumental and expressive violence modes differentiated in family violence attacks. And while battered women may contribute to reinforcing their own abuse, it is usually unwittingly in the attempts to calm down the batterers and minimize their pain and injuries, as shall be described later (Walker, 1984a).

The impact of gender and violence against women on personality development is only beginning to be addressed in the psychological literature. Walker and Browne (in press) have used social and clinical psychological theories to hypothesize that female and male sex-role assignments are a mediating factor in passing on the skills to permit the use of abusive rather than peaceful means to end family conflicts. In fact, the family is seen as a microcosm of the larger society where women, not men, are better able to look for peaceful solutions to world conflict (Walker, 1984b).

Clinical psychology theories that explain the impact of family violence on the thinking, feeling, and behavior of its members have provided more information than those that speculated on its causation from a clinical population. It has been the application of social-learning theories that yields the most information consistent with the available empirical and clinical data. Violence is seen as learned aggressive behavior which continues because it is reinforced and is not stopped because adverse consequences are not consistently applied. Abuse causes psychological injury to its victims which can be measured and diagnosed using the traditional *Diagnostic and Statistical Manual of Mental Disorders (DSM–III), Third Edition* (APA, 1981) under the Post-Traumatic Stress Disorder (308.21 Acute or 309.80 Chronic or Delayed, pp. 236–238). Subcategories of responses have been developed, and there are unique characteristics ascribed to the battered woman syndrome, battered child syndrome, rape trauma syndrome, and so on.

Less is known about the impact of violence on the aggressor. At this time, spouse-abuse advocates disagree with the clinical pathology model developed by many child-abuse advocates (see Helfer & Kempe, 1974, for example) and instead, rely on a skill deficit social-learning theoretical model. Male violence, it is postulated, is simply an extreme extension of socialized male aggressive behavior. Women who are violent learn that behavior from imitation of male violent behavior. Skill training to control their violent behavior, accompanied by external controls and enhancement of nonviolent conflict resolution skills then becomes the obvious antidote. Unfortunately, it is not quite that simple.

The apparent random and unpredictable nature of family violence seems to foster the development of psychological coping skills to minimize pain but not terminate the violence or the relationship. Seligman's (1975) theory of learned helplessness is consistent with the clinical (Walker, 1978, 1979) and empirical (Walker, 1984a) data from the battered women studied. These battered women lose their ability to predict that their responses will have an effect on what happens to them. Battered women develop similar distorted perceptions in their cognitive, affective, and behavioral processes as did the animals and college students subjected to the same noncontingent response/outcome events in Seligman's laboratory. Like other trauma victims, battered women concentrate on survival and when the danger from repeated violence is still present, their thoughts, feelings, and actions are regulated by the need to reduce the violence threat (Browne, in press a).

The measurement of learned helplessness outside of the laboratory has proved problematic because of the difficulty in direct observations of the aversive stimuli (usually beatings) that plague the design of such research (Walker, 1984a). However, scaled items measured were found to be consistent with the learned-helplessness theory indicating that battered women who demonstrate signs of learned helplessness at the time of testing report sufficient factors in their childhood and their battering relationships to have produced the current psychological symptoms using the laboratory findings as outcome measures (Walker, 1984a).

Although the description of battering incidents indicate that they appear to be in no particular predictable pattern to the victim, those who work with battered women have found that the abuse occurs within a measurable cycle which has three phases. The first phase is a period of *tension building* in which discrete abuse incidents occur but are quickly resolved to keep them from escalating out of control. Usually, the battered woman makes some intervention which causes this particular battering incident not to get worse. These continue to occur with the tension continuing to escalate until it reaches a period of inevitability and the second phase, the *acute battering incident*, occurs.

This second phase is the time when the violence is most severe and, therefore, most likely to come to someone else's attention. It usually is brief, a few minutes to less than 24 hours in duration, and can cause serious injury which may not be reported. In those cases where there is police involvement (approximately one-third of those in the Walker [1984a] study), most were called during this dangerous explosive stage. It stops when the batterer is finished, causing a drop in tension, which is physiologically reinforcing.

Most acute battering incidents are followed by a *period of calm, kind, loving contrition*. In some cases, just the absence of tension provides the reinforcement. It is not unusual to hear during this time reports of gifts, sweet talk, and promises never to do it again. The apparently variable and random expressions of violence and pleasure cause noncontingent experiences of success in predicting behavioral responses. Over time the third phase tends to grow shorter and less rewarding (Walker, 1984a). The ratio of costs and benefits of the relationship changes at some point in time which is when the prediction of contingent outcomes becomes possible again and termination of the relationship is often attempted. When the men or women learn their cycle, they are most likely to take control of the reinforcement schedule and are more likely to move to terminate the relationship. If the abusive partner is threatened by psychological abandonment issues, at the point of separation increased violence, suicide, and/or homicide are most likely to occur. This fear of further harm also reinforces the maintenance of the relationship. The protection offered by the battered-woman shelter can interrupt such a reinforcement schedule and allow the woman to seek her freedom.

The need to psychologically cope while in the battering relationship creates survival skills for the victim which often persist after the violence stops. Those most well-recognized include manipulation of the environment to keep everything smooth for the man, indirect expression of anger because of fear of further abuse should her anger be expressed directly at him, splitting of the mind and body to help tolerate the great pain these beatings cause, denial of danger, and desire for continued feelings of protectedness, specialness, and nurturance. Although some abused women do find themselves in more than one battering relationship, it is more likely that battered women are so sensitized to cues of potential harm that they remain out of relationships with all men, especially those who could be violent. Some women do not have the ability to be without a man for economic or emotional support. These women may indeed be at risk for further victimization.

There are some theories of causation that stress the high rate of victimization that certain women experience. Studies of rape victims suggest that women are often sexually abused more than once (Burgess & Holmstrom, 1978; Kilpatrick, Veronen & Resick, 1979). Almost half the sample in one research project on battered women had been sexually molested as children (Walker, 1984a). It is known that many prostitutes were sexually and physically abused as children (James, 1978). However, the feminist-political and sociocultural theorists would caution interpretations from these observations without the intervening gender theories. Members of the oppressed class, as women are considered to be, will by definition be more likely to be victimized. That some women are more vulnerable than others may simply be due to factors in the patriarchal structure of society and not clinical differences in the women.

## EMPIRICAL STUDIES

There has been an increase in empirical research during the last 10 years in the field of domestic violence, replacing the previous anecdotal case studies. Much of the data have been descriptive, self-report information gathered from adult victims and, less frequently, from the offenders. Attempts at using psychological measurement have been less than successful at yielding data consistent with the self-report interviews. Battered women, like rape and other assault victims, are in such distress when in crisis that they appear to have more serious psychological disorders as measured by traditional standardized tests. Erroneous interpretations are frequent, especially by those unfamiliar with the stress disorder literature. Corroboration of self-report data from the victim has been difficult, but when available it suggests that the battered woman is the best observer and can recall details better than those studying memory would predict. Some studies have used direct observational methods that yield good data about individual and interaction effects but rarely get to observe physical or sexual abuse. The use of inferential analysis empirical data to understand domestic violence is still in the infancy stage. This is partially because of the difficulties in obtaining nonabused samples but also because such analysis will most likely be nonlinear and all of the variables have not yet been identified. Longitudinal studies are most obviously absent.

There is no doubt that the study of domestic violence has produced some of the most difficult psychological conundrums to resolve. Logical assumptions which have provided underpinnings for research do not hold up in this field of study. It is usually accepted that when two people give different versions of a dispute, the truth is somewhere between both stories. In family violence the truth is almost always worse than either party's version. We expect our own personal beliefs that love and violence can't coexist to prevail. Yet, there is a strong love-bond in most battering relationships and the abuse tends to be viewed as an appendage rather than a systemic part of the relationship. There is an expectation that men and women both have free will to enter into and terminate interpersonal relationships. Yet, years of sex-role socialization condition women to believe that they are not valued unless they are someone's wife. Economic and legal structures of society discriminate against single women making any marriage seem more attractive and less stigmatizing than none. Free will, then, is an illusion given the environmental realities.

It is expected that personality is fairly stable and measurable by psychological instruments relatively impervious to the variability of environmental influences. However, personality measures taken during one period, say the tension-building phase, will markedly differ from those completed during the loving-contrition stage. Measures of anxiety, coping skills, depression, and general psychological strength will vary depending on where a person is in the cycle of violence and on his or her views of the seriousness or dangerousness of the situation. Also problematic is the male view of personality which permeates most of the psychometric measurement tools. Although Rosewater (in press b) argues that feminist interpretation of standardized tests can remediate the sexist influence, others argue strongly that the potential for harm is too great to justify using them (Rawlings & Carter, 1977).

It is possible that psychologists who have not dealt with their own fear of and vulnerability to potential abuse find comfort in labeling a victim as having an emotional disorder to explain her victimization. The attempt to look for pathology in the victim has encouraged similar patterns between victims, seen on psychometric tests without regard for underlying theoretical analysis. Starr (1978) has used the California Personality Inventory (CPI) to demonstrate a consistent battered-woman response set and has excluded other known battered women who do not fit her categories in forensic analysis. Such a narrow definition is inaccurate and can be harmful to battered women. It is more likely that psychometric testing will be useful in measuring the impact of the violence on the victim as is being done in the national crime studies in the Netherlands (Steinmetz, 1984) and England (Hough, 1984), and for rape victims in the United States (Burt & Katz, 1984; Kilpatrick et al., 1979). There have been difficulties in using psychometrics to measure impact in domestic violence victims. Conte (1984) discusses some of these problems in studies of psychological impact of incest. He points out the unique nature of repeated abuse by a significant person in the child's environment. Our current psychometric tests do not account for the ambivalence raised by such abuse.

Walker (1984a) used the CES Depression Inventory and found her sample were all clustered on the upper end of the scale indicating major depression risk with little room for variance. In fact, those out of the battering relationship for more than a year showed significantly more depression as measured on that instrument than those still in the relationship. Other indicators of depression, including self-report, did not match the high scores on that test. Rosewater (1982, in press a) has empirically demonstrated a battered-woman composite profile on the Minnesota Multiphasic Personality Inventory (MMPI) which closely resembles the schizophrenic and borderline profiles. Unless the Harris-Lingoes subscale analysis is used and a complete abuse history is obtained, she cautions against misdiagnosis using only the test data. In fact, some computerized analyses of the MMPI do send out erroneous profiles without accounting for the repeated experience of violence. For example, it is not paranoid for a severely battered woman to believe someone is out to get her. A woman who is involved with an insensitive legal system may well be having very unusual experiences and may be responding temporarily by measurable confusion. Rosewater found that those women who had the most serious violence documented by the court also were the most depressed on the MMPI.

Self-esteem is another often measured variable which yields little consistent results. In the Walker (1984a) study, her women responded to a semantic differential constructed for that research as believing they were better than most women in general on all items except sexual attraction. Rosewater, however, found low ego-strength as measured by the MMPI. Most clinicians would agree that battered women demonstrate the clinical signs of low self-esteem yet there is no evidence that the signs can be measured psychometrically.

Fear and anxiety are other variables which are said to be results of living with violence. The Modified Fear Survey (Kilpatrick et al., 1979) has been used with rape victims and has promise for use with battered women. Currently, it is being revised and field-tested in doctoral dissertation research at the University of Kansas. There is benefit for therapeutic intervention if an instrument measures specific fears rather than generalized anxiety.

*Clinical and structured interview* studies have, to date, yielded most information about battered women and domestic violence. Although some have used particular population samples, when put together we have learned that some variables are found across groups.

*Incidence and frequency levels* have been measured by the most comprehensive epidemiological study by sociologists Murray Straus, Richard Gelles, and Suzanne Steinmetz (1980). They conclude that 28% of the respondents they randomly chose to be interviewed had experienced at least one physically violent incident in the year for which they requested information. Approximately 5% were seriously abused, often with weapons and threats to kill. They indicate that they believe violence in the home may occur at twice the rate they have found (60% of all homes) while others including Walker (1979) estimate 50% of all women will be abused by someone who loves them at some time in their lives. The FBI reports that most homicides occur between those who have known one another and a high number of those are with family members. Browne (in press b) has analyzed those homicides that seem to have occurred in self-defense. Attempts to gather incidence data from the new police mandatory arrest orders is still in an exploration phase. All who have tried to measure incidence and frequency agree that those reported cases are a serious underestimate of its true occurrence.

*Demographic variables* have been studied in a variety of research projects. The Straus et al. (1980) study found that spouse abuse occurs in all socioeconomic classes, races, religions, ethnic groups, and educational levels. The Walker (1984a) study had a similar finding as did Fagan, Stewart and Hansen (1983), Pagelow (1981), and Hanneke and Shields (1981). Disagreement about the incidence rate in poor families has been found with Walker's self-volunteered research sample having higher incidence of professional and upper class victims than the others report. Women with less access to other resources are more likely to use shelters. It may be that a preponderance of reported violence is seen in lower class, less educated, and poorer families because they are less sophisticated in the need to hide it and most likely will use public agencies for assistance. Hanneke and Shields found that middle class offenders tended to use less overt violence that rarely was visible outside the home. The tendency for a battered woman to protect the batterer and not expose his violence may interact with those who are also class conscious to produce greater invisibility. Thus, visibility is a problem in establishing a true incidence rate, particularly in those with greater resources.

Some studies have found that the women have more family-of-origin status, education, religious training, and verbal ability than do their abusers (Fagan et al., 1983; Straus et al., 1980; Walker, 1984a). Others have seen a higher proportion of couples with dissimilar religious, racial, and ethnic backgrounds (Berk et al., 1983). These factors may reflect the difference in power within such relationships or may simply be an artifact of the samples used to study. Study findings agree that the woman seems to be emotionally stronger than the male, at least initially, although he dominates in almost every area of decisionmaking (Giles-Sims, 1983; Pagelow, 1981; Walker, 1984a).

Most of the researchers have examined the family-of-origin backgrounds of abusers and their victims. All have found that over three-quarters of the batterers studied (Boyd, 1978; Fagan et al., 1983; Ganley & Harris, 1978; Giles-Sims, 1983; Hanneke & Shields, 1981; Roy, 1982; Sonkin & Durphy, 1982; Straus et al., 1980) and perhaps half of the battered women studied (Fagan et al., 1983; Giles-Sims, 1983; Roberts, 1981; Straus et al., 1980; Walker, 1984a) have grown up experiencing or witnessing interpersonal violence. The percentages grow larger if perceived emotional abuse or rejection are included. It is not known, of course, if their reported childhood homes actually contained battering experiences that could be measured objectively. Psychologists believe, however, that the perception of being battered is sufficient to cause damage although degree of harm cannot easily be assessed. Also absent from evaluating the impact of these data is knowledge of whether the battering was labeled as it was being experienced or if it is only in retrospect that the experienced events appear to have been abusive. Such cognitive labeling will have a mitigating influence on the injury from the experience.

*The details of violence* which occur in battering relationships have been analyzed in many of the recent empirical studies (Browne, 1983, in press b; Dobash & Dobash, 1981; Fagan et al., 1983; Frieze, 1980; Giles-Sims,

1983; Hilberman & Munson, 1978; Pagelow, 1981; Roberts, 1984; Roy, 1982; Sonkin & Durphy, 1982; Straus et al., 1980; Walker, 1979, 1984a). Most of the information concerning such details comes from the victim; batterers deny, minimize, can't remember, or lie more often than do the victims. In fact, although women used to be considered hysterical and prone to exaggerate tales of abuse, most empirical data that have been verified by outside observers demonstrate that the victim is most likely to minimize and it is her terror which lies behind the strong emotional response. Hospital emergency room personnel remark at the high pain tolerance of domestic violence victims (Klingbeil & Boyd, 1984). Police are often fooled into believing the battered woman is all right because her desperate need to believe it is not so bad convinces the police, too. Others, of course, simply invalidate the victim's litany of complaints by reasoning that she wouldn't have stayed in the situation if it were so horrible. In fact, battered women, like other violence victims, are struggling to maintain control and will only discuss the details of violence when they feel safe and are with a nonjudgmental interviewer. The women studied say they are sensitive to the interviewer's potential reaction and will adjust their report if they sense there is not enough time or the interviewer won't hear their version of the abuse. They admit giving partial and incomplete information at such times. All evidence purporting to be details of domestic violence must be scrutinized to see if the data are valid and were appropriately collected.

Straus et al. (1980) tried to categorize the numbers of violent acts on a scale of which increased as acts were more likely to cause injury or death to the victim. By using this Conflict Tactics Scale, which does not account for antecedents or consequences, they found a high number of mutually violent men and women. They do caution against interpreting these findings to mean that women are as violent as men because most of the women's violent acts seemed to be defensive (like biting) rather than retaliatory or offensive. Since they did not collect data that could provide such a definitive interpretation their findings have generated much controversy, especially among those who do not accept the feminist-political perspective. Berk et al. (1983) provided their own analysis of data to demonstrate that mutual violence is a myth. No matter how the data are analyzed, however, it is clear from all empirical evidence to date that women are more frequently and more severely hurt than men.

The Walker (1984a) study asked battered women to give details of four specific battering incidents while measuring antecedents and consequences for each incident. Those reported were the first incident recalled, the second, one of the worst, and the last one prior to the interview. The escalation of violence between each of these incidents as well as measurement of the consequences provide a fairly good estimate of its potential dangerousness.

It was found that the violence almost always escalated. The specific details about battering yield many physical, sexual, and psychological abusive acts and injuries. They include slaps (back-handed, open-handed) shoves, pushes, hits, punches, being thrown across the room or down stairs, backed into walls and objects, tripped, kicked (with and without shoes or boots), stomped on, arms and legs twisted or held behind the back, forced to kneel or crawl on the floor, sexual abuse of all varieties, hit with objects, choked, smothered, burned, attempts to drown, stabbed, shot at, dragged by auto, thrown out of a moving or stationary car, genital mutilation, and various threats or attempts to be killed. Women are humiliated, and degraded by name-calling, attacks on their personal worth and competency, and repeatedly reminded of their previous mistakes. Most of this psychological and physical torture is accompanied by anger expressed in a variety of ways including yelling, sarcasm, sharp movements, or cold stony silence. Threats of harm are often made towards family, friends, pets, and treasured objects. There is a recitation of details explaining how each person will be tortured which terrifies the victim both because she fears for each person's safety but also because the batterer's ability to describe the horrible torture increases her fear of his dangerousness. These threats are sometimes carried out, on a random and variable basis, so that the battered woman believes she must be ever-vigilant. Much of the victim's energy goes to reducing the likelihood that the abuser will ever harm these other people. It explains why violence victims are always relieved it wasn't worse at the end of a battering incident. They had been told what more could have happened.

The description of violence details is similar in most studies which actually collect such data. This is true for shelter populations that are studied (Berk et al., 1983; Fagan et al., 1983; Pagelow, 1981), women who are seeking medical help (Klingbeil & Boyd, 1984; Hilberman & Munson, 1978) or legal assistance (Fields, 1978). Recitation of details that were previously limited in court testimony by women requesting protective or restraining orders against their batterers has educated attorneys and judges willing to listen. As women learn that their experiences are not unusual in battering relationships, they have been more likely to share their particular stories. The amount of violence so detailed is staggering.

*Sexual abuse* within battering relationships has been another area subjected to empirical study. Diana Russell (1982) in her survey of 900 randomly selected women in California found that approximately 12% had been raped by their husbands. In the Walker (1984a) study, 59% of the women reported being forced to have sex with the batterer as compared to only 7% being forced to have sex with a nonbatterer. Not surprisingly, 84% of those women found sex with the batterer to be unpleasant. Frieze (1980) found that 34% of the battered women in her sample were the victims of marital rape, although they may not have defined it using those terms. Finkelhor and Yllo (1983) report that Spektor's survey of 10 Minnesota battered women shelters found 36% were sexually abused in their primary relationships and Pagelow (1981) found that 37% were sexually abused by their husbands or cohabitating partner. Russell found that sexual assaults by husbands were reported as having occurred over twice as often as sexual assault by a stranger. "If these data can be generalized to the population at large, then battered women have three to five times the risk of being sexually assaulted by their partners than non-battered women" (Walker, 1984a, p. 49).

Sexual jealousy, another form of expressing power and control, is one of the most commonly reported features of the battering relationships. Hilberman and Munson (1978) label it pathological jealousy and describe its use to isolate and limit the woman's movements. Giles-Sims (1983), Pagelow (1981), Frieze (1980), Straus et al. (1980), Walker (1979, 1984a), Roy (1978) and Martin (1982) all describe the jealousy that is usually unfounded and excessive in its expression. Most often it is the violent man who is jealous of the woman but it has also been reported that the women demonstrate jealousy towards the men. In those reported cases, the woman's jealousy was more likely to be an accurate reflection of the man's affair with another woman.

There has been clinical evidence that abusive males are likely to sexually abuse their children but there are no known empirical reports. Conte (1984) and Finkelhor and Browne's (1984) review of the literature on sexual assault on children suggest a high incidence of incest fathers who also batter their wives. Reports of sex offenders who are obsessed with sexuality, have strong power and control needs, and impulsively act out under stress (Wolf, 1984) match reports about some samples of batterers (Harris & Bologh, 1984; Sonkin, Martin & Walker, 1985) and women's reports of batterers (Walker, 1984a).

*The impact of spouse abuse on children* has generated some empirical data which seem to support the clinical data indicating that such children are at higher risk for their own physical or psychological abuse. In the Walker (1984a) study, 87% of the women reported that the children were aware of the violence in their homes. While together in the battering relationship, over one-half of the men also abused the children. Further, one-third of the batterers threatened to abuse the children causing the women to modify their behavior to try to prevent them from venting their anger towards the children. In that study, about one-quarter of the women said they abused the children when living with a batterer. It went down to 5% of the women who admitted still battering the children when living with a nonviolent partner. Thus, battered women are eight times more likely to batter their children when they live in a violent home.

Straus et al. (1980) found that the rate of marital violence increased in direct proportion to the amount of physical punishment experienced as children. The Walker (1984a) study also supported social-learning theory which predicts that modeling of parents' behavior is a powerful way to pass violence as a strategy down to the next generation. Patterson (1982) and his colleagues (Reid, Taplin, & Lorber, 1981) have been studying aggressive boys and their families for the past 15 years. They use observational coding schemes while visiting the homes to collect data on family and individual interactions. In the dysfunctional and abusive families, they found a significantly higher ratio of negative interactions than positive ones. In homes where there was no identified aggressive boy, the ratio was balanced in favor of positive to negative acts. In abusive homes, the negative acts came in clusters, separated by positive acts. These clusters of nasty acts were described as beads on a chain, one following the other, creating a fogging effect which made an effective response less likely to occur. The chaining and fogging described by Patterson and his colleagues is similar in description to the three phases in the battering cycle of violence; the slow tension-building leading up to the inevitable phase two acute battering incident followed immediately with a period of loving-contrition or absence of tension (Walker, 1979, 1984a).

Burgess (1984) has also been analyzing observational data on reported child abuse families. In sifting through the numerous variables often discussed in other empirical studies, Burgess found that one common factor seemed to be the lack of social competence evidenced in the parents and some of the abused children. He postulates the mediating factor which determined whether or not an abusive style continued from parent to child is the peer socialization that child experiences. If the abused child is rejected by peers then he or she is unlikely to have any models from which to learn social skills. Studies of battered women would suggest that their social competence is greatly affected by the other situational factors which regulate their lives. Violence in the home may limit the expression of social competence.

There has been some interest in empirically measuring children's personality development. Giles-Sims (1983) discusses the dependency bonds that a closed system such as an abusive family can foster. Hughes and Barad (1983) measured the psychological functioning of children who accompanied their mothers to a shelter in Arkansas. They found the children were jumpy, frightened, nervous, and showed impaired academic performance. At Chiswick Women's Aid Refuge in London, Pizzey (1974) found fear, poor academic performance, confusion, withdrawal, and fantasies of a different home life. Preschool children are most likely to be disrupted by the violence in their homes and show signs of developmental delay (Hughes & Barad, 1983). Boys tended to show more aggressive behavior while girls were more likely to worry, become anxious, and oversensitive. Davidson (1978) cites the tendency of the adolescent girls in the Minneapolis/St. Paul shelter to identify with their fathers and also abuse their mothers. Others have noted that adolescent girls are at risk to enter into abusive relationships of their own (Hilberman & Munson, 1978). There is a greater risk of fathers abusing their teenaged daughters (Martin, 1982), which is a high risk factor for later emotional and behavioral disturbance. Time spent in the battered-woman's shelter was associated with the likelihood that mothers would continue to adopt the no-hitting rule in their child discipline even after they left the shelter.

The association between alcohol and drug dependencies and violence has a limited empirical base. Most researchers report a high degree of alcohol abuse for the batterer. Less is known about other drugs. Straus et al. (1980), Frieze (1980) and Walker (1984a) found approximately 60% of the abusers were reported to frequently drink alcohol. Labell (1979) found 72% of the partners of the battered women seeking shelter frequently abused alcohol and 28.9% had drug problems. Roy's (1978) study of 150 battered women who called the New York City Hotline for help reported 85% of their abusers had alcohol or drug problems. Less than one-fifth of battered women studied said they had an alcohol or drug problem. In most cases, if the woman drank to excess, so did her abusive partner. Eberle (1982) analyzed the Walker data to measure alcohol abuse across the four battering incidents and found that only 20% were intoxicated at all four times. Preliminary analysis indicated that the most serious injuries were associated with alcohol abuse. Browne (1983) found that alcohol abuse was frequently associated with those cases in which a homicide occurred. Thus, although no causal effects can be found, alcohol abuse is associated with greater risk of harm.

Empirical data on intervention techniques for the victims is limited at this time. However, clinical data indicate that individual and group counseling or therapy for abuse victims are helpful. Supportive therapy and crisis intervention were seen by the battered women in the Walker (1984a) study to provide the most help. Long-term treatment issues need to deal with survival as a single woman (and parent) in a couple's world as well as issues about victimization (Walker, 1984d). Children who have been abused also make good use of individual play therapy while adolescents find individual and group therapy most helpful to them. Reintegrating abuse victims' sense of mastery and control over their bodies and their lives is the goal of the intervention. This, then, deals with environmental situations as well as intrapsychic issues. Couples or family therapy has been found to be less useful for the violence victims although it is sometimes used as a means of getting the abuser into treatment. A more complete discussion of therapy options can be found elsewhere (Walker, 1984a, 1985).

*Policy research* has been an important contribution to the knowledge base in this field of study. In 1977 the U.S. Civil Rights Commission undertook a study to determine if the legal system was adequate to deal with spouse abuse in Denver, Colorado, and found that police do not make arrests, district attorneys do not prosecute, judges do not sentence, and battered women have little civil rights protection. This study led to a nationwide consultation in Washington, D.C., held by the U.S. Civil Rights Commission in 1978, which explored data from a variety of institutions on their effectiveness in protecting the rights of battered women. Several senate and congressional committees also requested testimony from researchers and activists to guide policy in scientific inquiry, service provisions, and legal alternatives. The President appointed a Task Force on Victims of Crime which chose to eliminate family violence from its study but recommended another Attorney General's Task Force on Family Violence which recently recommended the criminalization of spouse and child abuse. Changes in the legal system have made important social policy changes (Walker, 1984c).

### GAPS IN KNOWLEDGE

Although a number of empirical studies were reported in the previous section, it is clear that there are still many questions yet to be answered before we truly understand the multiple causes of domestic violence. Most of the empirical data to date are descriptive, not inferential studies, based on limited population samples. These survey-type studies typically use self-report on questionnaires or interviews to gather their information. Psychometric studies are limited by the tests available to be used. And there are no longitudinal studies, a most serious gap. However, despite the fact that behavioral observation studies have not been directly used to measure spouse abuse, the few reported have made important contributions to the understanding of causes of child abuse and have implications for battering relationships. These descriptive studies have provided a more accurate picture of the nature of family violence in a way that has caused most researchers and clinicians to revise their thinking, methodology, and intervention strategies. It is necessary to begin a new generation of inferential studies to look for relationships and cause and effect sequences.

Sample selection has been a limiting factor in the design of experiments. It is almost impossible to find a matched sample of women who have not experienced violence (Frieze, 1980). The extent to which childhood violence experiences are potentiators of greater impact should adult violence be experienced is not known. This is an important area to study especially as we begin to look at the impact of abuse of the elderly and other forms of crime on victims. Walker (1984a) found that learned helplessness could develop equally from childhood or relationship factors. Yet, as children, 50% of that sample had been sexually abused and 66% reported having grown up in homes where battering occurred.

One attempt to control for battering in the relationship to be studied was used by Walker (1984a) when she had each woman respond to the same set of questions about a nonviolent intimate relationship. One-half of the sample (200) had both battering and nonbattering relationships allowing them to serve as their own controls. Although a nonbattered group might also have provided additional information, it was not feasible or cost-effective to use when the psychological impact on the victim was being examined.

Special populations have provided the greatest source of empirical data at this time. Although shelter women are able to give important insights, only a small percentage of all battered women use the shelter. Battered women underutilize clinics, hospitals, and the police as well. Walker (1984a) found that as many as 50% of that research sample may not have used any public institution for help. One-third said they used friends, family, or religious leaders. Fewer than that sought medical attention for injuries related to the battering although there are some data to suggest battered women do seek medical help for other problems. Only about 10% have had contact with the police, although now that many jurisdictions have enacted mandatory arrest laws and regulations, it is anticipated that more violent families will receive legal attention.

## IMPLICATIONS FOR RESEARCH, SERVICES, AND SOCIAL POLICY

It seems that much of the research in the next decade needs to concern itself with understanding the basic causes of all family violence. Longitudinal studies, as well as those that test specific hypotheses arising out of the previous decade's knowledge base, offer the most promise. All research should integrate the factor of gender as it tests out its specific questions.

Specific program evaluation would be helpful provided the goals are formulated out of the service-based ideology. For example, in measuring a shelter's effectiveness, evaluation research needs to see if there are lowered rates of violence against women and children who were served, rather than concentrate on whether or not battered women return to their mates. Community impact of a shelter and strong criminal prosecution programs also need to be empirically studied. One study in Minneapolis (Sherman & Berk, 1984) found that if police made an arrest and put the batterer in jail overnight it was most likely to stop the violence (as measured by no further reports by the woman) compared to two other options, to do nothing or to mediate the dispute. The study is to be replicated in other cities.

The battered-woman's shelter, which developed out of a grassroots woman's movement, has proved itself to be the most beneficial addition to a community interested in lowering the rate of violence against women. The hotlines usually field other crisis calls, including those from women and children who were sexually assaulted. The shelter provides safety for women and children, access to counselors, and time for a woman to decide what to do with the rest of her life. Close networking with other community agencies usually provides women with a wide choice of options. Access to trained therapists in the community, usually women who consider themselves feminist therapists, helps the battered woman reverse the years of conditioning that occurs when she has lived with abuse. The goal is to stay safe, free from further violence. Most often that can only be accomplished by terminating the relationship. But, even divorce does not end the psychological harassment and sometimes perpetuates the physical and sexual abuse.

Many communities have begun to provide special counseling programs for abusive men. Some accept court-ordered treatment referrals; others will only work with voluntary men. Some of the most established, well-known programs are the men's program at Marin Abused Women Shelter (MAWS) in California, RAVEN in St. Louis, AMEND in Denver, Colorado (Ewing, Lindsey & Pomerantz, 1984), EMERGE in Boston (Adams & McCormick, 1982), AWAIC (Roy, 1982) in New York City, Sonkin & Durphy's (1982) groups in San Francisco and Ganley's (1981) treatment approach at American Lakes Veterans Hospital in Tacoma. There is little empirical data yet to come from these programs, although most report between 25% and 50% success rate in stopping the violence in a new relationship the man might enter (not the same abusive relationship which earned him his referral to the program). The general theoretical approach is a behavioral one: The violent behavior must stop. Then other issues, including analysis of male socialization patterns, are examined. Most counselors say that the work is hard and their clients are dangerous, and they are personally touched by their successes and failures.

These special programs, which mostly use a group-treatment modality, need empirical validation even though their proponents believe that they are successful. Particularly important is the development of guidelines for deciding which men will benefit from post-adjudication diversion into these programs and which men need to go to jail, either for their own or their partners' safety. The Walker (1984a) study found that over 70% of the women reported that their men were arrested for other criminal acts and about half of them were found guilty. Browne (1983, in press b) found that the factors that predicted lethality in the 40 homicide cases she studied were all in the man's frequency and severity of violent threats and behavior. Similar findings were noted by Rosenbaum and O'Leary (1981) in their study of abusive couples. More empirical data on the abusive men are needed to design effective intervention programs.

The abuse that continues following divorce often occurs around child custody and visitation issues. It is not unusual for batterers to fight for sole or joint custody of their young children, and frequent intimidation and harassment accompany these bitter custody disputes. Typically, the batterer puts on his charming face and the battered woman becomes hysterical and frightened. Custody evaluators, particularly in states that have adopted presumption of joint custody rules, do not recognize battering or, even more likely, do not understand its impact on the man's parenting ability. The children often respond to two totally different lifestyles, one of which they recognize as potentially harmful and to which they overadapt and protect each parent's needs while not meeting their own. Study of the outcomes of these disputes and the effect on children is critical.

Some women respond to living in violence by behaving in a violent manner, usually in self-defense. Although it is very rare for a woman to kill (Jones, 1980), battered women have killed their abusers in self-defense. Many women were thought to be retaliating in anger, some were found insane and others felt guilty about killing the man they loved. Rarely did these women receive justice or understanding in the legal system. More recently, however, expert-witness testimony has educated attorneys, judges, and juries so that a battered woman who kills her abuser while trying to stop him from seriously injuring or killing her gets a fair trial. The attention paid to this once-neglected area of the law has made profound changes in legal and social policy (Walker, 1984c). Bochnak (1981) has explored the legal implications when women use self-defense in sexual assault, battering, and other situations. Browne (in press b) has looked at the possibility of predicting lethality in battering relationships by analyzing those cases which did result in homicide. Little is known about the women who are killed or driven to commit suicide. The newspapers often report murder/suicide cases resulting from a "domestic dispute." As violent offenders become better identified in the community, many more deaths will be better understood.

Another neglected area of study and intervention has been the relationship between battering and subsequent criminal acts committed by women. New programs taking place in the women's prisons in Evanston, Wyoming; Jefferson City, Missouri; Framingham, Massachusetts; Philadelphia, Pennsylvania; and Canon City, Colorado are providing supportive counseling and self-help groups for incarcerated battered women. Estimates are that as many as 90% of women prison inmates have been abused. Many committed the crime for which they are serving time as a result of a batterer forcing or coercing them into doing it under threat of further abuse, but never received a duress defense. Some did not tell their attorneys because they did not realize the relevance. Others simply did not define themselves as battered women. And many more poor women of color did not even get much of a defense. This is an area where much intervention is needed and to which feminists are beginning to pay some attention.

Training of professionals who can provide adequate services to those affected by family violence should be a high priority in the legal and mental health professions. To date, neither profession mandates standards on training in any area of women's issues. Thus, it may be unrealistic to expect that systematic attention be paid to a specialized issue such as violence against women and children. Yet, many graduate students in psychology are choosing to learn intervention skills and do research projects in this area. Perhaps they will force their professors to retrain themselves to be a resource to their students. As feminist women become more involved in policy-making positions within their respective associations, greater attention will be focused in this area.

Finally, the work to date in the area of child abuse, sexual abuse, and battered women can be looked to as a model for the developing victims right's movement in this country. Many European countries have developed support schemes for victims that only recently have begun to be addressed in the United States. Shelters, crisis counseling, and supportive services can at the very least prevent a victim from being revictimized at the hands of an ignorant, uncaring, or inflexible system. Perhaps, as the data presented here suggest, psychology has much to offer domestic violence victims to lessen their pain and help them move from being a victim to becoming a survivor.

## REFERENCES

Adams, D. C., & McCormick, A. J. (1982). Men unlearning violence: A group approach based on the collective model. In M. Roy (Ed.), *The abusive partner* (pp. 170–197). New York: Van Nostrand Reinhold.

American Psychiatric Association, (1981). *Diagnostic and statistical manual of mental disorders (3rd ed.). (DSM-III).* Washington, DC: Author.

Berk, R., Berk, S. F., Loeske, D. & Rauma, D. (1983). Mutual combat and other family violence myths. In D. Finkelhor, R. Gelles, G. Hotaling & M. Straus (Eds.), *The dark side of families* (pp. 197–212). Beverly Hills, CA: Sage.

Berkowitz, L. (1983). The goals of aggression. In D. Finkelhor, R. Gelles, G. Hotaling, & M. Straus (Eds.), *The dark side of families* (pp. 166–181). Beverly Hills, CA: Sage.

Blum, H. P. (1982). Psychoanalytic reflections on the "beaten wife syndrome." In M. Kirkpatrick (Ed.), *Women's sexual experiences: The dark continent* (pp. 263–267). New York: Plenum.

Bochnak, E. (1981). *Women's self defense cases.* Charlottesville, VA: The Michie Law Publishers.

Bograd, M. (1984). Family systems approaches to wife battering: A feminist critique. *American Journal of Orthopsychiatry, 54*(4), 558–568.

Boyd, V. D. (1978). Domestic violence: Treatment alternatives for the male batterer. Paper presented at the APA meeting, Toronto.

Browne, A. (1983). *Battered women who kill.* Unpublished dissertation, The Union of Experimental Colleges and Universities.

Browne, A. (in press a) Assault and homicide at home: When battered women kill. In L. Saxe & M. J. Saks (Eds.), *Advances in applied social psychology* (Vol. 3). Hillsdale, NY: Lawrence Erlbaum Associates.

Browne, A. (in press b) *Battered women who kill.* New York: The Free Press.

Brownmiller, S. (1975). *Against our will: Men, women and rape.* New York: Simon & Schuster.

Burgess, A. W., & Holmstrom, L. L. (1978). Recovery from rape and prior life stress. *Research in Nursing and Health, 1*(4), 165–174.

Burgess, R. L. (1984). *Social incompetence as a precipitant to and consequence of child maltreatment.* Paper presented at the Third International Victimology Conference, Lisbon, Portugal, November 10–18.

Burt, M. R., & Katz, B. L. (1984). *Rape, robbery, and burglary: Responses to actual and feared criminal victimization with a special focus on women and the elderly.* Paper presented at the Third International Victimology Conference, Lisbon, Portugal, November 10–18.

Constantine, L. L. (1981). The effects of early sexual experience. In L. L. Constantine & F. M. Martinson (Eds.), *Children and sex: New findings, new perspectives* (pp. 217–246). Boston: Little, Brown & Company.

Conte, J. R. (1984). *The effects of sexual abuse on children: A critique and suggestions for future research.* Paper presented at the Third International Victimology Conference, Lisbon, Portugal, November 10–18.

Davidson, T. (1978). *Conjugal crime: Understanding and changing the wife-beating pattern.* New York: Hawthorne.

Dobash, R. E., & Dobash, R. P. (1981). *Violence against wives.* New York: The Free Press.

Dobash, R. P., & Dobash, R. E. (1983). The context-specific approach to theoretical and methodological issues in researching violence against wives. In D. Finkelhor, R. Gelles, G. Hotaling & M. Straus (Eds.), *The dark side of families* (pp. 261–276). Beverly Hills: Sage.

Douglas, M. A., & Der Ovanesian, M. (1984). *Attributional style and depression for battered and nonbattered women in crisis*. Unpublished manuscript.

Eberle, P. (1982). Alcoholic abusers and non-users: A discriminate function analysis. *Journal of Health and Social Behavior, 23,* 260.

Ewing, W., Lindsey, M., & Pomerantz, J. (1984). *Battering: An AMEND manual for helpers*. Denver: AMEND.

Fagan, J. A., Stewart, D. K., & Hansen, K. V. (1983). Violent men or violent husbands? Background factors and situational correlates of severity and location of violence. In D. Finkelhor, R. Gelles, G. Hotaling, & M. Straus (Eds.), *The dark side of families* (pp. 49–67). Beverly Hills: Sage.

Fields, M. (1978). *Wifebeating: Government intervention policies and practices*. In U.S. Civil Rights Commission (Ed.), *Battered women: Issues of public policy*. Washington, DC: U.S. Government Printing Office.

Finkelhor, D., & Browne, A. (1984). *The traumatic impact of child sexual abuse: A conceptualization*. Paper presented at the Second National Family Violence Research Conference, University of New Hampshire, Durham, N.H.

Finkelhor, D., & Yllo, K. (1983). Forced sex in marriage: A sociological view. In D. Finkelhor, R. Gelles, G. Hotaling, & M. Straus (Eds.), *The dark side of families* (pp. 119–130). Beverly Hills: Sage.

Frieze, I. H. (1980). *Causes and consequences of marital rape*. Paper presented at the APA meeting, Montreal.

Ganley, A. (1981). *Participant and trainer's manual for working with men who batter*. Washington, DC: Center for Women Policy Studies.

Ganley, A., & Harris, L. (1978). *Domestic violence: Issues in designing and implementing programs for male batterers*. Paper presented at the APA meeting, Toronto.

Gelles, R. J. (1972). *The violent home: A study of the physical aggression between husbands and wives*. Beverly Hills: Sage.

Gelles, R. J. (1981). Violence and the family: A review of the research in the seventies. *Journal of Marriage and the Family, 42*(4), 873–885.

Gelles, R. J. (1983). An exchange/social control theory of intrafamily violence. In D. Finkelhor, R. Gelles, G. Hotaling, & M. Straus (Eds.), *The dark side of families* (pp. 151–164). Beverly Hills: Sage.

Giles-Sims, J. (1983). *Wife battering: A systems theory approach*. New York: Guilford Press.

Gondolf, E. W. (1984). *Anger and oppression in men who batter: Empiricist and feminist perspectives and their implications for research*. Paper presented at the Third International Victimology Conference, Lisbon, Portugal, November 10–18.

Greenblatt, C. (1984). *"Don't hit your wife . . . unless . . . ": Preliminary findings on normative support for the use of physical force by husbands*. Paper presented at the Third International Victimology Conference, Lisbon, Portugal, November 10–18.

Hanneke, C. R., & Shields, N. M. (1981). *Patterns of family and non-family violence: An approach to the study of violent husbands*. Paper presented at the First National Conference of Family Violence Researchers, University of New Hampshire, Durham, July.

Harris, R. N., & Bologh, R. W. (1984). *The dark side of love: Blue and white collar wife abuse*. Paper presented at the Third International Victimology Conference, Lisbon, Portugal, November 10–18.

Helfer, E. R., & Kempe, C. H. (1974). *The battered child* (2nd ed.). Chicago: University of Chicago Press.

Herzberger, S. D. (1984). *Identifying cases of child abuse: A social psychological phenomenon*. Paper presented at the Third International Victimology Conference, Lisbon, Portugal, November 10–18.

Hilberman, E., & Munson, L. (1978). Sixty battered women. *Victimology: An International Journal, 2*(3-4), 460–471.

Hough, M. (1984). *The impact of victimization: Findings from the British crime survey*. Paper presented at the Third International Victimology Conference, Lisbon, Portugal, November 10–18.

Hughes, H. M., & Barad, S. J. (1983). Psychological functioning of children in a battered woman shelter: A preliminary investigation. *American Journal of Orthopsychiatry, 53*(3), 525–531.

James, J. (1978). The prostitute as victim. In J. A. Chapman & M. Gates (Eds.), *Victimization of women* (pp. 175–201). Beverly Hills: Sage.

Jones, A. (1980). *Women who kill*. New York: Holt, Rinehart & Winston.

Kilpatrick, D. G., Veronen, L. & Resick, P. A. (1979). Assessment of the aftermath of rape: Changing patterns of fear. *Journal of Behavioral Assessment, 1*(2), 133–148.

Klingbeil, K., & Boyd, V. D. (1984). Emergency room intervention detection, assessment, and treatment. In A. R. Roberts (Ed.), *Battered women and their families* (pp. 7–32). New York: Springer.

Labell, L. S. (1979). Wife abuse: A sociological study of battered women and their mates. *Victimology, 4*, 258–267.

Martin, D. (1982). *Battered wives* (rev. ed.). San Francisco: Volcano Press.

Pagelow, M. (1981). *Women battering: Victims and their experience*. Beverly Hills: Sage.

Patterson, G. (1982). *Coercive family processes*. Eugene, OR: Castaglia Press.

Pizzey, E. (1974). *Scream quietly or the neighbors will hear*. London: Penguin.

Rawlings, E. I. & Carter, D. (Eds.). (1977). *Psychotherapy for women: Treatment toward equality*. Springfield: Charles C Thomas.

Reid, J. B., Taplin, P. S., & Lorber, R. (1981). A social international approach to the treatment of abusive families. In R. B. Stuart (Ed.), *Violent behavior: Social learning approaches to prediction, management and treatment*. New York: Brunner/Mazel.

Roberts, A. R. (1981). *Sheltering battered women*. New York: Springer.

Roberts, A. R. (Ed.). (1984). *Battered women and their families*. New York: Springer.

Rosenbaum, A., & O'Leary, D. (1981). Marital violence: Characteristics of abusive couples. *Journal of Consulting and Clinical Psychology, 49*, 63–71.

Rosewater, L. B. (1982). An MMPI profile for battered women. Doctoral dissertation for the Union of Experimenting Colleges and Universities, *Dissertation Abstracts*, Ann Arbor, MI.

Rosewater, L. B. (in press a). Schizophrenic or battered? In L. B. Rosewater & L. E. A. Walker (Eds.), *Handbook of feminist therapy: Psychotherapy with women*. New York: Springer.

Rosewater, L. B. (in press b). Feminist interpretations of tests. In L. B. Rosewater & L. E. A. Walker (Eds.), *Handbook of feminist therapy: Psychotherapy with women*. New York: Springer.

Roy, M. (1978). *Battered women: A psychosocial study*. New York: Van Nostrand Reinhold.

Roy, M. (1982). Four thousand partners in violence: A trend analysis. In M. Roy (Ed.), *The abusive partner* (pp. 17–35). New York: Van Nostrand Reinhold.

Russell, D. E. (1982). *Rape in marriage*. New York: Macmillan.

Schechter, S. (1982). *Women and male violence: The visions and struggles of the battered women's movement*. Boston: South End Press.

Seligman, M. E. P. (1975). *Helplessness: On depression, development, and death*. San Francisco: W. H. Freeman.

Shainess, N. (1979). Vulnerability to violence: Masochism as a process. *American Journal of Psychotherapy, 33*(2), 174–189.

Sherman, L. W., & Berk, R. A. (1984). *The Minneapolis domestic violence experiment*. Washington, DC: Police Foundation Reports.

Sonkin, D., & Durphy, M. (1982). *Learning to live without violence: A book for men*. San Francisco: Volcano Press.

Sonkin, D., Martin, D., & Walker, L. (1985). *The male batterer*. New York: Springer.

Snell, J. E., Rosenwald, R. J., & Robey, A. (1964). The wifebeater's wife: A study of family interaction. *Archives of general psychiatry, 2*, 107–112.

Stahley, G. (1978). A review of select literature of spouse abuse. *Victimology, 2*,(3–4), 591–607.

Starr, B. (1978). Comparing battered and non-battered women. *Victimology, 3*,(1–2), 37–44.

Steinmetz, C. (1984). *Bystanders of crime: Some results from a national survey*. Paper presented at the Third International Victimology Conference, Lisbon, Portugal, November 10–18.

Straus, M. A., Gelles, R. A., & Steinmetz, S. K. (1980). *Behind closed doors: Violence in American families*. Garden City, NY: Anchor/Doubleday.

Walker, L. E. (1978). Battered women and learned helplessness. *Victimology, 2*(3–4), 525–534.

Walker, L. E. (1979). *The battered woman*. New York: Harper & Row.

Walker, L. E. (1981). A feminist perspective of domestic violence. In R. Stuart (Ed.), *Violent behavior: Social learning approaches to prediction, management and treatment* (pp. 102–115). New York: Brunner/Mazel.

Walker, L. E. (1983). Victimology and psychological perspectives of battered women. *Victimology, 8*(1–2), 82–104.

Walker, L. E. A. (1984a). *The battered woman syndrome*. New York: Springer.

Walker, L. E. A. (1984b). *Eliminating sexism to end battering relationships*. Presented in Symposium L. E. A. Walker (Chair), Making peace at home: Models for ending family violence. The APA Annual meeting, Toronto.

Walker, L. E. A. (1984c). Battered women, psychology, and public policy. *American Psychologist, 39*(10), 1178–1182.

Walker, L. E. A. (Ed.). (1984d). *Women and mental health policy*. Beverly Hills: Sage.

Walker, L. E. A. (1985). Feminist forensic psychology. In L. B. Rosewater & L. E. A. Walker (Eds.), *Handbook of feminist therapy: Psychotherapy with women*. New York: Springer.

Walker, L. E. A., & Browne, A. (in press). Gender and victimization by intimates. *Journal of Personality*.

Wardell, L., Gillespie, D. L., & Leffler, A. L. (1983). Science and violence against wives. In D. Finkelhor, R. Gelles, G. Hotaling, & M. Straus (Eds.), *The dark side of families* (pp. 69–84). Beverly Hills: Sage.

Wolf, S. C. (1984). *A multi-factor model of deviant sexuality*. Paper presented at the Third International Victimology Conference, Lisbon, Portugal, November 10–18.

# 5

# *Social and Structural Factors in Family Violence*

## George J. McCall and Nancy M. Shields

Violence is, properly speaking, an irreducibly social fact, about which disciplines such as physiology and psychology can have little to say. It is only regarding a simpler but related phenomenon—the use of physical force—that these latter disciplines can join in a dialogue with the social sciences. After all, by violence is meant the illegitimate use of force. Thus, society alone determines violence, by negotiating those social norms which define the limits of legitimate force within various social relationships, and by creating motives and reasons for individuals to press those limits. Violence—quite like crime, sin, or madness—is socially determined, in that it is socially defined, against a backdrop of shared meanings and normative understandings, and socially induced, through defined roles, situations, and interpretations.* Violence of all kinds is, then, an essentially sociological phenomenon.

Yet, it was not until around 1970 that "family violence" achieved distinct recognition as a puzzling theoretical problem within sociology: Given that family members are key social supports and significant others, how is intrafamily violence possible? What are the social dynamics through which an individual manages to bring himself to murder, assault, or brutalize a needed and loved member of his own family?

The general public's recognition of "family violence" as constituting a social problem is even more recent, substantially derivative, and a bit soft around the edges. The lengthy process of public recognition actual-

---

*It is important to note that human society is not unique in this matter. Students of animal social behavior have shown that among virtually all social-living mammals, intraspecific uses of physical force are overwhelmingly conventionalized, taking the form of ritualized mock combat. Violations of these conventions regarding who can be attacked, when, and how, constitute violence, and as such, usually lead to social control episodes.

ly began in 1962 with the "discovery" of the battered-child syndrome, leading gradually into a broader concern with child abuse and, most recently, child sexual abuse, including incest. During the 1970s, battered wives came into the public eye, a discovery which slowly widened to point to spouse abuse and, finally, marital rape. Similarly, the ugly phenomenon of "granny-bashing" came to light, paving the way for a broader concern with elder abuse. Research on the phenomenon of premarital or courtship violence is only now beginning to emerge. Only out of these separate, and fundamentally independent, concerns did the rubric of "family violence," injected by sociologists, slowly but inexorably emerge in public discussion as a strategic umbrella under which advocates of these separate concerns could usefully, if uneasily, join forces.

For a single term, in this case, "family violence," to refer at once to both a sociological problem and a social problem is not at all uncommon (Bash, 1983; McCall, 1984). And as so often occurs, the inevitable interplay between the sociological and the social problem has induced considerable research and theorizing, much of it valuable, all of it bearing quite unmistakably the distinctive saw marks of its origin in one or another mill of social advocacy, as we shall show in the next two sections.

## SOCIAL AND STRUCTURAL THEORIES OF FAMILY VIOLENCE

Relatively few of the theories reviewed here were actually developed as theories of family violence. Rather, most were developed as theories about some single type of family violence, such as child abuse or wife battering.

As a second limitation, many of these theories are essentially only attempts to conceptualize the nature of some single type of family violence in such a way as to show that the nature of the phenomenon contains within it certain implications regarding its causation. For example, if rape is reconceptualized as an exercise of power rather than of sexuality, different causal factors are suggested.

Third, most of these theories are, then, not technically well-developed to afford answers to any specific questions about family violence (e.g., differential incidence across socioeconomic strata), but rather remain largely oriented toward casting some light on how intrafamily violence is possible.

Fourth, these theories rarely display much sociological self-consciousness in characterizing the sort of social or structural phenomena they adduce as explanans. Therefore, these theories are grouped in a sociologically meaningful way.

## Social Structure

Macrosociologists regard social structure as being defined by the relations between and among social categories of individuals. To the extent that these relations define inequality, subordination, and superordination, the aspect of social stratification figures prominently in any account of social structure.

Of the major theories of family violence, only *feminist theory* (Dobash & Dobash, 1979; Russell, 1982; Straus, 1980c; Walker, 1981) points to the social structure, in this sense, as a causal factor in family violence. An assumption of virtually all feminist analyses is that most violence, at least most serious violence, is perpetrated by men against women. From this view, violence emanates from the patriarchal organization of society, in which men dominate and control women. The use of violence on the part of men reflects their greater relative power, authority and status in society. Women are devalued and are essentially the property of men; therefore, a man has the right to do what he wants with his own property. In fact, rape is seen as a violation by one man of another man's property. And a man taking a stick to his wife or child is no more unreasonable or offensive than a man taking a stick to his obstreperous cow.

Many feminist analyses of family violence, especially wife beating, have involved an in-depth analysis of the history of family violence, and a critique of the culture in which it takes place. A feminist approach nearly always emphasizes that any reduction or elimination of family violence must involve a basic restructuring of the nature of the power relationship between men and women.

## Culture

According to Kroeber and Kluckhohn (1952), "the essential core of culture consists of traditional (i.e., historically derived and selected) ideas and especially their attached values" (p. 181). Numerous analysts of family violence (e.g., Gil, 1970; Huggins & Straus, 1980; Steinmetz, 1977a; Straus, 1980b) point importantly to the cultural centrality (and the glorification) of force and violence in society, generally arguing that the cultural approval of violence in the larger society legitimates, inspires and reinforces the use of violence in the family. Some analysts, though, have also noted the inconsistent nature of some societal norms regarding the use of violence. For example, boys are taught that they should not hit girls, yet violence against women is often glamorized and sexualized in advertisements. However, some have argued that norms prohibiting the use of violence in the family are often only the "official" rather than the actual operating norms, or are limited to specific situations or classes of persons. For example, a little boy may discover that it is acceptable to hit his sister, but not the little girl who lives next door.

The *culture of violence* thesis rests on the assumption that a large segment of our society accepts the use of interpersonal violence (e.g., Stark & McEnvoy, 1970). However, Greenblat (1983) has pointed to the interesting fact that there is actually little empirical support for the notion that most people approve of the use of violence against family members. Greenblat's (1983) own research showed only minimal approval of such violence. Likewise, Huggins and Straus (1980) note that although interpersonal violence is a common theme in children's books, rarely is violence *between* family members actually depicted.

Another group of family violence analysts have argued that family violence is encouraged or discouraged by the norms of various subcultural groups. The subcultural argument is based on Wolfgang and Ferracuti's (1967) *subculture of violence* thesis, which states that rates of violence among certain segments of the population are higher or lower due to differential acceptance and approval of the use of violence by these subpopulations. Wolfgang and Ferracuti suggested that violence is more common among the lower class, given greater lower class emphasis on force and violence. Likewise, most family violence applications of the subculture of violence thesis have emphasized the idea that violence is more acceptable, even valued, in lower class culture (Brown, 1965; Toby, 1966).

Other family violence researchers have investigated subcultural differences in the use of family violence (including incest) among various ethnic and religious groups (Bagley, 1969; Carroll, 1980; Garbarino & Ebata, 1983). Similarly, battered wives have often reported that their husbands' violence against them is often supported (and perhaps suggested) by the husband's immediate peer network and workmates.

## Social Institutions

Only those most fundamental foci of social organization, which deal with universal problems of social life and are therefore found in all societies, are considered to be social institutions. The family is certainly one such institution, focused on regulating the reproductive, sexual, and nurturant relations between individuals and generations.

Traditionally, the family has been thought of as a unit within which love, nurturing, and comfort occur spontaneously and naturally. In contrast, some family violence analysts have proposed that the very nature of the social organization of the family actually makes the use of violence more probable than in other kinds of social groups (Farrington, 1980; Foss, 1980; Hotaling & Straus, 1980; Straus, 1980d). Ironically, the intense levels of love within the family often give rise to unusually high levels of hate and resentment. Spending large amounts of time together, the very private nature of the family, involuntary membership, and ascribed roles within the family, regardless of interest and competence, are all features of family organization which make the eruption of conflict, and sometimes subsequent violence, more likely than in other kinds of organizations, e.g., work groups. The high levels of disclosure typical of some family relationships also provide other family members with knowledge which can be used against the family member later. No one knows better than a family member how to hit a nerve of another family member (Hotaling & Straus, 1980).

*Social Systems*

According to *systems theory*, a system is an interdependent group of components, with a distinguishable boundary (Giles-Sims, 1983). Systems involve positive and negative feedback processes, and thresholds of viability that require a certain amount of change and a certain amount of stability. The family, a system composed of individual family members, is seen as a system within a larger system—society. The family is affected by the larger society and as such constitutes an open system.

Systems theories of family violence have been advanced by several family violence analysts (Elbow, 1977; Giles-Sims, 1983; Steinmetz & Straus, 1974; Straus, 1973). Of importance to the development of family violence is the idea that a disturbance in one aspect or part of the system affects the rest of the system. For example, a child's illness and the parental care it entails can affect the parents' sex life. Thus, a family is a system in which, when tension builds, violence is one method of coping with the built-up tension, as when the family strain resulting from a husband's being laid off from work may eventuate in the wife taking a belt to their small child.

A more specialized social-systems account is that provided by the several *resource and exchange theories* of family violence (Brown, 1980; Gelles, 1974, 1983; Hornung, McCullough, & Sugimoto, 1981; Straus, Gelles & Steinmetz, 1980). The exchange relationship is usually conceptualized as dyadic, either between spouses, or between parent and child. In this context, violence is seen as a failure of "normal" family exchange relations; violence is used as a resource to restore a threatened dominant status. When the perpetrator does not receive the rewards he expects, or he feels that his status is threatened, he resorts to the use of violence. Indeed, Allen and Straus (1977) have referred to the use of violence in such family exchange systems as the "ultimate resource."

A related conceptualization of a family exchange system involves a comparison of the statuses of family members *within* the family with statuses *outside* the family in the larger society (Gelles, 1978). A husband whose status outside the family system is inconsistent with his status inside the family is thought to be more likely to resort to the use of violence to restore the family system to equilibrium (Gelles, 1978). The husband's status outside the family is evaluated relative to that of his wife, and is expected to be higher. It is taken for granted that the husband holds the dominant, more powerful position within the family.

The concept of a dynamic social system is likewise central to various *interactionist theories* of family violence (Chatterton, 1976; Gelles, 1974; Hotaling, 1980; Pagelow, 1981; Reid, Taplin, & Lorber, 1981; Straus, 1973). Several of the interactionist theories draw directly from labeling theory (Pagelow, 1981; Straus, 1973), and attribution theory (Hotaling, 1980). Interactionist theories based on labeling theory are concerned with issues such as whether or not the batterer is labeled "deviant," whether or not an identity of "violent person" has emerged for the batterer and those processes by which violence escalates.

Other interactionist theorists have been primarily concerned with how conflict arises out of social interaction (Goode, 1971; Hepburn, 1973; Straus et al., 1980). Conflict is seen as an inevitable aspect of social relationships, and the more the conflict, the more likely it is that violence will be used as a problem-solving tactic.

A third group of interactionists have emphasized the importance of meaning to both parties involved in the violent interaction (Chatterton, 1976; Ferraro, 1984). Major concerns have to do with how people decide when a line of conduct is violent, how the threat is perceived, etc.

Finally, interactionist theories have also focused on interactional breakdowns. For example, violence may be seen as resulting from the parents' inability to discipline the child (Reid et al., 1981), or as an inability to communicate effectively in a nonviolent way (Watkins, 1982).

## Social Roles

Those patterns of action and sentiment expected of persons by virtue of their occupying a particular social position constitute social roles and powerfully influence the orderliness of social life.

Several versions of role theory have been developed to account for family violence. Perhaps the most common application of role theory has been *sex-role theory*. The argument is that traditional childhood sex-role socialization prepares boys to become aggressive and violent, and girls to become submissive and victims of men (Fox, 1980; Walker, 1979). Boys are taught that it is good to be aggressive and dominant and that violence is an acceptable problem-solving strategy—an acceptable way to demonstrate authority. Girls are taught that their eventual roles as wife and mother will be their most important roles in life, and that it is their responsibility to maintain their marriages at all costs. Girls are taught that it is their job to serve and take care of the rest of the family, and that their main identities will be defined in relation to the men whom they marry. Such sex-role socialization is seen as compatible with the husband's use of violence against his wife.

A second application of role theory, *family-role theory*, focuses on failures of role performance within the family. For example, a parent's violence against a child may be interpreted as resulting from inadequate parenting skills. Or, incest might be seen as resulting from *role confusion* (Finkelhor, 1979; Russell, 1984), where the wife and daughter enact the other's role within the family. *Role reversal* has also been noted among violent parents (Steele & Pollock, 1974), where the parent expects the child to behave as an adult and to nurture the parent.

A final way in which role theory has been used to explain family violence involves the argument that once a person has been victimized, the identity and role of victim is likely to develop, making the person more vulnerable to further victimization (MacFarlane, 1978; Shields & Hanneke, 1984a).

## Interpersonal Influences

Of course, not all the effects of one person upon another are so clearly mediated by socially defined role expectations. For example, the *intergenerational transmission theory* of family violence is based on the idea that violence is learned in the home through the mechanism of modeling, in which one person emulates the behaviors of someone he or she admires or respects. Exposure to family violence as a child is hypothesized to be a factor in the development of adult family violence, bringing about through this modeling mechanism an increased likelihood of adult victimization and participation in family violence (Gayford, 1975; Gelles, 1976; Gil, 1970; Herrenkohl, Herrenkohl, & Toedter, 1983; Sears, Maccoby, & Levin, 1957; Steinmetz, 1977a; Straus et al., 1980).

As more research on the intergenerational transmission hypothesis has been conducted, researchers have begun to address more refined questions about the ways in which family violence is passed from one generation to the next. For example, Owens and Straus (1975) studied the relationship between experiencing violence as a child and adult attitudes toward the use of violence, and Kalmuss (1984) investigated the extent to which the transmission of violence is role- and sex-specific. Although the exact mechanism of transmission is unknown or unspecified, it is generally believed that victims of domestic violence model the behavior they have been exposed to as children (Bandura, 1973), learning both the role of aggressor (Carroll, 1980) and that of victim (Post, Willett, Franks, & House, 1984).

A second theory of family violence having to do with interpersonal influence is *victim-precipitation theory*. The notion of victim precipitation was originally presented by Wolfgang and Ferracuti (1967) and referred to fatal violent interactions in which the victim was the first to use physical force. The application of victim-precipitation theory to the area of family violence involves a less literal sense of precipitation. The use of actual physical force on the part of the victim prior to victimization has been of little interest.

One version of victim-precipitation theory involves viewing the victim as masochistic, in the sense of making oneself more vulnerable to victimization by communicating to others, mainly nonverbally, that one expects to be victimized (Shainess, 1977, 1984). According to Shainess, this masochistic process does not involve the victim *enjoying* the violence directed toward her. Such a demurral notwithstanding, this version of victim-precipitation theory, which places immediate blame on the victim, has not been well received by most family violence researchers, especially the more feminist analysts.

The other main version of victim-precipitation theory focuses on characteristics or behaviors of the victim that appear to trigger victimization or to make the individual more vulnerable to victimization (Block & Sinnott, 1979; Finkelhor, 1979; Steinmetz, 1977a; Watkins, 1982). Such characteristics typically include extreme dependency, unusual levels of demands on caretakers or provocative behaviors such as the alleged nagging of the battered wife or the seductive behavior of the incest victims.

## Desocializing Influences

Finally, some theories explain family violence as being due to circumstances that attenuate or overwhelm internal and external social constraints against intrafamily violence.

For example, proponents of *stress theory* have argued that family violence arises out of the stresses and strains that certain families and certain family members must bear. When stresses and pressures become too great, violence results. Stress has been defined in several ways, as referring to normative life changes, both positive and negative (Makepeace, 1983; Straus et al., 1980; Watkins, 1982), and to a host of individual variables that are thought to bring about tensions within the family: pregnancy (Gelles, 1975), child rearing (Steinmetz, 1977a), and poverty and lower socioeconomic status (Gil, 1970; Straus et al., 1980). Stress has even been defined as change of any kind (Justice & Justice, 1976). When the particular stress stems from some characteristic of the victim that is stressful to the caretaker, such as a handicap, stress theory essentially reduces to victim-precipitation theory. Similarly, much of the research attributing the use of violence to stress has focused largely on socioeconomic variables such as unemployment, employment status, income, and education.

Analysts of family violence have also argued that *social isolation* of the family increases the likelihood of family violence (Allan, 1978; Finkelhor, 1979, 1983, 1984; Russell, 1982). Social isolation has been conceptualized as actual geographical isolation, such as rural location (Finkelhor, 1984; Russell, 1982), as well as limited social interaction with others (Gelles, 1974).

## Multifactor Theories and Theoretical Integrations

Now that the major theories of family violence have been reviewed, it should be noted that several leading family violence analysts have argued that family violence is a multidimensional phenomenon and that multifactor causal models are necessary to explain family violence (Finkelhor, 1979, 1984; Gelles, 1973, 1974, 1978; Gil, 1970; Straus et al., 1980). Some have even attempted theoretical integrations, both intradisciplinary (Straus, 1977) and interdisciplinary (Harris, 1982).

Virtually all the individual theories discussed in this chapter have been represented in these various multifactor models. However, most of these models have been developed to explain one particular form of family violence, such as wife abuse or child sexual abuse. Straus's (1973) general systems model has been the only comprehensive model proposed to explain all forms of family violence.

## APPLICATIONS OF THEORIES
## TO FORMS OF FAMILY VIOLENCE

The term *family violence* is too often used to refer only to spousal violence (mainly violence against wives) and child abuse. However, although their literatures are not large, several other forms of family violence have been investigated: sibling violence, violence against parents and elders, and most recently, courtship violence. Crosscutting these relationship types is the distinction between sexual and nonsexual modes of violence.

In this section is an examination of each of the main theories of family violence as these have been or might be applied to all the various forms of family violence. Gaps in the application of various theories will be noted, and suggestions for novel, promising applications will be discussed.

## Feminist Theory

Feminist theory views violence as an expression of social power. The patterns of family violence therefore follow pecking order: husbands are more powerful than wives, parents are more powerful than their young children, and the middle-aged are more powerful than the elderly. Such unequal relationships may be formalized in the larger social structure as reflecting legitimate authority, or even property rights. That women are seen as the sexual property of their husbands is evident in the fact that marital rape remains legal in most states; that children are seen as the property of their parents is evidenced by the reluctance of the criminal justice system to prosecute parents for violence, especially sexual violence, against their children.

Thus, feminist theory has been a popular explanation for husbands' violence against wives, both sexual (Russell, 1982) and nonsexual (Dobash & Dobash, 1979; Straus, 1980c; Washburne, 1983); for violence of parents against children, both sexual (Densen-Gerber, 1983; Finkelhor, 1984; Herman, 1981; Rush, 1980; Russell, 1984) and nonsexual (Marsden, 1978; Washburne, 1983); and, to a limited extent, adult children's violence against their elderly parents (Block & Sinnott, 1979).

Research on sibling violence has generally not been concerned with measuring a power dimension in any meaningful sense apart from age, and thus might present a promising area of application for feminist theory. For example, the little research that has been done does suggest that sibling violence is related to the overall power structure in the family (Felson, 1983).

Application of feminist theory to the newly emerging area of courtship violence would appear to be even more straightforward. Because most victims seem to be female and most perpetrators male, courtship violence might be seen as another form of violence that can be explained as the result of male-dominated society. Even in premarital relationships, males might be seen as using violence to control and to maintain superior status.

The great gap in the applicability of feminist theory is, of course, those forms of family violence which run counter to the usual pecking order of power within the family, in particular, wives' violence against their husbands. Since most husbands are viewed as the dominant member of their marital relationships, feminist theory would have grave difficulty in explaining husband battering. In practice, however, most feminist researchers and theorists have been almost exclusively concerned with those violent relationships in which the perpetrator is male and the victim is female.

## Culture of Violence Theory

The *culture of violence* thesis has often been presented in a very broad way as it applies to family violence in general (Walters, 1975). For example, Watkins (1982) points out that violence is widespread in American culture, and enumerates several areas of cultural support for the use of violence.

This culture of violence thesis has played an important role in several theoretical accounts (notably Gil, 1970) of the parental use of violence against children. A cultural explanation for child sexual abuse has also recently been presented by Finkelhor (1984), who argues that the sexual abuse of children is legitimated in our society by several cultural processes: the existence and increasing prevalence of child pornography; relatively weak criminal sanctions against the sexual abuse of children; general social toleration of sexual interest in children; an absence of sex education for children; cultural sexual valuation of the characteristics of smallness, youth, and submissiveness; and a tendency in our society for males to eroticize all affectionate relationships.

The culture of violence thesis has also been a popular explanation for wife abuse. Straus (1980b) has argued that in our society, there is at least implicitly some approval and support for the use of violence on the part of husbands against wives: "the marriage license is a hitting license" (p. 39). Others (e.g., Russell, 1984) have argued that both the media and the law encourage, or at least permit, sexual violence against wives.

Similar cultural explanations have been put forward for courtship violence, both sexual (Goodchilds & Zellman, 1984) and nonsexual (Olday & Wesley, 1984); elder abuse (Block & Sinnott, 1979); and sibling violence (Steinmetz, 1977a).

Prospectively, it might also be argued that cultural support exists for sexual violence between siblings. Young children are expected to experiment sexually, and such behavior is viewed as normal, even for siblings. Conversely, there would not appear to be much cultural support for the sexual abuse of elders and parents, but again, this problem is itself little documented.

The most serious difficulty in all applications of the culture of violence theory is that such studies tend to presume rather than test its truth (Greenblat, 1983) and selectively emphasize only those aspects of culture that are supportive of violence. The existence of counternorms (e.g., that boys are not supposed to hit girls, or that one is not supposed to beat up on those who are much smaller than oneself) is too seldom acknowledged. To be persuasive, studies of cultural factors in family violence need to be demonstrably evenhanded in weighing out those cultural elements which support and those which contravene violence. Indeed, some recent data do call into question the extent to which there actually is widespread cultural support for violence against wives (Greenblat, 1983), and the extent to which the use of violence in intimate relationships does increase with marriage (Yllo & Straus, 1980).

## Subcultural Theory

Subcultural explanations of family violence probably have been most frequently advanced for parental violence against children. Garbarino and Ebata (1983) have noted that American subcultural groups differ significantly in their values and practices regarding the use of physical force against children. Further, their research indicates that ethnic subcultural groups differ in both the rates and the forms of such uses of force. Results from the Straus et al. (1980) national survey also suggested some subcultural variation—both ethnic and social class—in parental use of violence against children.

The sexual abuse of children has also been explained in subcultural terms. Pierce and Pierce (1984) review race as a factor in child sexual abuse. Russell (1984) has noted that it has often been suggested that within certain subcultures, notably the rural, "Tobacco Road" type, parents are more likely to become involved in the use of sexual violence against children, and especially incest. Finkelhor (1979, 1984) has also noted that sexual abuse of children is more common in the lower classes and among descendents of French, Canadian, and English populations. Finkelhor (1984) has also suggested that, compared with the "female subculture," the "male subculture" may be more tolerant of the sexual abuse of children.

Carroll (1980) contends that there are also subcultural differences regarding spouse abuse, particularly between contrasting ethnic groups. There is at least limited support for these conclusions in the findings of the Straus et al. (1980) national survey of family violence on ethnic and social class differences in rates of spousal violence.

Subcultural differences in the incidence of marital rape, elder and parent abuse, and courtship violence are largely unknown and represent areas in which research is needed. Essentially all the research on courtship violence has been conducted among relatively homogeneous college and high-school student populations; therefore, data on subcultural variation are not available. Cornell and Gelles (1982a) found essentially no adolescent-parent violence in rural areas. However, elder abuse (Block & Sinnott, 1979) and marital rape (Russell, 1982) have been found to be slightly more common among Protestants, compared with other religious groups.

With few exceptions, epidemiological studies of the incidence and prevalence of various forms of family violence have thus far lacked the scope and representativeness to permit strong comparisons among subcultural groups—ethnic, religious, geographic, or socioeconomic (Hampton & Newberger, 1985). The future utility of subcultural theory will depend largely on whether or not reliable subgroup differences in the rates and forms of various types of family violence can be established.

### Family Social Organization Theory

Unique social organizational features of the family have been suggested as reasons why rates of family violence might be expected to be relatively high (Farrington, 1980; Foss, 1980; Hotaling & Straus, 1980) compared with other kinds of organizations. For example, Hotaling and Straus argue that the following 11 features of family organization contribute to family violence: high time at risk (because family members spend so much time together, they are at substantial risk of becoming victims of violence); a wide range of activities and interests among members of the family; great intensity of involvement with family members; competing and infringing activities of various family members; family membership rights to influence; age and sex discrepancies leading to conflict; ascribed roles; family privacy; involuntary membership; high levels of stress; and extensive knowledge of social biographies.

Organizational features such as these have not yet been analyzed in terms of how well they can explain different forms of family violence, and thus they present an area where further theoretical and empirical work are greatly needed. Not all of the 11 features are highly relevant to each form of family violence. For example, although the primary caretaking parent may be with the child almost around-the-clock, most spouses may actually spend more time with their co-workers than they do with their spouses. Furthermore, extensive knowledge of the others' social biographies may be limited to only certain family relationships: While spouses may have very extensive knowledge, children may know relatively little about their parents' backgrounds and experiences. Similarly, the feature of involuntary membership does not really apply to courtship relationships and perhaps not to many cohabiting and marital relationships. Of the eleven features listed by Hotaling and Straus, perhaps it is *family privacy* that will prove the most generally applicable and useful.

## Systems Theory

Perhaps the most thoroughly developed application of systems theory to family violence is Giles-Sims's (1983) six-stage model of wife battering, from establishment of the family system through assessing the impact of the wife's leaving and resolving whether it is to be a permanent state of the system.

Systems theory has also been applied to child sexual abuse (Finkelhor, 1984) and to nonsexual violence against children (Erchak, 1981, 1984; Justice & Justice, 1976). Finkelhor notes that from a systems perspective, incest is seen as related to the breakdown of the marital relationship in the family. Hence, a problem in one relationship within the family (husband-wife) affects another relationship (e.g., father-daughter). Erchak's (1981, 1984) analysis of the use of nonsexual violence against children has emphasized the role that victim plays within the family, and how patterns of abuse are maintained in the family through regenerative feedback.

Systems theory has not been extensively applied to the phenomena of marital rape, courtship violence, elder and parent abuse, or sibling violence. Felson's (1983) work on violence between siblings might be described as a systems model, since the actions of the parents are seen as central to whether or not violence occurs between siblings. Elder abuse would seem a fruitful area for application of systems theory, analyzing how the presence of an elderly person affects the family as a whole and how resulting problems and stresses contribute to elder abuse.

## Resource and Exchange Theories

Some principles of exchange theory, applied to family violence in general, have been discussed by Gelles (1983) and Straus et al. (1980). Gelles notes that in the family, as in any social organization, violation of the *principle of distributive justice* can result in resentment, conflict and violence. The perpetrator of violence will be more likely to continue to use violence when the rewards of doing so exceed the costs. However, a family member may also resort to violence when his or her investment in the relationship is greater than the rewards. According to most family analysts, the use of violence is a last resort, a final alternative when other methods to influence family members have failed. Violence may be used as a resource to reaffirm one's status within the family and will follow definite lines of power and authority.

As applied specifically to spousal violence, the idea of status consistency between husband and wife has been emphasized (Gelles, 1978; Hornung et al., 1981). More violence against the wife is expected when the wife's status outside the family is higher than her husband's. Parental violence against the child (Steinmetz, 1977a) has been viewed as a last resort to control the child and is more likely to be used when other disciplinary methods have failed. Regarding elder abuse, Lau and Kosberg (1979) have proposed the operation of a possible exchange relationship between the abusing child and the abused elder, that is to say, those abused as dependent children grow up, and eventually may abuse their now dependent elderly parents.

Exchange and resource theories have not yet been explicitly applied to marital rape, to sexual abuse of either children or elders, or to courtship violence. There is now some evidence (Hanneke, Shields, & McCall, in press) that within marriage sexual violence and nonsexual violence serve similar purposes for the perpetrator—power and control, rather than sexual gratification—and as such, exchange theories could treat sexual and nonsexual violence as different, but essentially equivalent commodities. Similar research comparing the use of sexual and nonsexual violence against children, elders and dates is needed to determine whether there, too, these forms of violence could serve as equivalent or distinct commodities in exchange models of these family relationships.

## Interactionist Theory

Interactionist theories of family violence, of a quite general character, have been presented by Chatterton (1976), Goode (1971), Hepburn (1973), and Hotaling (1980). As applied to more specific forms of family violence, interactionist theory has given greatest attention to *wife battering* (Ferraro, 1984; Pagelow, 1981; Straus et al., 1980; Watkins, 1982). The roles of the child and the parent in the interaction process leading to the nonsexual abuse of children have been analyzed by Reid et al. (1981). An interactionist approach to the occurrence of sexual violence against children has also been suggested by Finkelhor (1979), who notes that the behavior and appearance of a child may symbolize a sexual object to the adult, while the child's interaction orientation is quite different.

Interactionist approaches to marital rape, elder abuse, courtship violence, and sibling sexual violence have not been developed. An interactionist approach to these problems would emphasize the respective roles that each party plays in the interactions, the meaning of the situations to the participants, and the ways in which the rules concerning the use of force in the relationship discourage or encourage such use of physical force. For example, an interactionist approach to sibling sexual abuse might note the ways in which some sexual acts emerge from a process of play and sexual experimentation among siblings.

*Sex-Role Theory*

One version of role theory, feminist in orientation, argues that childhood sex-role socialization is conducive to wife battering (Fox, 1980; Walker, 1979; Watkins, 1982). According to this theory, traditional sex-role socialization has the effect of socializing girls to become victims and boys to become perpetrators of violence. Boys are taught that males are supposed to be strong, in control, and the primary wage earners in the family. Girls learn that their major adult jobs will be maintaining their marriages, domestic work, and child care. Watkins (1982) has also proposed that similarly, sexual childhood socialization is supportive of later sexual abuse of women. Boys are taught to be the sexual aggressors and girls are taught to be submissive. Girls are taught also that an important goal is to be physically and sexually attractive to men. These traditional male and female sex roles are held to be linked to the later roles of aggressor and victim.

For the most part, however, empirical research has yet to provide much support for these stereotyped notions. Male batterers have not been found to hold extremely traditional sex role orientations (Rouse, 1984), and battered women have not been found to hold traditional female role identities (Fox, 1980).

As applied to the use of violence against children, role theory has instead focused on various types of role failures. For example, sexual abuse of children has been thought to result from *role confusion* (Finkelhor, 1979; Russell, 1984); the incestuous father, for instance, may treat the child as if she were his wife rather than his daughter. Similarly, Steele and Pollock (1974) have claimed that nonsexual abuse of children often results from a parent-child *role reversal*. The parent may expect the child to behave as an adult and to satisfy the parent's needs. When the child fails, the parent is outraged and becomes physically violent with the child.

Sex-role theory, in either vein, has not yet been applied to the areas of marital rape, elder and parent abuse, or courtship violence. However, research that is still in progress on marital rape (Shields & Hanneke, 1984b) is investigating a possible relationship between traditional sex-role attitudes and victimization. Preliminary results suggest that victims of both battering and marital rape do not hold traditional sex-role orientations.

## Intergenerational Transmission Theory

Of all the theories of family violence, intergenerational transmission theory has probably been applied more widely than any other. The idea that patterns of violence are learned in childhood from one's parents has been evaluated in relation to spousal violence (Straus et al., 1980); adolescent violence toward parents (Cornell & Gelles, 1982a); elder abuse (Lau & Kosberg, 1979; Rathbone-McCuan, 1980); child abuse (Straus et al., 1980); and courtship violence (Bernard & Bernard, 1983; Makepeace, 1983; Olday & Wesley, 1984; Plass & Gessner, 1983). Regarding sexual family violence, the intergenerational transmission hypothesis has also been applied to marital rape (Shields & Hanneke, 1984a); the sexual abuse of children (Russell, 1984); and date rape (Murphy, 1984). Although almost all theoretical statements of the intergenerational transmission hypothesis involve the transmission of violence from the parent to the child, one study (Gully, Dengerink, Pepping, & Bergstrom, 1981) has also suggested that involvement in sibling violence as a child is a predictor of involvement in family violence as an adult.

Besides an emphasis on the way in which violence is passed from one generation to the next, many of these family violence analyses have also been concerned with the way in which one form of violence generalizes to another. For example, Straus et al. (1980) found that violent husbands and wives were also more likely than nonviolent partners to use violence against their children. They also found that in families where a parent uses violence against a child, there is likely to be more sibling violence as well.

A related research interest centers on the differential effects of having witnessed violence as a child versus having experienced violence as a child. Overall, it appears (Straus et al., 1980) that both facets contribute to later involvement in family violence, and that those who have both witnessed and experienced violence as a child are the most likely to use violence as an adult.

Although intergenerational transmission theory has been fruitful, in the sense of generating much empirical research on many forms of family violence, its explanatory value is not yet clear. Herzberger (1983) rightly cautions against the dangers of overinterpreting small differences in adult violence rates between those who have been exposed to violence as children and those who have not.

## Victim-Precipitation Theory

As applied to child abuse and to elder abuse, victim-precipitation theory has focused on identifying those characteristics and behaviors of such victims which may have made them vulnerable to victimization. Difficult development stages, provocative behavior (e.g., being seductive, daring the parent to use violence), a difficult personality, and dependency have been noted as characteristics of many abused children (Watkins, 1982). Characteristics of abused elders that have been related to their abuse include physical impairments, poor health, extreme age, handicaps and senility (Block & Sinnott, 1979). Steinmetz (1977a) has noted that small children and elders share two main characteristics that make both groups vulnerable to abuse—dependency, and being a source of family stress.

Application of victim-precipitation theory to wife battering is rare (Shainess, 1977), for it is widely regarded among feminists as a form of blaming the victim that feeds on those public stereotypes (e.g., the insufferably nagging wife) that are sponsored by male-dominated cultures.

## Stress and Social Isolation

The relationship between *stress* and family violence has received much research attention. Some connection between stress and violence either has been suggested or established for nonsexual elder abuse (Block & Sinnott, 1979; Watkins, 1982), spouse abuse (Steinmetz, 1977a; Straus, 1980d; Straus et al., 1980; Watkins, 1982), nonsexual courtship violence (Makepeace, 1983), and nonsexual child abuse (Gil, 1970; Straus et al., 1980; Watkins, 1982). For the most part, the relationship found between stress and violence has been a positive one, with only minor specifications of form. Straus et al. (1980) found that in the case of spouse abuse, the relationship of stress and violence seems to be stronger among women than men; Makepeace (1983) found that the relationship between stress and courtship violence held only among men.

Curiously, the relationship between stress and sexual forms of family violence has yet to be investigated.

Another desocializing influence—*social isolation*—is similarly widely considered to be related to family violence in the forms of wife battering

(Finkelhor, 1983), marital rape (Russell, 1982), both sexual and nonsexual abuse of children (Allan, 1978; Finkelhor, 1979, 1983, 1984; Russell,
1984), sibling sexual abuse (Loredo, 1982), and adolescent to parent violence (Cornell & Gelles, 1982a). In every case but the latter, there has been
found a positive relationship between isolation and violence. Only Cornell and Gelles (1982a) found the opposite: Adolescent-to-parent violence
was actually nonexistent in the rural areas.

## Summary of Applications

As Figure 1 shows quite graphically, virtually none of the major theories
of family violence has yet managed to address anything approaching even
one-half of the various forms of family violence. Each theory seems to
have been tailored to, at most, two or three of these forms of violence.

Conversely, as Figure 1 also shows, there are quite a few forms of family
violence that almost entirely escape any theoretical attention whatsoever.
In general, sexual forms of family violence have received very little attention, and the virtual absence, apart from Steinmetz (1977b) and Straus
et al. (1980), of serious research concerning wives' violence against their
husbands must strike the uninvolved outsider as most curious indeed. Of
course, the emerging areas of sibling violence, elder abuse, and courtship
violence are only just beginning to bid for analytic attention (Gelles & Cor
nell, 1985), and it is in these areas that fruitful applications most readily
suggest themselves.

### CONCLUSIONS AND IMPLICATIONS

This chapter began by noting that family violence represents both a
theoretical problem within sociology and a social problem recognized
within the body politic. It concludes by noting that, although each of these
problems has served to fuel and energize the other, they still remain
distinct and even divergent problems.

The loose social movement that emerged to define family violence as
a social problem is, like many, a marriage of convenience—linking but
not uniting a variety of special interest groups, each rather single-mindedly
concerned about a specific form of family violence. This fractionated
character of the movement has adversely affected pursuit of the theoretical problem of family violence, as the centrifugal tugs of all the special-
interest groups have tended to overpower the centripetal force exerted
by the sociological formulation. "Theories of family violence" is almost
a misnomer, for most of the theories reviewed in this chapter clearly were
framed to address only one or another form of domestic violence.

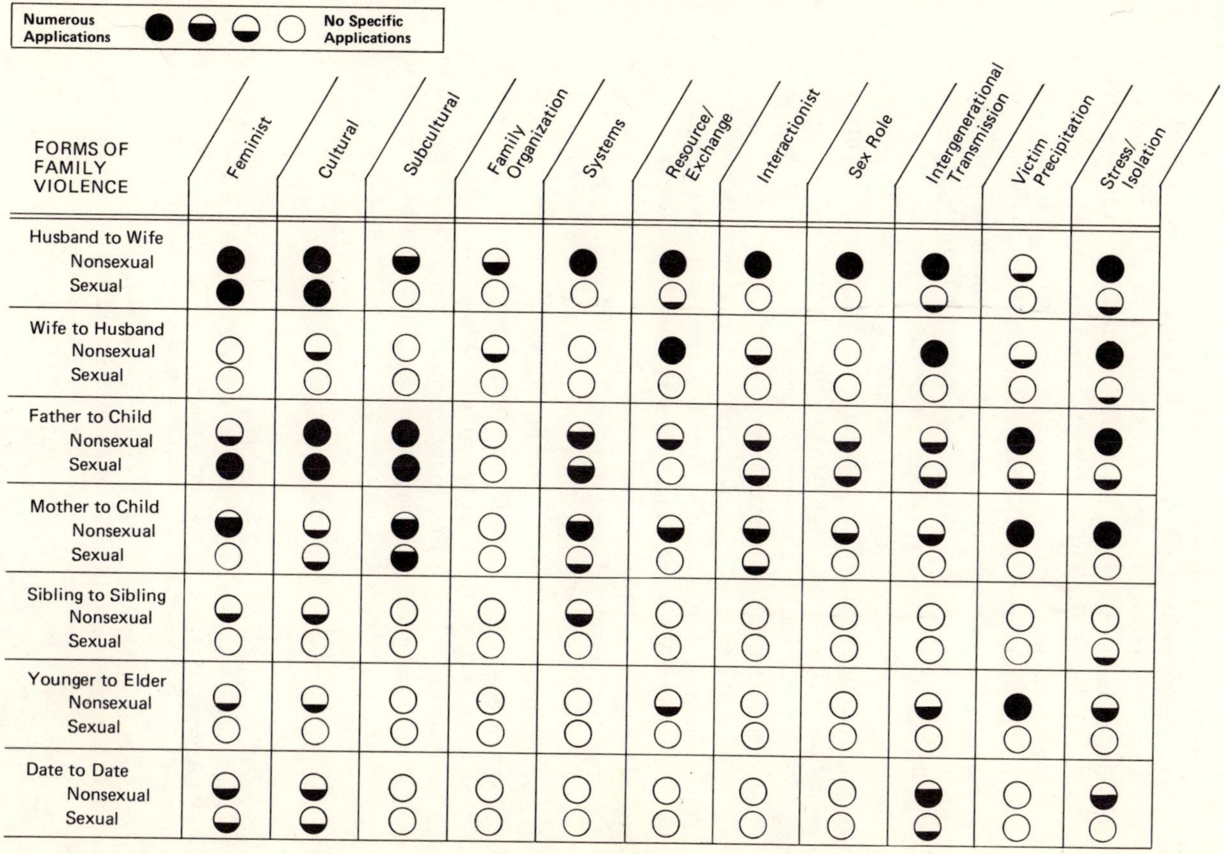

**Numerous Applications** ●   ◐   ○ **No Specific Applications**

FORMS OF FAMILY VIOLENCE

Theories (columns): Feminist, Cultural, Subcultural, Family Organization, Systems, Resource/Exchange, Interactionist, Sex Role, Intergenerational Transmission, Victim Precipitation, Stress/Isolation

Forms of family violence (rows):
- Husband to Wife — Nonsexual, Sexual
- Wife to Husband — Nonsexual, Sexual
- Father to Child — Nonsexual, Sexual
- Mother to Child — Nonsexual, Sexual
- Sibling to Sibling — Nonsexual, Sexual
- Younger to Elder — Nonsexual, Sexual
- Date to Date — Nonsexual, Sexual

*Figure 1.* Extent of applications of theories to specific forms of family violence

On the other hand, sociology's theoretical problem of family violence —apt though it is for purposes of the discipline—has tended actually to deflect attention from the key applied research questions. The theoretical problem, once again, is how it is that family violence is even thinkable; research is thus directed to a search for causes of family violence. The policy problem of family violence, on the other hand, is to refine or revise societal norms defining the limits of legitimate force within families; a search for causes of violence is of little direct relevance. Rather, policy-relevant research should seek to 1) explore and explain variations in such norms and 2) identify those aspects of family functioning which serve to dampen, constrain, and direct the uses of force within families.

American society, in the last couple of decades especially, has been uneasy in its approach to revising norms regulating uses of force—witness the grave ambivalence regarding capital punishment, police brutality, corporal punishment in schools, prisons, and the military. Revising norms limiting uses of force within the almost sacred institution of the family seems vastly more troubling to the American public.

Family policy of any kind has always proved most nettlesome for any national government, but especially for libertarian polities in pluralistic societies. Our own child abuse legislation serves to show clearly how the existence of subcultural and community standards for child rearing enormously complicate, if not foil, well-intended legislative attempts to revise family norms about uses of force (Giovannoni & Becerra, 1979). Consequently, many influentials within the family violence movement have begun to ask whether poorly informed policy might be worse than no policy at all (Newberger, 1983). Accordingly, one implication we derive for federal research policy is that higher priority ought to be placed on studies of subcultural and family-organizational variations in family functioning and in norms regarding the proper uses of physical force.

## REFERENCES

Allan, L. J. (1978). Child abuse: A critical review of the research and the theory. In J. P. Martin (Ed.), *Violence and the family* (pp. 43–80). New York: John Wiley & Sons.

Allen, C. M., & Straus, M. A. (1977). Resources, power and husband-wife violence. In M. A. Straus & G. T. Hotaling (Eds.), *The Social Causes of Husband-Wife Violence*. Minneapolis: University of Minnesota Press.

Bagley, C. (1969). Incest behavior and incest taboo. *Social Problems, 16,* 505–519.

Bandura, A. (1973). *Aggression: A social learning analysis.* Englewood Cliffs, NJ: Prentice Hall.

Bash, H. H. (1983). Sociology as discipline and as profession: A sociological scratch for every social itch? *International Journal of Sociology and Social Policy, 4,* 15–28.

Bernard, M. L., & Bernard, J. L. (1983). Violent intimacy: The family as a model for love relationships. *Family Relations, 32,* 283–286.

Block, M. R., & Sinnott, J. D. (1979). Methodology and results. In M. R. Block & J. D. Sinnott (Eds.), *The battered elder syndrome: An exploratory study*. College Park, MD: University of Maryland.

Brown, B. W. (1980). Wife-employment, marital equality and husband-wife violence. In M. A. Straus & G. T. Hotaling (Eds.), *The social causes of husband-wife violence* (pp. 176–187). Minneapolis: University of Minnesota Press.

Brown, C. (1965). *Manchild in the promised land* (pp. 263–271). New York: Macmillan Co.

Carroll, J. C. (1980). A cultural-consistency theory of family violence in Mexican-American and Jewish ethnic groups. In M. A. Straus & G. T. Hotaling (Eds.), *The social causes of husband-wife violence* (pp. 69–81). Minneapolis: University of Minnesota Press.

Chatterton, M. R. (1976). The social contexts of violence. In M. Borland (Ed.), *Violence in the family* (pp. 26–49). Atlantic Heights, NJ: Humanities Press.

Cornell, C. P., & Gelles, R. J. (1982a). Adolescent to parent violence. *Urban and Social Change Review, 15*(1), 8–14.

Cornell, C. P., & Gelles, R. J. (1982b). Elderly abuse: The status of current knowledge. *Family Relations, 31*, 457–465.

Densen-Gerber, J. (1983). *Medical aspects of human sexuality*. New York: Hospital Publications.

Dobash, R. E., & Dobash, R. (1979). *Violence against wives*. New York: Free Press.

Elbow, M. (1977). Theoretical considerations of violent marriages. *Social Casework, 58*, 515–526.

Erchak, G. M. (1981). The escalation and maintenance of child abuse: A cybernetic model. *Child Abuse and Neglect, 5*, 153–157.

Erchak, G. M. (1984). The escalation and maintenance of spouse abuse. *Victimology: An International Journal, 9*(2), 247–253.

Farrington, K. M. (1980). Stress and family violence. In M. A. Straus & G. T. Hotaling (Eds.), *The social causes of husband-wife violence* (pp. 94–114). Minneapolis: University of Minnesota Press.

Felson, R. B. (1983). Aggression and violence between siblings. *Social Psychology Quarterly, 46*(4), 271–285.

Ferraro, K. J. (1984). *An existential approach to battering*. Paper presented at the Second Conference for Family Violence Researchers, Durham, NH.

Finkelhor, D. (1979). *Sexually victimized children*. New York: Free Press.

Finkelhor, D. (1983). Family abuse. In D. Finkelhor, R. J. Gelles, G. T. Hotaling & M. A. Straus (Eds.), *The dark side of families: Current family violence research* (pp. 17–28). Beverly Hills, CA: Sage.

Finkelhor, D. (1984). *Child sexual abuse: New theory and research*. New York: Free Press.

Finkelhor, D., & Hotaling, G. T. (1984). Sexual abuse in the national incidence study of child abuse and neglect: An appraisal. *Child Abuse and Neglect, 8*, 23–33.

Foss, J. E. (1980). The paradoxical nature of family relationships and family conflict. In M. A. Straus & G. T. Hotaling (Eds.), *The social causes of husband-wife violence* (pp. 115–135). Minneapolis: University of Minnesota Press.

Fox, S. B. (1980). *Response to spousal violence as a function of sex-role identity and family role salience*. Doctoral dissertation, St. Louis University.

Garbarino, J., & Ebata, A. (1983). The significance of ethnic and cultural differences in child maltreatment. *Journal of Marriage and the Family, 45*(4), 773–783.

Gayford, J. J. (1975). Wife battering. A preliminary survey of 100 cases. *British Medical Journal, 25*, 194–197.

Gelles, R. J. (1973). Child abuse as psychopathology: A sociological critique and reformulation. *American Journal of Orthopsychiatry, 43*(4), 611–621.

Gelles, R. J. (1974). *The violent home*. Beverly Hills, CA.: Sage.

Gelles, R. J. (1975). Violence and pregnancy: A note on the extent of the problem and needed services. *The Family Coordinator, 24*, 81–86.

Gelles, R. J. (1976). Abused wives: Why do they stay? *Journal of Marriage and the Family, 38*, 659–668.

Gelles, R. J. (1978). Violence in the American family. In J. P. Martin (Ed.), *Violence and the family* (pp. 169–182). New York: John Wiley & Sons.

Gelles, R. J. (1983). An exchange/social control theory. In D. Finkelhor, R. J. Gelles, G. T. Hotaling, & M. A. Straus (Eds.), *The dark side of families: Current family violence research* (pp. 151–165). Beverly Hills, CA.: Sage.

Gelles, R. J. & Cornell, C. P. (1985). *Intimate violence in families*. Beverly Hills, CA: Sage.

Gil, D. G. (1970). *Violence against children: Physical child abuse in the United States*. Cambridge, MA: Harvard University Press.

Giles-Sims, J. (1983). *Wife battering: A systems theory approach*. New York: Guilford Press.

Giles-Sims, J., & Finkelhor, D. (1984). Child abuse in stepfamilies. *Family Relations, 33,* 407–413.

Giovannoni, J. M., & Becerra, R. M. (1979). *Defining child abuse*. New York: Free Press.

Goodchilds, J. D., & Zellman, G. L. (1984). Communication and sexual aggression in adolescent relationships. In N. Malamuth and E. Donnerstein (Eds.), *Pornography and sexual aggression*. New York: Academic Press.

Goode, W. (1971). Force and violence in the family. *Journal of Marriage and the Family, 33,* 624–636.

Greenblat, C. S. (1983). A hit is a hit . . . or is it? Approval and tolerance of the use of physical force by spouses. In D. Finkelhor, R. J. Gelles, G. T. Hotaling, & M. A. Straus (Eds.), *The dark side of families: Current family violence research* (pp. 235–260). Beverly Hills, CA: Sage.

Gully, K. J., Dengerink, H. A., Pepping, M. & Bergstrom, D. (1981). Research note: Sibling contribution to violent behavior. *Journal of Marriage and the Family*, May, 333–337.

Hampton, R. L., & Newberger, E. H. (1985). Child abuse incidence and reporting by hospitals: Significance of severity, class, and race. *American Journal of Public Health, 75,* 56–60.

Hanneke, C. R., Shields, N. M., & McCall, G. J. (in press). Assessing the prevalence of marital rape. *Journal of Interpersonal Violence*.

Harris, O. C. (1982). Toward an integrative approach to child abuse. *Urban and Social Change Review, 15*(1), 3–7.

Hennessey, S. (1979). Child abuse. In M. R. Block & J. D. Sinnott (Eds.), *The battered elder syndrome: An exploratory study* (pp. 19–32). College Park: University of Maryland.

Hepburn, J. R. (1973). Violent behavior in interpersonal relationships. *Sociological Quarterly, 14,* 419–429.

Herman, J. (1981). *Father-daughter incest*. Cambridge, MA: Harvard University Press.

Herrenkohl, E. C., Herrenkohl, R. C., & Toedter, L. J. (1983). Perspectives on the intergenerational transmission of abuse. In D. Finkelhor, R. J. Gelles, G. T. Hotaling, & M. A. Straus (Eds.), *The dark side of families: Current family violence research* (pp. 305–316). Beverly Hills, CA: Sage.

Herzberger, S. D. (1983). Social cognition and the transmission of abuse. In D. Finkelhor, R. J. Gelles, G. T. Hotaling, & M. A. Straus (Eds.), *The dark side of families: Current family violence research* (pp. 317–329). Beverly Hills, CA: Sage.

Hornung, C. A., McCullough, B. C., & Sugimoto, T. (1981). Status relationships in marriage: Risk factors in spouse abuse. *Journal of Marriage and the Family, 43*(3), 675–92.

Hotaling, G. T. (1980). Attribution process in husband-wife violence. In M. A. Straus & G. T. Hotaling (Eds.), *The social causes of husband-wife violence* (pp. 136–156). Minneapolis: University of Minnesota Press.

Hotaling, G. T., & Straus, M. A. (1980). Culture, social organization and irony in the study of family violence. In M. A. Straus & G. T. Hotaling (Eds.), *The social causes of husband-wife violence* (pp. 3–22). Minneapolis: University of Minnesota Press.

Huggins, M. D., & Straus, M. A. (1980). Violence and the social structure as reflected in children's books from 1850 to 1970. In M. A. Straus & G. T. Hotaling (Eds.), *The social causes of husband-wife violence* (pp. 51–67). Minneapolis: University of Minnesota Press.

Justice, B., & Justice, R. (1976). *The abusing family*. New York: Human Sciences Press.

Kalmuss, D. (1984). The intergenerational transmission of marital aggression. *Journal of Marriage and the Family, 46*(1), 11–19.

Kroeber, A. L., & Kluckhohn, C. (1952). *Culture: A critical review of concepts and definitions.* Cambridge: MA: Harvard University Peabody Museum of American Archeology and Ethnology.

Lau, E. E., & Kosberg, J. I. (1979). Abuse of the elderly by informal care providers. *Aging,* Sept.–Oct., 11–15.

Loredo, C. M. (1982). Sibling incest. In S. M. Sgroi (Ed.), *Handbook of clinical intervention in child sexual abuse* (pp. 177–190). Lexington, MA: Lexington Books.

MacFarlane, K. (1978). Sexual abuse of children. In J. R. Chapman & M. Gates (Eds.), *The victimization of women* (pp. 81–110). Beverly Hills, CA: Sage.

Makepeace, J. M. (1981). Courtship violence among college students. *Family Relations, 30,* 97–102.

Makepeace, J. M. (1983). Life events stress and courtship violence. *Family Relations, 32,* 101–109.

Marsden, D. (1978). Sociological perspectives on family violence. In J. P. Martin (Ed.), *Violence and the family* (pp. 135–168). New York: John Wiley & Sons.

McCall, G. J. (1984). Social science and social problem solving: An analytic introduction. In G. J. McCall & G. W. Weber (Eds.), *Social science and public policy: The roles of academic disciplines in policy analysis* (pp. 3–18). Port Washington, NY: Associated Faculty Press.

Murphy, J. E. (1984). *Date abuse and forced intercourse among college students.* Paper presented to Midwest Sociological Society, Chicago, IL.

Newberger, E. H. (1983). The helping hand strikes again: Unintended consequences of child abuse reporting. *Journal of Clinical Child Psychology, 12,* 307–311.

Olday, D., & Wesley, B. (1984). *Premarital courtship violence: Family of origin and dating correlates.* Paper presented at the 1984 Annual Meeting of the Midwest Sociological Society.

Owens, D. M., & Straus, M. A. (1975). The social structure of violence in childhood and approval of violence as an adult. *Aggressive Behavior, 1,* 193–211.

Pagelow, M. (1981). *Woman-battering: Victims and their experiences.* Beverly Hills, CA: Sage.

Pierce, L. H., & Pierce, R. L. (1984). Race as a factor in the sexual abuse of children. *Social Work Research and Abstracts, 20,* 9–14.

Plass, M., & Gessner, J. (1983). Violence in courtship relations: A Southern sample. *Free Inquiry in Creative Sociology, 11,* 198–202.

Post, R. D., Willett, A. B., Franks, R. D., & House, R. M. (1984). Childhood exposure to violence among victims and perpetrators of spouse battering. *Victimology, 6* (1–4), 156–166.

Rathbone-McCuan, E. (1980). Elderly victims of family violence and neglect. *Social Casework, 61*(5), 296–304.

Reid, J. B., Taplin, P. S., & Lorber, R. (1981). A social interactional approach to the treatment of abusive families, In R. B. Stuart (Ed.), *Violent behavior: Social learning approaches to prediction, management and treatment* (pp. 68–82). New York: Brunner/ Mazel.

Rosenberg, M. S. (1984). *Intergenerational family violence: A critique and implications for witnessing children.* Paper presented at the 92nd Annual Convention of the American Psychological Association, August: Toronto, Canada.

Rouse, L. P. (1984). *Conflict tactics used by men in marital disputes.* Paper presented at the Second Conference for Family Violence Researchers, Durham, NH.

Rush, F. (1980). *The best kept secret: Sexual abuse of children.* Englewood Cliffs, NJ: Prentice-Hall.

Russell, D. E. H. (1982). *Rape in marriage.* New York: Macmillan.

Russell, D. E. H. (1984). *Sexual exploitation: Rape, child sexual abuse, and workplace harassment.* Beverly Hills, CA: Sage.

Sears, R., Maccoby, E. E., & Levin, H. (1957). *Patterns of child rearing.* New York: Harper & Row.

Shainess, N. (1977). Psychological aspects of wifebeating. In M. Roy (Ed.), *Battered women: A psycho-sociological study of domestic violence* (pp. 111–119). New York: Van Nostrand Reinhold.

Shainess, N. (1984). *Sweet suffering: Woman as victim*. New York: Bobbs-Merrill.

Shields, N. M., & Hanneke, C. R. (1984a). *Multiple sexual victimization: The case of incest and marital rape*. Paper presented at the Second Conference for Family Violence Researchers, Durham, NH.

Shields, N. M., & Hanneke, C. R. (1984b). *Victim reaction to marital rape and battering*. Progress report to the National Institute of Mental Health, Rockville, MD.

Stark, R., & McEnvoy, J. (1970). Middle class violence. *Psychology Today, 3* (Nov.), 52–54, 110–112.

Steele, B. F., & Pollock, C. B. (1974). A psychiatric study of parents who abuse infants. In R. E. Heffer & C. H. Kempe (Eds.), *The battered child* (2nd ed.) (pp. 103–148). Chicago, IL: University of Chicago Press.

Steinmetz, S. K. (1977a). *The cycle of violence: Assertive, aggressive and abusive family interaction*. New York: Praeger.

Steinmetz, S. K. (1977b). Wife beating, husband beating—A comparison of the use of physical violence between spouses to resolve marital fights. In M. Roy (Ed.), *Battered women: A psycho-sociological study of domestic violence* (pp. 63–72). New York: Van Nostrand Reinhold.

Steinmetz, S. K., & Straus, M. A. (Eds.). (1974). *Violence in the family*. New York: Harper & Row.

Straus, M. A. (1973). A general systems approach to a theory of violence between family members. *Social Science Information, 12* (June), 105–125.

Straus, M. A. (1977). Determinants of violence in the family: Toward a theoretical integration. In W. Burr, R. Hill, I. Nye, & I. L. Reiss (Eds.), *Contemporary theories about the family*. New York: Free Press.

Straus, M. A. (1978). Wifebeating: How common and why? *Victimology, 2*(3–4), 443–458.

Straus, M. A. (1980a). The marriage license as a hitting license: Evidence from popular culture, law and social science. In M. A. Straus & G. T. Hotaling (Eds.), *The social causes of husband-wife violence* (pp. 39–50). Minneapolis: University of Minnesota Press.

Straus, M. A. (1980b). Sexual inequality and wife beating. In M. A. Straus & G. T. Hotaling (Eds.), *The social causes of husband-wife violence* (pp. 86–93). Minneapolis: University of Minnesota Press.

Straus, M. A. (1980c). Social stress and marital violence in a national sample of American families. *Annals of the New York Academy of Sciences, 347*, 229–250.

Straus, M. A. (1980d). A sociological perspective on the causes of family violence. In M. R. Green (Ed.), *Violence and the family* (pp. 7–31). Boulder: Westview Press.

Straus, M. A., Gelles, R. J., & Steinmetz, S. K. (1980). *Behind closed doors: Violence in the American family*. Garden City, NY: Doubleday.

Toby, J. (1966). Violence and the masculine ideal: Some qualitative data. In M. Wolfgang (Ed.), *Patterns of violence, the annals of the American academy of political and social science, Vol. 364* (pp. 20–27).

Walker, L. E. (1979). *The battered woman*. New York: Harper & Row.

Walker, L. E. (1981). A feminist perspective on domestic violence. In R. B. Stuart (Ed.), *Violent behavior: Social learning approaches to prediction, management and treatment* (pp. 102–115). New York: Brunner/Mazel.

Walters, D. R. (1975). *Physical and sexual abuse of children: Causes and treatment*. Bloomington, IN: Indiana University Press.

Washburne, C. K. (1983). Analysis of child abuse and neglect. In D. Finkelhor, R. G. Gelles, G. T. Hotaling, & M. A. Straus (Eds.), *The dark side of families: Current family violence research* (pp. 289–292). Beverly Hills, CA: Sage.

Watkins, C. R. (1982). *Victims, aggressors and the family secret: An exploration into family violence*. Minnesota Department of Public Welfare.

Wolfgang, M. E., & Ferracuti, F. (1967). *The subculture of violence*. London: Tavistock Publications.

Yllo, K. A., & Straus, M. A. (1980). Interpersonal violence among married and cohabiting couples. *Family Coordinator*, April, 30, 339–347.

# 6

# *Sociocultural Aspects of Domestic Violence*

## David G. Gil

### INTRODUCTION

Studies of violence throughout human history and across different cultures suggest that violent feelings, attitudes and acts are moments in processes of social relations, rather than independent events. Violent episodes may often seem senseless when studied in isolation, apart from their societal and historical contexts. However, when viewed in these contexts their internal logic and meanings are easily unravelled.

Domestic violence should therefore be studied as phases in cycles of societal violence and personal counterviolence in everyday life, rather than, as is often done, as a discrete phenomenon reflective of individual deviance or pathology. From such a perspective, domestic violence is a multidimensional phenomenon, related to sociocultural and historic dynamics whose impacts on people tend to trigger diverse reactions, including violent eruptions among members of families and households.

### THE CONCEPT OF VIOLENCE:
### BASIC HYPOTHESES AND DEFINITION

A main thesis of this chapter is that violence in human relations, including its domestic version, is rooted in socially evolved and institutionalized inequalities of status, rights and power among individuals, sexes, ages, classes, races, and peoples. All social formations which involve such inequalities as a basis for domination and exploitation, from patriarchy and slavery to feudalism, capitalism, colonialism, imperialism, and authoritarianism, are therefore intrinsically violent societies. They

124

violate the individual development of their members and they bring forth violent reactions from oppressed individuals and groups.

Inequalities in human relations and social institutions certainly did not come about as a result of free choice by individuals and groups to be victimized. Rather, inequalities are likely to have been established by means of coercive events and processes. Only then did they become institutionalized as "law and order," rationalized and justified through mythology, religion, philosophy, ideology, history, social sciences, and legal theory, and transmitted and stabilized through processes of socialization and social control. Once established, social-structural inequalities required continuous application of overt or covert and subtle force for their perpetuation, maintenance, expansion, and defense.

A corollary of this thesis is that the coercive processes by which social inequalities are established and conserved tend to induce violent responses from individuals and groups who are exploited, deprived, and oppressed within inegalitarian social structures. In turn, violent reactions from oppressed groups tend to lead to intensified repressive reactions on the part of privileged and dominant groups and their collaborators, that, in turn, create vicious circles of ever-escalating violence, counterviolence and repression. It seems that the only course for humankind to overcome these violent interactions on every level of social existence is to transcend socially originated and maintained inequalities, and to evolve, in their place, social orders shaped consistently by egalitarian and democratic principles.

Social phenomena may be defined descriptively or dialectically. Descriptive definitions usually lead to fragmented, symptom-oriented conceptions and programs while dialectic definitions are intended to reveal relations of phenomena to social and historical contexts. They are, therefore, well-suited to generate source-oriented intervention strategies. Viewed dialectically, *violence means human-originated acts, relations, processes, practices, and conditions which obstruct free and spontaneous unfolding of innate human potential, the intrinsic human drive toward growth, development and self-actualization, by interfering with the fulfillment of fundamental biological, psychological, and social needs. Development obstructing, i.e., violent acts, relations, processes, practices, and conditions may occur between individuals as well as between individuals and social institutions, between social groups within societies, and between entire societies.*

Implicit in the foregoing dialectic concept and definition of violence is the assumption that humans are self-propelled toward becoming what they are intrinsically capable of becoming and that a tendency toward spontaneous growth and development is inherent in humans in the same way it appears to be inherent in the seeds of plants. Seeds will grow into healthy, mature plants only when embedded in nutritious soil, and when rain and sunshine correspond in timing, quality, and quantity to their unique developmental requirements. Similarly, human development will be inhibited, i.e., violated, unless humans live in natural and social environments compatible with their developmental needs.

A further assumption underlying this concept and definition is that humans are not compelled by nature to relate to other humans in violent, domineering, exploitative, and oppressive ways, although, of course, they have ample capacity to do so. Yet, they also have the alternative capacity to relate to others nonviolently, cooperatively, caringly, supportively, and lovingly. Which of these capacities will emerge as the dominant tendency among a group of humans will depend on the social patterns and ideology they have evolved for themselves throughout their history (Benedict, 1970).

Erich Fromm, a noted social scientist and psychoanalyst who studied the sources and dynamics of violence in Europe during the early decades of this century, reached similar conclusions to those suggested here:

> It would seem that the amount of destructiveness to be found in individuals is proportionate to the amount to which expansiveness of life is curtailed. By this we do not refer to individual frustrations of this or that instinctive desire, but to the thwarting of the whole of life, the blockage of spontaneity of the growth and expression of man's sensuous, emotional, and intellectual capacities. The more the drive toward life is thwarted, the stronger is the drive toward destruction; the more life is realized, the less is the strength of destructiveness. Destructiveness is the outcome of unlived life. (Fromm, 1941)

*Violence*, according to Fromm, *is not a primary human tendency but a reaction to a prior blocking of spontaneous, constructive life energy.*

## LEVELS OF MANIFESTATION AND DYNAMICS OF VIOLENCE

Violent, i.e., development-obstructing, acts, processes, relations, practices, and conditions may occur among individuals in their homes and also between individuals, groups, social institutions, and entire societies. Individuals may violate one another's integrity and development by physical and psychological means or by creating and maintaining conditions which interfere with the development of others through deprivation, exploitation, and oppression. Institutions such as schools, health and welfare systems, and business corporations may, through their policies and practices, disregard developmental needs of people and may thus subject them to conditions that harm their development. Finally, entire societies may, through their values, policies, and practices, evolve and sanction phenomena such as: poverty; discrimination by class, race, sex, or age; unemployment and inflation; and foreign conquests, domination and exploitation, which inevitably interfere with the development of many individuals and groups, at home and abroad.

Violence inherent in societal conditions and processes may be thought of as social-structural violence because it is a consequence of inegalitarian social structures. Social-structural violence is usually a "normal" condition, inherent in established social patterns and legitimate practices, while "personal violence" involves acts which usually conflict with prevailing social norms or laws. Personal and social-structural violence cannot, however, be understood apart from one another. Rather, they interact with and reinforce one another. They are merely different manifestations of the same underlying social context: the same social values, mentality, institutions, and dynamics.

Personal violence as suggested in Fromm's conclusion is usually reactive violence rather than initiating violence. It is one way in which people react to stresses and frustrations caused by structural violence they encounter in everyday life. Personal violence appears to be fueled by developmental energy which has been transformed into destructive behaviors when blocked by social-structural violence. Social-structural violence is, therefore, the source or trigger of personal violence which, in turn, may lead to chain reactions as successive victims become agents of further violence. The usual focus of government agencies and the media on sensational cases of personal violence, and their consistent disregard of the roots of personal violence in social-structural violence, disguises the causal links and precludes understanding and effective, preventive intervention. However, emphasis on personal violence and neglect of social-structural violence tend to serve the interests of dominant and privileged classes in society, for they deny by implication the nexus between personal and societal versions of violence. Society is thus absolved of guilt and responsibility and the necessity of structural change toward nonviolent institutions, while individuals are scapegoated.

## FAMILIES AS AGENTS AND ARENAS OF VIOLENCE

Why does personal violence occur more frequently within families and in homes rather than in settings where people confront structural violence more directly? In modern, industrial, urbanized societies, the family and the home are expected to restore the emotional stability of individuals who encounter unsettling experiences outside their homes, at places of work and in other formal settings where people are often treated in an impersonal, dehumanizing, and alienating manner (U.S. Department of HEW Task Force, 1973). Families and homes serve often as balance wheels or lightning rods for the stresses of everyday life. They are used as settings for uninhibited discharge of feelings of hurt, insult, frustration, anger, and reactive violence, feelings that originate mostly outside the family, but can usually not be discharged at their places of origin, as such direct discharge would lead to social sanctions including dismissal from jobs, arrest, and prosecution for unlawful acts. Discharging these feelings in the privacy of one's home is relatively safe since it is hidden from public view, and the risk of social sanctions is usually lower than for similar behavior in the public domain.

There is one further, subtle link between family life and structural violence, namely, the family's socialization function, its responsibility for preparing children for roles as adults, and for adaptation to societal patterns with which they will have to live. In societies such as ours, in which submission to structural violence is a "normal" aspect of adult everyday life, families along with schools, the media, and other agents of socialization tend to prepare children to adjust to, and participate in, these practices and experiences. This preparation for living with violence is not intentional, but occurs automatically through "normal" child rearing and educational processes: play, sports, stories, art, cognitive and experiential learning, quality of human relations and emotional milieu, rewards and punishments, and especially, an ample measure of corporal punishment. Hierarchical structures, male dominance, and irrational, arbitrary authority are frequent attributes of home life in such societies, all of which are relevant to the task of preparing children for adjustment to a lifetime with structural violence. Male dominance and hierarchy are, of course, particular forms of socially structured inequalities, rooted in and maintained by coercion and violence and tending, in turn, to induce counterviolence.

## SOCIAL-STRUCTURAL VIOLENCE IN THE UNITED STATES

Having clarified the meaning, manifestations, and dynamics of social-structural and domestic violence, and links between them, we need now to examine social-structural violence in the prevailing institutional and ideological context of the United States. In accordance with the concept of violence presented here, the scope of structural violence in any human society reflects the extent to which fundamental human needs tend to be frustrated and human development tends to be inhibited, as a result of the normal workings of society's institutions. We begin this analysis by first identifying fundamental, developmental and existential human needs. Next, we will examine whether these needs can be fulfilled in our society, given the workings and values of prevailing social institutions.

## Human Needs

Knowledge concerning human needs may be imperfect. However, many students of human development consider fulfillment of the following related needs essential to healthy development:

1) regular access to life-sustaining and life-enhancing goods and services;
2) meaningful social relations and a sense of belonging to a community, involving mutual respect, acceptance, affirmation, care and love, and opportunities for self-discovery and for the emergence of a positive sense of identity;
3) participation in meaningful and creative ways, in accordance with one's innate capacities and stage of development, in productive processes of one's community and society;
4) a sense of security derived from fulfillment of needs for life-sustaining and life-enhancing goods and services, meaningful relations, and meaningful participation in socially valued productive processes; and
5) becoming what one is capable of becoming, or, in Maslow's terms, self-actualization through creative, productive work. (Dewey, 1935; Fromm, 1955; Maslow, 1970)

## Culture and Human Needs

The extent to which people are able to meet fundamental needs, to develop, and to realize their innate capacities depends in many ways on the conditions in which they live and on the quality of their human relations. Living conditions and human relations, in turn, are shaped largely by the social, economic, and political institutions, and by the corresponding ideologies of societies. In continuing this analysis, it is important to keep in mind that institutional orders and ideologies of societies evolve from cooperative and antagonistic interactions among individuals and groups in pursuit of survival and out of people's relations to their natural environments. This means that humans themselves, rather than extra-human forces, are the originators and shapers of their ways of life and of the ideological systems that explain and justify these ways. It also means that humans, at any stage of social development, have the capacity to transform their established ways of life when they realize that they cannot fulfill their fundamental needs within the context of a prevailing institutional order and ideology. The foregoing assumptions and principles, by the way, are enshrined in the Declaration of Independence of the United States.

Institutional orders and ideologies vary from place to place and over time. Some variations are more applicable than others to the realization of fundamental human needs and the requirements of human development. Or, in terms of the dialectic concept of violence discussed above, some social orders may be nonviolent, i.e., compatible with requirements of human development, while others may involve varying degrees of social-structural violence, i.e., human-originated obstacles to meeting fundamental needs and developing innate potential.

Implicit in the proposition that humans themselves, in pursuit of survival, originate and shape their societal institutions and ideologies, are important insights from biology. Biologically, the human species is perhaps the least programmed species in nature. Human genes do not transmit set patterns of life as do the genes of insects, birds, and many other species. Rather than transmitting set patterns of life, human genes transmit capacities, possibilities, ranges, and limits. As a consequence, humans not only can, but must make choices as they develop the specifics of their personal and social life-patterns. The transmission of ways of life and thought among generations of humans is therefore largely a sociocultural process, rather than a biological one.

The relative openness of the human genetic program makes possible the amazing creativity, productivity, and adaptability of our species. Humans can and do live all over the globe. However, the fact that human biology requires us to create our own patterns of individual and social existence means also that certain solutions to existential imperatives, i.e., cultures, are more compatible with human development than others, and that some cultures are actually incompatible with the fulfillment of nearly all human needs and hence with growth and development (Turnbull, 1972).

A further difficulty inherent in the human condition is the tendency to conserve and perpetuate patterns of existence once they are established and to actively resist changes in these patterns. This tendency has social, psychological, and biological aspects. Cultural continuity provides a sense of relative security, while cultural innovation tends to generate anxiety and insecurity, especially when change involves perceived or real challenges to the vested interests of privileged groups in a society. However, the tendency to conserve established ways of life reflects not only the defense of perceived interests of advantaged groups and the anxieties and insecurities aroused by the prospect of relinquishing known patterns and facing the unknown, but also the biological reality that established ways of life are learned and internalized early in life when humans are highly dependent on adult care in a material and psychological sense, and when capacities for critical consciousness are, as yet, underdeveloped or easily suppressed by agents of socialization into established cultures.

These brief observations on the human condition in nature and on the origins and inherent opportunities and limitations of human cultures should serve as backdrop for an analysis of the prevalence of social-structural violence in the institutional order and ideology of the United States and for the subsequent discussion of social and cultural change aimed at the reduction and elimination of structural violence as a precondition for overcoming domestic violence.

## Human Needs and Social Structure in the United States

To gauge the level of social-structural violence in a society, one must examine the extent to which its members can meet their fundamental human needs and thus realize their innate potential in the context of the prevailing institutional order and ideology. Such an examination involves studying the normal workings of the following related key processes of social organization and their consequences for the quality of life, circumstances of living, and human relations of people:

1) control, use, conservation, and development of natural and human-created resources;
2) organization, definition, and design of work and production; and
3) exchange and distribution of life-sustaining and life-enhancing goods and services, and of social, civil, and political rights. (Gil, 1973)

## Resource Management

In the United States, a minority of the people, individually or as corporations, own and control most means of production, exchange, and distribution: land and other natural resources; factories and machinery; banks and commercial and service establishments; transportation and communication; and knowledge and technology. A fraction of productive resources is owned collectively by all the people and is administered by government agencies, supposedly in the "public interest." However, administration of the "public sector" tends to be influenced by interests of individual and corporate enterprises, the "private sector."

The majority of the people do not own and control sufficient resources to survive by working with what they control. Hence, they depend for survival on selling their labor, knowledge, and skills to owners and managers of means of production at the discretion and in the interest of those in control of resources. The propertyless working classes differ among themselves by origin, race, history and culture; by sex and age; by education, skills, and attitudes; and by occupation and income. These differences tend to divide them as they compete for employment, goods and services, and rights.

Owners and managers tend to use the resources they control toward production of goods and services for sale with the intent of realizing profits. Profits, in turn, are largely reinvested to expand control over means of production and markets. The competitive drive among enterprises toward accumulation of capital and control over resources and markets tend to shape the logic of everyday life and to affect the consciousness, behavior and mutual relations of people. The quality and quantity of products, the extent to which production corresponds to actual needs of the population, the quality of the labor process, the effects of production on people, communities, the environment, and the conservation of resources —all these considerations are less important in shaping production decisions than criteria of profitability and accumulation and concentration of capital.

## Work and Production

In the prevailing work system of the United States, "work" does not mean activities geared to the satisfaction of human needs, but activities which directly or indirectly contribute to the generation of profits for individuals or corporations who own and control most productive resources. The paradoxical consequences of this concept of work are illustrated by the fact that "profitable" activities, such as professional sports and "spreading illusions" (also known as advertising), are considered work while "nonprofitable" activities such as rearing one's children, caring for one's home or for disabled relatives and providing services as a volunteer, are not considered work. The former are routinely included in the gross national product (GNP), the official measure of the aggregate of activities generating goods and services, and are rewarded materially and socially, while the latter are excluded from the GNP and from material rewards and social prestige.

The organization of work in the United States reflects the profit motive of enterprises and the foregoing concept of work shaped by that motive. It reflects also the division of the population in terms of ownership, control, and management of means of production. The propertied, controlling, and managerial classes, a powerful minority, rely on the labor of the relatively powerless majority of propertyless workers who, in turn, are dependent for their livelihood on employment by, and in the interest and at the discretion of, individual and corporate owners. In general, the higher the ratio of employment-seeking workers to available jobs, the lower will be the average level of wages and the higher the average rate of profits. Owners and managers of enterprises tend, therefore, to welcome an oversupply of workers relative to available jobs. This tendency results usually in varying degrees of unemployment and underemployment which forces workers and potential workers to compete fiercely for available positions.

The constant exclusion of many people from work and the related competition for jobs result not only in personal rivalries, but also in intergroup conflicts and discrimination by race, sex, and age. Competition results not only from job scarcities but also from the drive for advancement in pyramidal, bureaucratic organizations, and corresponding wage and prestige systems. Hierarchical structures, in turn, seem necessary to supervise and control workers whose innate capacities for self-direction have not had opportunities to develop and who usually lack incentives to maximize productivity since the fruits of their labor do not belong to them. Competition for jobs and for advancement to more desirable positions tends to reduce opportunities for meaningful human relations in work places and throughout society since individuals who are forced to compete for the same scarce positions and opportunities are unlikely to develop close, caring, and meaningful relationships. It also tends to inhibit the development of solidarity among workers and unemployed individuals, and it gives rise to loneliness, frustration, and alienation, which, in turn, may lead to depression, alcoholism, drug addiction, domestic violence, crime, and suicide (U.S. Congress Joint Economic Committee, 1976; U.S. Department of HEW Task Force, 1973).

Unemployment, which seems a regular feature of capitalist economies, has many destructive consequences. It holds down the general level of wages, depresses the self-image of unemployed workers, and induces insecurity among employed workers who may lose their jobs at the discretion of employers. The emotions of unemployed workers usually affect the milieu of their families, who suffer emotionally along with actual or threatened material deprivation. Furthermore, unemployment has consequences far beyond households directly involved, since reduced household incomes affect the economic realities of communities and society.

While unemployment dehumanizes its victims, and sooner or later leads to systemic crises, employment under prevailing conditions is, at best, a mixed blessing as it usually does not provide opportunities to actualize one's innate potential. Workers are usually considered and treated as means to the ends of employers, and they have little say in shaping and directing their work. They are not perceived as whole and unique individuals, but as functions or components of production processes—"hired hands." When one is treated as a replaceable attachment to a machine, one's self-esteem suffers and one's development as a whole person with multifaceted capacities is inevitably stunted.

As a result of employers' efforts to increase efficiency, productivity, and profits, the tasks of most workers have been reduced to simple routines, small steps in complex production processes of which workers usually possess only limited knowledge. Consequently, workers are no longer competent and knowledgeable masters of production in their fields, but are, in the revealing jargon of economists, mere "factors of production." Beyond their earlier enforced separation from material means of production, workers, since the Industrial Revolution, have been separated from nonmaterial means, the knowledge component of production—the ultimate stage of expropriation—depriving workers of their human essence—their sense of dignity, integrity and autonomy—thus completing their transformation into easily marketable and replaceable commodities (Braverman, 1974; Pope John Paul II, 1981; U.S. Department of HEW Task Force, 1973).

The transformation of most work into routines requiring little or no initiative, creativity, and intellectual effort, and of workers into uncritical performers of routine tasks within authoritarian work settings, has inevitably affected child rearing, socialization, and formal education, the interrelated processes which prepare the young to fit into established patterns of adult life and to take their place in the prevailing organization of work. Since established patterns of life and work in the United States require mainly conforming and apathetic workers, such workers are produced through prevailing modes of life and human relations in homes, schools, churches, and neighborhoods. These destructive, "violent" consequences of current patterns do not result from conscious, intentional practices of parents, teachers, and educational authorities; rather, they result automatically from growing up in homes, schools, and neighborhoods segregated by social, economic and occupational class, and by race, attitudes, expectations and aspirations. Consequently, though not intentionally so designed, child rearing, socialization and formal education in the contemporary United States result in massive underdevelopment of the rich potential of most children and youth (Bowles & Gintis, 1976; Gil, 1979a).

Most individuals in the United States are not expected, nor do they have opportunities, to use their innate capacities in the normal course of employment. Therefore, many individuals either fail to fully develop their capacities or allow developed capacities to atrophy from lack of use. The result is a society in which most people function below their potential. This underdevelopment progressively reduces the capacity of culturally and developmentally damaged generations to nurture those following them.

Moreover, ongoing efforts to enhance efficiency and productivity through further refinements in the subdivision of labor will intensify social and psychological conditions and processes that result inevitably in developmental deficits. This trend will be reversed only when the prevailing capitalist organization of work is transformed into one in which people are expected, and have the opportunity, to integrate their innate intellectual, physical, and emotional capacities in their work and in other domains of everyday life—when they will no longer be factors but rather masters of production and of their own existence (Baran & Sweezy, 1966; Fromm, 1955).

Further features of aggregate production in the United States that should be noted are irrationality and waste. Production tends to be planned, rational, and efficient in terms of profit considerations of individual firms. Yet, aggregate production is unplanned, irrational, inefficient, and wasteful in terms of the real needs of the population, the survival and development of communities and regions, and the conservation of resources and ecology. This internal contradiction of capitalist, "free market" production derives from the fact that individual firms and the economy as a whole are not oriented toward actual needs of people, but toward "effective demand" as reflected in purchasing decisions and toward maximizing profits of competing firms. The needs of people who lack adequate purchasing power are, therefore, neither considered nor met under prevailing patterns of production and distribution. Adam Smith's (1961) "self-regulation" of markets under conditions of "perfect competition" by means of a mythical "invisible hand" clearly does not work in the interest of the entire population, nor does it promote the general welfare as claimed by conservative economists (Hunt & Sherman, 1981).

The absence of planning geared to the needs of all people and to the long-range needs of communities and society results not only in severe underproduction in terms of people's needs, but also in wasteful over-production of unnecessary goods and services that people with surplus purchasing power are induced to buy by means of sophisticated, yet mind-less, advertising. Further aspects of irrationality and waste in capitalist production are frequent, arbitrary changes of models and fashions, and built-in obsolescence in many products, requiring premature repairs and replacements. The massive waste in production is a major, objective source of inflation, intrinsic to capitalist dynamics. Inflation, generated by waste, in turn, stimulates subjective, social and psychological tenden-cies, which reinforce the inflationary process.

Lack of planning geared to the needs of all people and communities, and waste-induced inflationary practices lead, inevitably, to periodic ec-onomic crises to which individual firms and the economic system respond by cutting back production and laying off employees. From the perspec-tive of powerful enterprises and the established economic order, such crises are necessary mechanisms to regulate the economy in the absence of planning. From the perspective of individuals, households, small enter-prises, and communities, these crises are usually severe disasters.

## Distribution of Goods and Services

In the United States, goods and services are available mainly through markets. Consequently, purchasing power, in the form of money or cred-it, is necessary to secure goods and services. The quantity and quality of the goods and services that people can obtain depends mainly, therefore, on their wealth and their incomes from wealth, work, and government grants and subsidies.

The distribution of wealth and income over time in the United States involves major inequalities among individuals, households, age groups, sexes, ethnic groups and social classes. The distribution reveals that pover-ty (defined as income insufficient to secure an acknowledged, minimally adequate standard of living) is built into the fabric of our society, since large segments of the population own little or no income generating wealth, nor are they assured access to gainful employment.

Propertyless people who never secured employment or lost their jobs, be they young, old, or in-between, are usually doomed to poverty. What-ever purchasing power they command derives from government transfer payments or from extralegal practices, i.e., crime. Transfer payments to poor persons tend to be very low. They usually do not even match the U.S. government's poverty index, a measure derived from a short-term, emergency food budget, that corresponds to less than two-thirds of the "low-level budget" for urban households as determined by the U.S. Bureau of Labor Statistics (1984). During 1983 over 35,000,000 individuals, more than 15% of the population, were living in households with incomes at or below the official poverty level, in spite of government assistance. Another 40,000,000 were "near-poor" in accordance with a 1980 report of the National Advisory Council on Economic Opportunity. "Near-poverty" corresponds to 125% of the official poverty index. The incidence of poverty and near-poverty is significantly higher among children, youth and aged persons; among women, especially in single parent families; and among racial minorities and native American tribes.

However, not only individuals who never secured employment, lost their jobs or retired from work, tend to exist in or near poverty. In the United States, many regularly employed workers live in or near poverty since the legal, minimum wage does not assure incomes above the poverty line, and since the prevailing wage structure generates an income distribution that leaves about one-third of the entire population in or near poverty.

## Social, Civil and Political Rights

In theory, everyone in the United States is entitled to equal social, civil and political rights. In reality, however, these rights too, tend to be distributed unequally, as they are subtly associated with material wealth and income, and with race, sex, age, occupation, education and social class. Economically powerful groups tend to acquire disproportionately large shares of social prestige and political influence. Public authorities often treat the well-to-do more politely and more favorably than poor people, especially when the latter are members of racial minorities. Even in courts of law and in the correctional system, wealthy and prestigious individuals and corporations are often able to secure preferential treatment with the help of expensive lawyers.

Theoretically, our society is a political, but not an economic, democracy. Throughout history we have secured important civil and political rights and liberties, though we do not always observe these in practice. Many insightful students have suggested, however, that our political system is, in fact, like all capitalist states, a subtle dictatorship of propertied minorities over majorities of expropriated and constantly exploited working classes (Miliband, 1969). They argue that majorities would never have chosen voluntarily nor would they consent to exist under conditions of oppression, exploitation, deprivation, and poverty, unless powerful, dominant minorities were able to maintain and defend the established, unjust order through ideological hegemony and socialization, and, as a last resort, through overt and covert "legitimate" force and coercion by the military, the police, and various secret services.

The fact that people in the United States periodically elect legislatures and executives does not mean that they can choose freely between the established capitalist system and egalitarian alternative systems which would assure everyone's right to realize intrinsic needs and innate capacities, participate in productive activities, and share, as equally entitled, in the nation's wealth. People decide now only who will govern the established order, not whether to maintain or to change that order. That latter issue is beyond our present political agenda, and groups that intend to place it on the agenda tend to encounter resistance and repression. Moreover, election campaigns are costly and candidates without personal wealth who dare to challenge the interests of propertied classes are unlikely to secure the necessary financial support to campaign for political office. Also, media of communication tend to be controlled by wealthy advertisers. Political groups opposed to capitalism face, therefore, severe obstacles to disseminate their ideas through the media.

The Constitution of the United States and our legal system are important tools towards preserving and reproducing the established, inegalitarian-violent social order and its skewed distribution of power and wealth. Property rights are guaranteed by the Constitution and protected by law, while no comparable guarantees exist for the fulfillment of people's material, relational, developmental, security, and self-actualization needs, except for the vaguely phrased preamble. Human rights to development and individuality are nowhere assured through law and the Constitution and certainly cannot be claimed in practice. Under prevailing conditions, for large segments of the population, these rights are nothing but abstractions—a fiction and a myth.

The admirable philosophy of equality and liberty of the Declaration of Independence did not shape the U.S. Constitution. Rather, our Constitution accepts and protects inequalities of wealth and of wealth-related rights—major sources of structural violence in our society. Symbolic of this shift in philosophy from the Declaration of Independence to the Constitution is article I, section II, 3 of the Constitution wherein slavery is acknowledged implicitly, and the value of "other persons" is set as three-fifths of "free persons." Though these dehumanizing and blatantly violent provisions are no longer in force, and though a Bill of Rights and other important amendments were added, the U.S. Constitution continues to uphold inequalities of wealth and associated social and political inequalities, and does not guarantee the fulfillment of people's developmental needs. Hence the Constitution and the legal system derived from it maintain structural violence, whether or not the framers intended these results.

## Ideology

Central to any ideology are positions on the following related value continua:

| | |
|---|---|
| equality ———————————————————— | inequality |
| affirmation of community and individuality ———— | selfishness |
| cooperation ————————————————— | competition |
| liberty ————————————————————— | domination |

Our paramount ideology seems oriented toward the right poles of these value continua although we tend to deny this. We proclaim that "all men are born equal"; but we seem to live by the premise that individuals, groups, classes, and peoples are intrinsically unequal in worth and are consequently entitled to unequal shares of resources, goods and services, and to unequal social, civil, and political rights. We affirm the sanctity of all life, pay lip service to "community spirit," and condemn selfishness in our religious and philosophical traditions; but we do not seem to value the lives and individuality of others, we easily disregard community concerns and interests and seem to accept selfishness as a commonsense, guiding principle for everyday life and human relations. We teach children at home and in school to share and cooperate; but nearly all domains of adult existence are permeated by acquisitive and competitive dynamics. We are enthusiastic advocates of liberty and "human rights" as abstract principles; but we do not hesitate to dominate and exploit other individuals, classes, races, and peoples and to use them as means to our ends.

## Realization of Fundamental Human Needs

Having reviewed the normal workings of key processes and major ideological tendencies of our social order, we can now examine whether fundamental human needs can be realized and innate human capacities can unfold freely within the prevailing ways of life in the United States. Such an examination serves as an "acid test" of structural violence in any society. As noted above, we are concerned with needs for basic, material goods and services; meaningful human relations conducive to the emergence of a positive sense of identity; meaningful and creative participation in socially valued productive processes; a sense of security; and self-actualization.

1) Analysis of our institutional and ideological context revealed that large segments of the population now lack access to an adequate level of basic goods and services since they do not own and control sufficient means of production or possess unconditional rights to gainful employment and adequate income. Unemployment and poverty and their debilitating, dehumanizing, and alienating consequences obstruct the satisfaction of the material needs and thus the healthy development of about one-third of our people.

2) Next, we found massive obstacles to meaningful, mutually caring human relations conducive to the development of a positive sense of identity in places of work, schools, and other public settings as well as people's homes. This is due largely to pervasive, structurally induced competition for employment and promotions, and for preferred positions, conditions, and opportunities in spheres of existence shaped by bureaucratic-hierarchical dynamics. Meaningful human relations are usually not possible among individuals who are unequal in prestige, status, and power, and who evaluate, use, and control one another as means in the pursuit of selfish ends. Also, meaningful relations are unlikely to develop when households tend to function as separate economic units, each trying to survive as best as possible in a noncooperative way of life. And finally, meaningful relations are undermined in the private domain when people's developmental energy is blocked in the public domain; people react to the frustrations and their own powerlessness in everyday life with interpersonal violence in intimate relations.

3) Meaningful and creative participation in socially valued productive processes is beyond the expectations of most people, when: (a) any kind of employment is not assured; (b) most available work is designed as fragmented meaningless routines, to be performed in alienating, oppressive and exploiting conditions; and (c) child care, socialization, and formal schooling result inevitably in massive underdevelopment of innate human capacities.

4) A sense of security tends to emerge when people's needs for goods and services, meaningful human relations, and meaningful participation in society's productive endeavors can be realized regularly. Since these needs were shown to be unrealizable for many people in the context of prevailing societal dynamics and values, few individuals can be expected

to develop a genuine sense of security; many suffer a nagging sense of insecurity.

5) Self-actualization is usually not pursued by people whose material, relational, developmental, and security needs are unrealizable (Maslow, 1970). Thus, with widespread frustration in meeting material, relational, developmental, and security needs, we are forced to conclude that few individuals may be expected to realize their innate need for self-actualization.

To summarize, the foregoing analysis strongly suggests that life in the United States involves now widespread frustration of people's fundamental needs. When people live under such conditions, their innate capacities usually do not unfold freely and fully and their development is inevitably stunted. Accordingly, our society appears to be a development-inhibiting or development-violating social environment, permeated with social-structural violence, reflective of and geared to the perpetuation of multiple, socially structured inequalities of statuses and rights. These circumstances are often acknowledged with respect to people living in poverty or near poverty. Paradoxically, however, this is equally true, though in different ways, for people living in middle income and affluent homes. For material adequacy and affluence do not by themselves lead directly to the realization of relational, developmental, security and self-actualization needs, as they cannot insulate people from the dehumanizing effects of inegalitarian, selfish, competitive, and exploitative-antagonistic patterns of everyday life.

## OVERCOMING VIOLENCE

Violence in our homes and on every level of human relations can be prevented. However, prevention cannot be accomplished merely by treating or punishing individuals who are trapped in cycles of violence. Rather, social-structural violence, the roots of personal and domestic violence, would have to be eliminated by thoroughly transforming social, economic, political, and cultural institutions in accordance with egalitarian, cooperative, and genuinely democratic values and principles. While such transformations would not eliminate all personal violence immediately, they are essential, though not sufficient conditions, toward its eventual prevention, as they seem compatible with the requirements of individual growth and development. Prevention of violence in our homes and lives is, therefore, primarily a political, rather than a professional and technical issue.

Regrettably, our society does not seem ready at present for major institutional and ideological changes without which structural and interpersonal violence cannot be overcome. It is nevertheless necessary to identify and work toward these changes and to build political movements committed to them.

Social transformations toward a nonviolent, egalitarian, democratic, and humanistic order are not a brief, cataclysmic event, but an extended process. Prevention of domestic violence, which depends on such fundamental social transformations, is, therefore, also an extended process. It involves many steps, each of which needs to challenge consistently the destructive elements of the prevailing violent social order: its values and ideology; its legal definitions of the rights of people and especially of children and women; and its inegalitarian institutional arrangements such as poverty and the prevailing organization of work and production which, as described, result inevitably in stunted human development, insecurity, frustration, and stress. Measures that treat victims of domestic violence and reduce the suffering of those involved but do not challenge its structural sources are not steps in a preventive strategy. Such measures are certainly necessary when violence and suffering are widespread. However, one ought to avoid the illusion that ameliorative measures in themselves can eliminate the sources of violence from the fabric of society.

## Prevention and Amelioration

Some clarification seems necessary regarding the concepts of prevention and amelioration before suggesting a set of social policies designed to combine these dimensions in dealing with domestic and social-structural violence. Prevention involves: identification and eradication of the sources of unwanted phenomena, such as disease-causing organisms in the environment; provision of clean water, air and healthy housing; and inoculation of people against disease.

Public health and social service professionals differentiate, however, between several levels of prevention. *Primary prevention* refers to the model of identification and eradication of causes or sources of phenomena as described above while *secondary prevention* refers to identification of early signs and stages of an wanted phenomenon and swift intervention, so as to keep it from reaching severe dimensions or to reduce the likelihood of recidivism. Cancer-screening programs illustrate this level of prevention. The goal in secondary prevention is to prevent or reduce serious consequences after the onset of an undesired process. *Tertiary prevention* refers to intervention after an undesired event has occurred in order to reduce or "ameliorate" the symptoms and consequences. Tertiary prevention is actually the same as amelioration. In practice, the three levels merge into one another and are not always readily differentiated. Thus, some arbitrariness is involved in these definitions.

Based on these notions, prevention and amelioration may be best thought of as polar positions on a continuum and particular intervention strategies may be thought of as points on this continuum. Source-oriented prevention and symptom-oriented treatment or amelioration are, therefore, not mutually exclusive approaches. Rather, they may be combined and integrated, as long as their functional distinction is kept in mind.

Under conditions of acute suffering, immediate amelioration and treatment are essential for humanitarian reasons. However, when a community or society invests all available resources and energy in treatment and amelioration of acute situations to the exclusion of primary and secondary prevention, or worse, when treatment and amelioration are misrepresented as primary preventive measures, then undesirable phenomena tend to become permanent features. In the opinion of many observers, the public response to domestic violence in the United States has been relatively ineffective because it involved mainly tertiary prevention or amelioration, some efforts at secondary prevention, but no primary prevention (Gil, 1979b).

Social problems such as domestic violence cannot be prevented through professional and administrative processes independent of political measures. Primary prevention of such problems is essentially a political issue, since it requires significant changes of the social, economic, and political context within which these problems are rooted. Accordingly, the measures suggested below concern political, social, and economic dimensions. They are designed to push for maximum feasible structural changes within the prevailing societal context, as well as for amelioration for victims of violence.

## Toward a Nonviolent Mode of Work

The organization and design of work and ideas concerning work are key aspects of social orders at any time and place. Depending on its goals, organization and design, work may or may not bridge gaps between fundamental human needs and possibilities of meeting these needs. Consequently, the organization and design of work are key factors concerning the scope of human development and the level of social-structural violence in society. Our analysis has revealed the essentially violent dynamics of the prevailing work system in the United States. Primary prevention of violence in our society and homes, therefore, requires transformation of the existing mode of work into a nonviolent one.

Based on the concept of violence developed in this chapter, a nonviolent mode of work would be one compatible with the development of everyone's innate capacities. Thus, it would be geared toward fulfilling everyone's biological, psychological and social needs. Furthermore, such a mode of work would be cooperative rather than competitive, and no one would be dominated and exploited—materially, psychologically, or socially. Everyone would share as an equal in determining, designing and implementing the goals and processes of work and in using the products. Finally, a nonviolent mode of work would be in harmony with nature; it would involve nondestructive and nonwasteful relations to natural resources, and a commitment to high-quality, durable products. In short, a nonviolent mode of work would be democratic, nonhierarchical, communal, and decentralized; egalitarian, humanistic, universalistic, and ecological; and rationally planned in the interest of everyone living now and in the future, here and elsewhere on the globe.

No doubt, we have a long way to go toward a genuinely nonviolent mode of work. Yet the concept can serve as a frame of reference as we develop policies to transform prevailing, violent ways of life and work into nonviolent alternatives. Reconceptualizing and redefining work would be a necessary, initial step. If the purpose of nonviolent work is the maintenance of life and the enrichment of its quality, then work ought to be defined as a combination of activities geared to meet the biological, social and emotional needs of people. Implicit in such a concept of work are criteria for a revised concept of the GNP: Activities necessary for and conducive to human development would be included and socially and materially recognized and rewarded; activities that obstruct or are harmful to development would be excluded, neither recognized nor rewarded, and eventually phased out.

As for transforming the prevailing organization of work, the primary goal should be elimination of the wasteful and irrational practice of excluding some people from participating in work through unemployment and underemployment, at the discretion and in the interest of owners and managers of means of production. This goal could be attained across the United States by way of a constitutional amendment such as the one introduced in the Congress in 1983 by Representative Owens of New York, which states: "The right to employment opportunity shall be guaranteed to each person in the United States. Congress shall have power to enforce this article by appropriate legislation" (U.S. House of Representatives, 1983). To implement such a guarantee, Congress could change periodically the legal length of the workday or workweek, so as to match the number of available workers with changes in the scope of production. A mandated reduction of the average work day by one hour would result in the absorption of all now officially unemployed workers, assuming the scope of current production were not changed (Gil, 1983). Congress, of course, also could establish appropriate and meaningful work programs in the public sector of the economy to fill major gaps in needs of the population in domains such as housing, health, education, transportation and conservation. States, too, could take initiative and amend their constitutions along similar lines.

Establishing an unconditional right to work for all is also an essential, though not sufficient, measure toward overcoming discrimination by race, sex, age, and handicap. It is also a precondition toward phasing out useless and harmful practices such as featherbedding, built-in obsolescence and military production, which workers understandably insist on doing in the absence of alternative work. In short, guaranteeing work to everyone who wants it is necessary if we aim to develop a rational, efficient, and effective economic system fostering human development and well-being, at home and abroad.

The above redefinition of work and a work guarantee would also open the way to considering and treating parental child-care, housework and similar tasks as integral components of our work system. This would entitle those opting to undertake this important work to adequate wages, paid out of federal revenues. Obviously, the federal government would have to raise the necessary transfer funds through appropriate tax reforms (Gil, 1973).

The foregoing policies can be enacted democratically even before a comprehensive transformation of capitalism. When implemented, these policies would not result in a decline of real income for working people as is sometimes assumed. Aggregate income is always a function of the scope, efficiency, productivity, and quality of production. The proposed measures would certainly not reduce, and are likely to enhance that scope, efficiency, productivity, and quality, and even may result in an increase in aggregate income. The distribution of that income will depend on the relative power of different groups, classes, and occupations, as it does now. However, the proposed measures would significantly increase the relative power of working people, since nothing weakens workers more than actual or threatened unemployment. Accordingly, once work is redefined and guaranteed to all, the income share of workers is likely to go up.

Furthermore, redefining work to include parental child care and similar tasks would also increase the relative power and prestige of people performing these tasks, and would thus assure them an adequate share of income. One additional benefit of this would be the phasing out of the controversial Aid to Families with Dependent Children (AFDC) Program. Altogether, the proposed policies when complemented by an adequate, guaranteed income for the elderly and other people who are unable to work for valid reasons, would, when fully implemented, eliminate poverty and its multiple correlates once and for all—no small feat, indeed, considering the limited success on this score of the New Deal, the War on Poverty, Model Cities, and several other well-intended, yet ineffective efforts.

The redefinition of work suggested above and constitutional guarantees of a right-to-work seem compatible with the Protestant work ethic (which supposedly is a basic value of our culture) and with progressive Catholic thought as reflected in recent statements by Pope John Paul II (1981). Thus, it should be possible to develop political support for such policies and to enact them eventually, in spite of intense opposition that is likely to come from propertied and managerial classes and their allies.

The shift in power from propertied and managerial minorities to working majorities and related shifts in social, psychological, and economic rewards (which should result from the proposed redefinition and reorganization of work) would gradually open up further opportunities for expanding democratic control and management by workers, consumers, and communities over society's productive resources and capacities. Of course, such social transformations will not happen automatically. They will require the emergence of broad-based liberation movements among working people which transcend conventional interest-group politics and promote instead a unifying, humanistic consciousness and corresponding political practice. The gradual unfolding of a genuine, democratic renaissance should facilitate further constructive steps to reorganize and redesign work processes and products toward humanistic ends, thus enhancing their quality and harmonizing work with ecological requirements and with developmental needs of people throughout the world. As we move to reduce the violent structures of the prevailing organization and relations of work that perpetuate a polarity of privilege and deprivation on local and global levels, and that require for their maintenance constant threats or actual use of coercive force, and in turn lead to violent feelings and reactions by oppressed and exploited individuals and peoples, we would set in motion countercycles reversing the dynamics of violence everywhere.

## Redefining Rights of Women and Children

A less comprehensive change than transforming work into a nonviolent process is the redefinition of the rights of children and women. This change is, however, an important component of cultural transformation toward nonviolent ways of life.

The rights of children and women should be redefined through appropriate legislation. Children ought to be viewed and treated as persons entitled to the full protection of the Constitution, including the integrity and inviolability of their bodies and minds. All forms of corporal punishment and physical coercion of children in the public domain ought to be outlawed as was recently done in Sweden, and cultural sanctions ought to be developed against such punishments and coercion in the private domain as well. This would reverse the cruel tradition reflective of a slave mentality: "spare the rod and spoil the child."

Concerning women's rights, the Equal Rights Amendment to the U.S. Constitution should be passed, and provisions should be enacted for open-minded, sensitive sex education, access to contraception, and elimination of legal and economic obstacles to personal choices concerning motherhood. Such laws would enhance the position of women in both the public and private domains and would reduce the alarming rise, especially among teenagers, in unintended pregnancies and unwanted children—prime targets of domestic violence.

## Rights to Health and Education

Eliminating obstacles to human development also requires prevention and treatment of physical and emotional ill health, which are often associated with poverty and domestic violence. In any case, access to adequate health maintenance and care is a necessary aspect of the elimination of social structural violence. An appropriate mechanism for promoting health and assuring care in case of ill health, accidents, and injury would be a universal, comprehensive health maintenance system focused both on prevention and cure, and maintained through general revenues. Such a system should also provide, on a voluntary basis, family planning services including contraception and abortions. Ameliorative care for victims of domestic violence would also be the responsibility of a comprehensive health care system.

A further essential component of a nonviolent, development-oriented way of life is a comprehensive system of education from nursery school through graduate school geared sensitively to the individual capacities of each individual. As part of such a system, parents should also have access to day care on a voluntary basis. This comprehensive education system also should be financed from general revenues to assure equal access for all.

## Tax Reform

To implement the set of policies sketched here, we would have to reform the existing tax system. What is needed is a simple, fair, loophole-free progressive tax on income, irrespective of source, above the level of the "low standard of living" as measured by the Bureau of Labor Statistics (1984). Income below that level ought to be defined as "basic" and should, therefore, be tax-free. There should also be taxes on income-producing capital once income from its use exceeds the basic income level, and there should be sales taxes on luxury goods but not on nonluxury goods. Income tax rates would have to be adjusted periodically upward or downward to assure a relatively balanced budget and avoid government borrowing and wasteful debt services.

## Epilogue

The work, income, rights, health, and education policies suggested here as initial steps to overcome social-structural violence in the fabric of our culture and to eliminate the roots of domestic violence are feasible within the Constitution of the United States. They do not require abolition of currently guaranteed rights, including rights to property. What is required are several amendments to the Constitution—a universal right to work, equal rights for women, and a right to inviolability of a child's body—and several pieces of legislation on work sharing, public works, universal health maintenance, comprehensive education, and tax reform. While presently, these proposals are likely to be resisted by privileged groups, they should nevertheless be actively pursued in the political arena by progressive forces committed to human rights and to comprehensive, rather than formal, democracy.

It should be stressed that the proposed policies do not involve "real" economic costs in terms of national wealth, but a significant redistribution of claims to the goods and services produced in our economy. Thus, the political argument which will certainly be raised—that we cannot afford these policies since they are too costly—is simply not valid. Not only do these policies cost nothing in aggregate economic terms, but they are also likely to generate, over time, considerable benefits in economic, social, and psychological terms. Their only costs are political, since the tax reforms implicit in them involve significant challenges to vested interests of privileged classes.

Social-structural violence as interpreted here, does not stop at international borders. The dynamics of inequality, domination, and exploitation are global in scope, and transformation toward nonviolent human relations at home will have to be matched by corresponding measures in our foreign policies and our global economic and social relations. All these relations will eventually have to be shaped by egalitarian, humanistic and democratic values if we wish to liberate ourselves from dynamics of violence on every level and in every sphere of our lives.

The policies and concepts suggested here are not final solutions to problems of domestic, societal, and global violence. They are, however, feasible and meaningful next steps of an extended process of an ideological and political struggle toward possible human liberation and fulfillment in egalitarian, nonviolent, cooperative communities and societies.

## REFERENCES

Baran, P. A., & Sweezy, P. (1966). *Monopoly capital.* New York: Monthly Review Press.

Benedict, R. (1970). Synergy: Patterns of the good culture. *American Anthropologist, 72*(2), 320–333.

Bowles, S., & Gintis, H. (1976). *Schooling in capitalist America.* New York: Basic Books.

Braverman, H. (1974). *Labor and monopoly capital.* New York: Monthly Review Press.

Dewey, J. (1935). *Liberalism and social action.* New York: Putnam.

Fromm, E. (1941). *Escape from freedom.* New York: Rinehart.

Fromm, E. (1955). *The sane society.* Greenwich, CT: Fawcett.

Gil, D. G. (1970). *Violence against children.* Cambridge, MA: Harvard University Press.

Gil, D. G. (1973). *Unravelling social policy* (3rd ed.). Cambridge, MA: Schenkman.

Gil, D. G. (1979a). The hidden success of schooling in the United States. *The Humanist, 39*(6), 32–37.

Gil, D. G. (Ed.). (1979b). *Child abuse and violence.* New York: AMS Press.

Gil, D. G. (1983). Rethinking strategies against unemployment. *Planners Network, #40, 3.* (also in *Socialist Forum, #5,* 1984)

Hunt, E. K., & Sherman, H. J. (1981). *Economics.* New York: Harper & Row.

Kropotkin, P. (1956). *Mutual aid.* (1902). Boston: Porter Sargent.

Maslow, A. H. (1970). *Motivation and personality.* New York: Harper & Row.

Miliband, R. (1969). *The state in capitalist society.* New York: Basic Books.

Pope John Paul II (1981). *On human work—Laborem exercens.* Boston: Daughters of St. Paul.

Smith, A. (1961). *The wealth of nations.* Indianapolis: Bobbs-Merrill.

Turnbull, C. M. (1972). *The mountain people.* New York: Simon & Schuster.

U.S. Bureau of Labor Statistics (1984). *Statistical abstract of the United States* (104th ed.). Washington, DC: U.S. Government Printing Office.

U.S. Congress (1976). Study for Joint Economic Committee, *Estimating the social costs of national economic policy.* Washington, DC: U.S. Government Printing Office.

U.S. Department of Health, Education & Welfare Task Force (1973). *Work in America.* Cambridge, MA: MIT Press.

U.S. House of Representatives (1983). Joint resolution, 202, March 16.

# Part III

# CLINICAL INTERVENTION PROGRAMS

# 7

# *Intervention Programs for Individual Victims and Their Families*

## Carol Nadelson and Maria Sauzier

### SPOUSE ABUSE

Violence has been estimated to occur in 50% of American families (Gelles, 1974; Straus, 1977–78). While generally, concerns about family violence focus on child abuse, more recently spouse abuse has been identified as a substantial problem. Spouse abuse is not limited to a particular social class or ethnic group. Although the highest reported incidence is among the poor, this is probably because they are more likely to come to the attention of public agencies and legal authorities. A study of 600 couples who were in the process of divorce bears this out: 40% of lower-class women and 23% of middle-class women reported physical abuse by spouses (Levinger, 1966). Stark, Flitcraft, and Frazier (1979) emphasized that physicians vastly underestimated the amount of battering in the patient population, thus, while Rounsaville and Weissman (1977–78) reported that 3.8% of the women presenting to an emergency trauma service and 3.4% of the women presenting to an emergency psychiatric service had been battered by men with whom they were intimate, Stark et al. put the figure from the same services reported by Rounsaville and Weissman at 25%. Other authors (Hilberman & Munson, 1977–78; Rosenfeld, 1979) confirm the tendency toward underreporting.

Of all the murders in this country, 20% to 50% occur within the family. One study reported that 40% of the homicides in a major U.S. city were between spouses (Kansas City Police Department, 1973), and the FBI estimates that one out of every four women who is murdered is killed by her husband or boyfriend (FBI, 1982).

153

Wife beating is often accompanied by physical and/or sexual abuse of the children (Gayford, 1975; Hilberman & Munson, 1977–78; Scott, 1974), and children who are abused often grow up to abuse their offspring. In addition, children who see violent interactions often have physically abusive relationships in adulthood.

Clinicians have been impressed with the frequency with which child abuse and spouse abuse occur together. Gayford (1975) reported that 37% of the women and 54% of the men who had been abused beat their children; Hilberman and Munson (1977–78) identified physical and/or sexual abuse of children in a third of the families they studied. Emotional neglect, abuse, alcoholism and frequent separations were the norms, and children in violent homes were witnesses and targets of abuse (Gayford, 1975; Gelles, 1974; Hilberman & Munson, 1977–78; Scott, 1974; Walker, 1979).

Thus, lifelong violence begins with early and repeated patterns in childhood for both men and women who are later involved in abuse (Gayford, 1975; Gelles, 1974; Hilberman & Munson, 1977–78; Pizzey, 1974; Rounsaville, 1978; Scott, 1974; Walker, 1979). Suicides and homicides among family members and neighborhood acquaintances occur frequently. Studies indicate that most of the women left home at an early age to escape from violent and seductive fathers. They tended to marry while teenagers and many were pregnant at the time of marriage or had had children before marriage. They viewed pregnancy as the only way they would be allowed to leave the family. Further, most women reported an increase in the pattern of violence during pregnancy (Hilberman & Munson, 1977–78), often leading to abortions and premature births (Gayford, 1975; Gelles, 1974; Hilberman & Munson, 1977–78; Walker, 1979).

In these families, violence often erupted when a husband felt that his needs were not gratified or when he was drunk. Frequently, this occurred after he had been with another woman. The assaults usually happened at night and on weekends, so children were witnesses and participants when they attempted to defend or protect the mother. An association between alcohol use and marital violence has been noted (Gayford, 1975; Gelles, 1974; Hilberman & Munson, 1977–78). Drinking accompanied by violence occurred in 22 to 100% of those reported and many spouse abusers who were alcoholics were also abusers when they were sober.

In looking at the predictors of future violence, Walker (1984) notes,

> The best prediction of future violence was a history of past violent behavior. This included witnessing, receiving and committing violent acts in their childhood home; violent acts toward pets, inanimate objects or other people; previous criminal records; longer time in the military; and previous expression of violent behavior toward women. If these items are added to a history of temper tantrums,

> insecurity, need to keep the environment stable, easily thr[e]
> by minor upsets, jealousy, possessiveness, and the abilit[y]
> charming, manipulative, and seductive to get what he wants, and
> hostile, nasty, and mean when he doesn't succeed—then the risk for
> battering becomes very high. If alcohol abuse problems are includ-
> ed, the pattern becomes classic. (pp. 10–11)

Walker (1984) indicates that a certain combination of factors seem to suggest higher risk potential. One, which is also mentioned by Straus, Gelles, & Steinmetz (1981), is the difference on sociodemographic variables between the batterers and the battered women. Batterers tend to be less educated than their wives and from lower socioeconomic classes as well as different ethnic, religious or racial groups. Men who are more traditional than women in their attitudes toward women's roles are potentially at higher risk; these men measure a woman's feelings for them by how well she meets the sex-role expectations they have defined.

These men are also in need of a great amount of nurturance and are very possessive of women's time (Hilberman & Munson, 1977–78; Martin, 1976). Extreme jealousy was reported in a large percentage of these marriages (Gayford, 1975; Gelles, 1974; Hilberman & Munson, 1977–78; Scott, 1974). Husbands made active efforts to keep their wives isolated. If the women left the house for any reason, they were often accused of infidelity and were assaulted. Friendships with women were discouraged and husbands often embarrassed their wives in the presence of their friends by asserting that they were lesbians, prostitutes or otherwise unacceptable.

The women often felt sorry for their husbands because of their histories of deprivation and abuse. Many women left their marriages for brief periods but returned because of economic and emotional dependence on husbands, and threats of further violence from which they had no protection (Hilberman & Munson, 1977–78; Scott, 1974). Some women were assaulted daily, while others were beaten intermittently and lived in constant anticipatory terror (Dewsbury, 1975; Fonseka, 1974; Gayford, 1975; Gelles, 1974; Hilberman & Munson, 1977–78; Martin, 1976; Scott, 1974; Walker, 1979). Guns were available in most of these homes and were constant threats (Hilberman & Munson, 1977–78).

Some women sought recourse through the criminal justice system, but these attempts were often frustrated by the unresponsiveness of officials, as well as by threats of retaliation by the husband (Chapman & Gates, 1978; Eisenberg & Micklow, 1976; Field & Field, 1973; Gates, 1977; Hilberman & Munson, 1977–78; Walker, 1979). While most women were passive and did not defend themselves, the few women who themselves resorted to violence did so in desperation when other options had failed.

They used violence in response to direct threats to their lives and their be-havior usually surprised them. They were often unaware of the extent of their rage and their capacity for violence (Hilberman & Munson, 1977–78).

## IMPACT OF ABUSE

Hilberman and Munson (1977–78) have described a response pattern among the battered women which is similar to that described for the rape-trauma syndrome. Terror was constant but since chronicity and unpre-dictability were also characteristic, severe agitation and anxiety with fears of imminent doom were also present (Burgess & Holmstrom, 1974a). These women were unable to relax or sleep, and at night they experienced violent nightmares. During the daytime they were passive and lacked energy. They experienced a pervasive sense of hopelessness, helplessness and despair. They often saw themselves as deserving abuse and as power-less to change their lives.

Frequently, there were somatic symptoms reported such as headaches, asthma, gastrointestinal symptoms, and chronic pain. More than half of these women had prior psychiatric histories. Depression was the most fre-quent diagnosis. They had often sought medical help and many had been treated for drug overdoses and suicide attempts. Although they had multi-ple medical contacts over many years, they did not tell their physicians of the abuse, nor were they asked (Dewsbury, 1975; Hilberman & Mun-son, 1977–78).

A high incidence of somatic, psychological, and behavioral dysfunc-tions have also been described in their children. These included head-aches, abdominal complaints, asthma, and peptic ulcer. Depression, suici-dal behavior, and psychosis were also reported (Gayford, 1975; Hilberman & Munson, 1977–78). For the preschool and young school children, somatic complaints, stuttering, school phobias, enuresis, and insomnia were frequent. Insomnia was often accompanied by intense fear, scream-ing and resistance to going to bed at night. Most children had impaired concentration and difficulty with school-work. Among older children, ag-gressive disruptive behavior, stealing, temper tantrums, truancy, and fight-ing with siblings and schoolmates were characteristic of boys, whereas girls were more likely to experience somatic symptoms.

## COUNSELING IMPLICATIONS

The response to family violence is often blame and disbelief. This is supported by the tendency of victims to deny the problem and by their difficulty in acknowledging anger about it. This occurs, in part, because they fear losing control especially because of their close relationship with the abuser. As a result, aggression may be directed against themselves or those who try to help.

Several studies provide evidence of the profoundly self-destructive behaviors that emerge after victimization. In comparing 59 abused and neglected children with 29 neglected children and 30 children who were neither abused nor neglected, Green (1978) found self-destructive behaviors exhibited by 40.6% of the abused, 17.2% of the neglected, and 6.7% of the controls. He concluded that "the abused child's sense of worthlessness, badness and self-hatred as a consequence of parental assault, rejection and scapegoating form the nucleus for self-destructive behavior" (p. 581).

Fear, especially in the presence of continuing threats, appears to be a major deterrent to activity (Martin, 1976; Symonds, 1978). Another reason for the reluctance to leave may be "learned helplessness," the inability to effect change, which has been described by many authors as a particular problem for women (Ball & Wyman, 1977–78; Seligman, 1975; Waites, 1977–78; Walker, 1977–78, 1984). Certainly, the reaction of hostages, the "Stockholm syndrome," where positive feelings, perhaps based on terror, dependence, and gratitude, is seen in captives and hostages. Further, some women experience what has been called "learned hopefulness," which leads them to think, "I hope he will change and get better," or "I hope I can change him." This may be a possible explanation for the behavior of battered women (Ochberg, 1980). These issues must be understood by those working with family violence.

Counselors working with these women often become frustrated and angry at their passivity, failure to follow through on suggestions and the frequency with which they return to the abusive situation (FBI, 1972, 1974; Hilberman & Munson, 1977–78; Walker, 1977–78, 1979). Attempts to rescue victims and overidentification with the helplessness and dependency may support and reinforce abusive behavior and prevent these women from acting on their own behalf (Ball & Wyman, 1977–78; Ridington, 1977–78).

⟨Women are often reluctant to reveal the extent of their problem because of their mistrust and of low self-esteem. It is difficult for them to establish trusting relationships, even with those who promise help, since they expect deception and they have no basis for trust. Further, they are often unaware of the rage they harbor because of long-standing suppression of these feelings and, as indicated above, fear of loss of control may become a predominant theme and increase the difficulty of achieving autonomy.⟩

While involvement of the abuser in counseling may be an important therapeutic goal, it may also be counterproductive in some cases, until individual psychotherapy has enabled the abused to establish some control and autonomy (Straus, 1974; Pizzey, 1975). In addition, interventions must be directed at the reality of the victim's life circumstances to provide necessary medical care, legal counseling and social supports. Services must be coordinated and the victim supported and educated.

Counseling usually involves a short-term issue-oriented crisis approach, with the goal of restoring the victim to her previous level of functioning as quickly as possible (Burgess & Holstrom, 1974b). Attention must also be paid to the possibility of long-term symptoms such as those seen in post-traumatic stress disorders. Symptoms such as those described above may be delayed in onset for months to years after the abusive situation has changed. At times, events later in life will trigger earlier traumatic experiences and foster symptom development. Walker (1984) has emphasized that these women are more successful at reversing helplessness when they leave the relationship than when they remain. Further, a Washington, DC Police Foundation study (1983) revealed that the most effective deterrent to repeated incidents of violence of men against wives or girlfriends is arrest.

## A MODEL PROGRAM FOR SEXUALLY ABUSED
## CHILDREN AND THEIR FAMILIES

The prevalence of sexual abuse of children in our culture is now well documented. As early as 1953, Kinsey (1953) gathered data about all aspects of human sexuality and revealed that 23% of women had had abusive sexual experiences in their childhoods. The prevalence of father-daughter incest, which represents only one kind of sexual abuse, is estimated to be 1%, on a par with schizophrenia and diabetes (Herman & Hirschman, 1981a).

In Massachusetts, there has been a major and steady increase of incidents reported to the Department of Social Services each year: 1,400 cases in 1981, 2,142 in 1982, 2,938 in 1983, and 5,325 in 1984 (Department of Social Services, 1981–1984). This increase is seen by most experts as representing a greater likelihood of revelation and report, rather than an increase in actual occurrence.

There are several prerequisites to reporting sexual abuse: an awareness of sexual abuse as a problem, knowledge about available resources, and trust that reporting will be beneficial. Public education has affected awareness and knowledge, but the benefits of revelation and reporting are often questioned by media accounts of inappropriate interventions. Among clinicians there is still no consensus about the effectiveness of reporting sexual abuse of a child. The absence of an established and tested intervention protocol, the paucity of clinicians trained in this field and the uneven quality of child welfare services offered by different states all combine to lower the incidence of reported sexual abuse.

At this time, it must be acknowledged that all varieties of interventions offered to sexually abused children and their families are experimental in the sense that none have been validated by long-term follow-up research. Eighteen-month follow-up data available from one major study reported here (Gomes-Schwartz, Horowitz, & Sauzier, 1984) have enabled us to develop the model intervention program described in this chapter.

## Background Data

Information about sexual abuse comes from case histories (Gutheil & Avery, 1977; Katan, 1973), small-scale psychological studies (Herman & Hirschman, 1981b; Tsai, Feldman-Summers, & Edgar, 1979), or large-scale sociological studies (Finkelhor, 1979; Kinsey, 1953).

One broad psychological research project has recently been conducted at New England Medical Center, using 181 cases of sexual abuse (156 confirmed, 25 unconfirmed) (Gomes-Schwartz et al., 1984). Concomitant with data collection was the provision of therapy for the child and his or her family, including the offender.

The children seen were between six months and 18 years old. Seventy-two percent were girls, 28% were boys; 29% were under six years of age, 37% were latency age (7 to 12), and 35% were adolescents (13 to 18) at the time of revelation of the abuse. The sexual abuse reported ranged from witnessing an exhibitionist to experiencing sexual intercourse, with some genital contact occurring in 88% of the cases. Ninety-four percent of the offenders were male, ranging from teenage babysitters to grandfathers. Their average age was 29. Only 3% of offenders were total strangers. Incest in the biological sense occurred in 41% of the cases seen. Incest, in the broader current definition, which includes parental figures such as live-in boyfriends, occurred in 62% of the cases. Only 21% of the abuse occurred as one single incident, either rape or incest. In most cases, incidents occurred over a period of time, some spanning more than five years, with a frequency varying between several times for the whole span of years to more than once a week. Most abuse incidents occurred in places familiar to the child, like his or her home or the perpetrator's home. The families studied were representative of the greater Boston population in terms of race, religion, and socioeconomic status. The only remarkable demographic difference found was a preponderance of single-parent households.

Emotional stress and psychopathology in the children seen was significantly greater than that found in a matched normal population, but less than that found in a matched psychiatric clinic population. Specific symptoms seen varied according to age. Preschool-age children showed age-inappropriate sexual activity and immaturity in their intellectual and prosocial development (e.g., acquiring socially valued behaviors, such as discerning between right and wrong). They also showed reactive symptoms such as anxiety, fears, and depression. School-age children also showed age-inappropriate sexual behavior, but less intellectual and social immaturity, and no prosocial deficit. Their presentation was marked by increased aggression, antisocial activity and fears. As a group, the school-age children showed more emotional disturbance than preschool-age children. Adolescents showed fears of being harmed, anxiety, depression, dependent-inhibited behavior and hostility. Teenagers who had already run away from home were hospitalized or in youth detention centers, and were not brought to this outpatient clinic. The study thus lacks information about the group of adolescents showing the most serious psychopathology related to sexual abuse experiences.

Research data relevant to the design of a treatment program include correlations between distress levels and various factors related to the abuse. Emotional distress and behavioral problems were related to the degree of violence associated with the abuse more than to any other characteristic of the sexual abuse (e.g., type of sexual acts performed, duration, etc.). This is consistent with the findings in the rape literature (Burgess & Holmstrom, 1974a, 1974b); the sexual assault is primarily an expression of aggression and a quest for power and only secondarily a sexual act.

Incest in the broader sense, perpetrated by nonbiological father figures (e.g., stepfathers, boyfriends of mothers), was related to poorer self-esteem and more behavioral problems than incest performed by biological fathers or other relatives. There was no difference in the degree of violence, but a significant difference in the way mothers reacted: They were, as a group, more likely to side with a boyfriend or stepfather/husband than with a husband who was the biological father of the victim. A negative (hostile, blaming and rejecting) reaction on the part of the victim's mother to the revelation of abuse was correlated to the level of emotional distress, low self-esteem and the symptoms seen. A positive reaction (caring, protecting and nonblaming), cannot mitigate the effects of abuse, but at least it does not compound them.

Forty-one percent of the mothers of sexual abuse and incest victims had been sexually abused in their own childhoods; 34% had been physically abused or neglected. Clinically, they presented a wide spectrum of diagnoses, which did not correlate with their reaction to the revelation of abuse. No significant differences between incest and nonincest mothers were found.

At the 18-month follow-up, most victims showed a significant decrease in psychopathology and an increase in self-esteem. Exceptions were those children who had exhibited few or no symptoms during crisis intervention, but were symptomatic 18 months later. Revictimization was rare (only 5%) in this sample.

Seventy-eight percent of the victims required more than crisis intervention. Those children who received prolonged treatment in a specialized program showed the highest rate of improvement.

These data were gathered between 1980 and 1983, supported by a grant from the Office of Juvenile Justice and Delinquency Prevention,* which mandated the provision of therapy concomitant with data collection. A specific model program—the Family Crisis Program (FCP) for Sexually Abused Children—was designed, responding to both the mandate of the grant and the need of the greater Boston community. When grant funding ended in 1984, the need for a specialized sexual abuse program was evident and the program continued on a fee-for-service basis.

## Literature Review

Designing a clinical sexual abuse program requires the adaptation of traditional child psychiatric treatment strategies to the special needs of sexually abused children and their families. There is little conclusive information about effective treatment strategies for these families to draw upon (Mrazek & Kempe, 1981). A review of the literature on incest reveals that a wide variety of treatment approaches has been advocated. Individual therapy sessions for the child are an essential component of many programs (Burgess, Holmstrom, & Sgroi, 1978; Peters, 1976; Sgroi, 1982). Those who view sexual abuse as a sign of pathology in the family system advocate traditional family therapy (Eist & Mandel, 1966). Some therapists have focused almost exclusively on father-daughter incest. For example, Browning and Boatman (1977) hypothesize that a failure in the mother-daughter relationship leaves the daughter vulnerable to sexual abuse. Therefore, they advocate treatment centering on the mother-daughter dyad. A "humanistic" approach to incest treatment developed by Giar-

*Grant No. 80-JN-AX-0001, S2

retto (1976) includes multiple treatment modes: individual treatment, mother-daughter therapy, marital therapy, father-daughter treatment, family sessions, group treatment for each family member, and self-help groups. One unifying theme in much of the previous literature is that the occurrence or revelation of sexual abuse presents a family with a crisis which cannot be handled with its usual coping mechanisms. Thus, numerous therapists have advocated an adaptation of classic crisis treatment for handling child sexual abuse (Burgess, Holmstrom, & Sgroi, 1978; Peters, 1976; Sgroi, 1982; Simrel, Berg, & Thomas, 1979).

The treatment approach developed by the FCP, drawing on classic crisis theory (Caplan, 1964; Lindeman, 1944), suggests that crises occur in people's lives when an individual is faced with a major obstacle to achieving important life goals which cannot be surmounted with ordinary coping mechanisms. As the person in crisis struggles ineffectively to apply old problem-solving strategies, she or he experiences increasing discomfort and helplessness, which may reach disorganizing proportions. However, during this period of mounting tension, the individual may be especially accessible to treatment strategies that focus on the quick development of new problem-solving approaches. Thus, crisis intervention not only may relieve the individual's current distress, but it may also modify and strengthen his or her capacity to withstand future stresses.

In sexual abuse situations, the assumption is generally made that the occurrence or the revelation of the sexual activity is the precipitant for some type of crisis in the family. The family's usual patterns of coping are disrupted by both the realization that their child has been victimized and the flurry of activity that often ensues as police or protective service workers attempt to investigate the allegations of sexual abuse. The goal of treatment is to restore equilibrium in each of the family members and to help them develop more adaptive coping mechanisms (especially when the sexual abuse has occurred within the family unit).

Crisis theory (Caplan, 1964) suggests that these goals are best met by intervening as soon as possible after the crisis situation develops. The objective is to engage the patient in the therapeutic work while she or he is most accessible to change. In crisis intervention, no attempt is made to alter basic personality structure. Treatment is brief and focused very specifically on helping to resolve the crisis at hand. Therapists take much more active roles then is customary in psychodynamic therapies. Sessions may be scheduled more often than once a week and may take place in settings other than the therapist's office. The therapist may intercede on the patient's behalf to help him or her resolve a practical problem (e.g., obtaining emergency social services or a restraining order against the perpetrator).

The FCP treatment model incorporated several of these fundamental tenets of crisis therapy into the crisis intervention aspect of the treatment. As stated above, less than one-quarter of the families seen required only crisis intervention. Most needed more long-term individual or group treatment after the initial crisis intervention.

## General Concepts

The FCP has conceptualized the effort needed to help sexually abused children and their families in a model that offers comprehensive clinical intervention and cooperation with all other agencies and systems involved. This model includes a four-pronged approach to the problem.

*Investigation*, substantiation, and case management performed by the state agency responsible for child welfare are the basis for any intervention geared to helping sexually abused children and their families. Most states mandate reporting abuse incidents to that agency.

*Clinical services* may be necessary at any stage of contact with sexually abused children and their families and will be described in greater detail below.

*Judicial system involvement*. Cooperation between the judicial and mental health systems is becoming increasingly important. Many states are in the process of reassessing their response to child victims from a child welfare as well as from a judicial point of view. In Massachusetts, a 1983 law (General Laws of Massachusetts) mandates reporting incest and serious sexual or physical abuse to the district attorney's office. The decision about whether to prosecute is made at a multidisciplinary conference, which ideally includes the mental health clinicians involved with the child and his or her family. Clinicians are also expected to provide written and verbal testimony in court, and to be expert witnesses.

*Advocacy*. A sexual abuse program has to be involved in a broad range of activities related to the issue. These include: 1) consciousness-raising with the public, the legislature, health care and human service providers on the existence and prevalence of the problem of sexual abuse of children; 2) increasing awareness of the problem in the legislature to improve funding for programs and to promote enactment of laws easing the victim's course through the legal system; 3) education regarding prevention, in schools, to groups of health care and human service providers, and through the media; 4) education of the public, especially parents and health care providers, regarding presenting symptoms, elucidation of suspicions, and the most helpful responses to revealed abuse; and 5) coordination of services for the individual families involved with the program, including medical, psychiatric, protective, legal, educational, and foster placement services as well as advocacy on their behalf.

## Countertransference Issues

Clinical work with sexually abused children, their families and offenders can be very stressful; crisis intervention in general requires a high level of activity and involvement; in addition, sexual abuse intervention raises a host of powerful feelings, ranging from disgust and rejection to identification with the victim or the aggressor, and from rage and retaliatory wishes to vicarious and unconscious sexual excitation. Disbelief, minimization and denial of the occurrence of abuse may represent attempts by the clinician to deal with his or her own feelings, but they have powerful deleterious effects on the presenting victim and family. Countertransference responses tend to become increasingly inappropriate as clinician burnout increases, and lead to ineffective or harmful interventions.

Safeguards against unbearable stress and burnout need to be debated and then incorporated into the concept delineated. Suggestions offered here cannot be exhaustive, as particulars such as case flow, number of staff, levels of expertise, and personal as well as interpersonal dynamics vary.

Teamwork is essential. The seductive power of incestuous family dynamics can easily overcome one clinician's evaluation or treatment of a family system. Team members need to remind each other that mental health professionals are trained to help people acknowledge their feelings, express them and use them in appropriate ways. Clinicians are not police investigators, child protective workers, prosecuting or defending attorneys, or judges. Interprofessional cooperation and teamwork are crucial, and boundaries are best kept clearly defined.

## Clinical Services

The services offered by the FCP include:

1) elucidation of the allegation by clinicians trained to elicit information from children of all ages, developmental stages, and levels of psychological functioning. Staff are experienced in the use of adjuncts such as anatomically correct dolls, doll houses, and drawings.

2) assessment of the immediate impact of the abuse and its revelation on the child and the family, including the risk for retaliation, further abuse or psychological harm as consequences of the revelation. History gathering (prior abuse or neglect in the presenting family or in the background of any family member) is a critical component of the risk assessment.
3) diagnostic assessment of the child, all family members involved and the offender, leading to DSM-III diagnoses, if applicable.
4) diagnostic assessment of the family dynamics as they pertain to the occurrence of abuse and the risk of reabuse.
5) medical exam, if indicated, by a pediatrician experienced with sexually abused children.
6) determination of the kind of intervention or therapy needed based on all the factors listed above. This includes the development of a comprehensive treatment plan for all family members involved, including the offender when applicable.
7) referral to and consultation with other specialty units for further assessment or treatment.
8) short-term or long-term therapeutic intervention tailored to the needs of each child and family: crisis intervention, short-term individual, sibling or couples therapy, group therapy (for latency age and adolescent victims, for mothers of incest victims and for fathers or grandfathers who committed the incest), and family therapy when appropriate.
9) periodic reassessment and termination of therapeutic intervention when specific individual and family goals have been met.

Therapy with an incest or sexual abuse victim and his or her family cannot and does not exist in a vacuum. Cooperation and consultation with other agencies involved are crucial and include the following: work with child protective workers (who in most states have case management responsibilities) investigating the allegation of sexual abuse or offering services after substantiation; and work with the judicial system in the form of verbal or written reports and testimony, as well as guidance and support to those victims and families who are testifying.

## CONCLUSION

The model program presented here is but one of several. Others are described in the literature (Burgess, Holmstrom, & Sgroi, 1978; Giarretto, 1976; Sgroi, 1982). As stated above, follow-up data about various kinds of interventions are not available. All interventions therefore should be regarded as experimental. This implies thoughtful and careful application of various models, permitting the best interests of the child to guide the choice of all procedures. Cooperation with other agencies and professionals is mandated and, increasingly, legislated. Thorough knowledge of the evolving state and federal laws regarding child abuse is required. Advocacy is needed to make interventions more accessible in order to protect the child from revictimization by offenders as well as by the medical, protective and judicial systems. Public and professional education regarding the revelation or early recognition of ongoing sexual abuse is vital. Prevention of child abuse needs to become a national and local priority.

## REFERENCES

Ball, P., & Wyman, E. (1977–78). Battered wives and powerlessness: What can counselors do? *Victimology: An International Journal, 2*(314), 545–552.

Browning, D., & Boatman, B. (1977). Incest: Children at risk. *American Journal of Psychiatry,* Jan. *134*, 1–10.

Burgess, A., & Holmstrom, L. (1974a). Rape trauma syndrome. *American Journal of Psychiatry, 131*(9), 981–986.

Burgess, A., & Holmstrom, L. (1974b). *Rape: Victims of Crisis.* Bowie, MD: Robert J. Brady.

Burgess, A., Holmstrom, L., & Sgroi, S. (1978). *Sexual assault of children and adolescents.* Lexington, MA: Lexington Books.

Caplan, G. (1964). *Principles of preventive psychiatry.* New York: Basic Books.

Chapman, J., & Gates, M. (Eds). (1978). *The victimization of women.* Beverly Hills, CA: Sage.

Department of Social Services. (1981–84). *Annual statistics reports.* Boston, MA: Department of Social Services.

Dewsbury, A. (1975). Family violence seen in general practice. *Review of Social Health Journal, 95*, 290–294.

Eisenberg, S., & Micklow, P. (1976). The assaulted wife: "Catch 22" revisited. *Women's Rights Law Reporter, 5*(3/4), 138–147.

Eist, H., & Mandel, A. (1966). Family treatment of ongoing incest behavior. *Family Process, 7*, 216–224.

Federal Bureau of Investigation. (1972, 1974, 1982). *Uniform crime reports.* Washington, D.C.

Field, M., & Field, H. (1973). Marital violence and the criminal process: Neither justice nor peace. *Social Service Review, 47*, 221–240.

Finkelhor, D. (1979). *Sexually victimized children.* New York: Free Press.

Fonseka, S. (1974). A study of wife beating in the Camberwell area. *British Journal of Clinical Practice, 28*, 400–402.

Gates, M. (1977). *The battered woman: Criminal and civil remedies.* Paper presented at the 130th Annual Meeting of the American Psychiatric Association, Toronto, Canada.

Gayford, J. (1975). Battered wives. *Medicine and Science Law, 15*, 237–245.

Gelles, R. (1974). *The violent home: A study of physical aggression between husbands and wives.* Beverly Hills, CA: Sage.

General Laws of Massachusetts. (1983). Amendment of Section 51B of Chapter 119, Chapter 288 of Acts of 1983. Boston, MA.

Giarretto, H. (1976). *The treatment of father-daughter incest: A psychosocial approach.* Washington, D.C., DHEW (pub. no. 76-30014).

Gomes-Schwartz, B., Horowitz, J., & Sauzier, M. (1984). *Sexually exploited children: Service and research project.* Washington, DC: Office of Juvenile Justice and Delinquency Prevention.

Green, A. (1978). Self-destructive behavior in battered children. *American Journal of Psychiatry, 135,* 579–582.

Gutheil, T., & Avery, N. (1977). Multiple overt incest as family defense against loss. *Family Process, 16*(1), 105–116.

Herman, J., & Hirschman, L. (1981a). Families at risk for father-daughter incest. *Journal of the American Psychiatric Association, 138,* 7–15.

Herman, J., & Hirschman, L. (1981b). *Father-daughter incest.* Cambridge, MA: Harvard University Press.

Hilberman, E., & Munson, M. (1977–78). Sixty battered women. *Victimology: An International Journal, 2*(3/4), 460–471.

Kansas City Police Department (1973). *Conflict management: Analysis resolution.* Kansas City, MO.

Katan, A. (1973). Children who were raped. *Psychoanalysis of School Children, 28,* 443–449.

Kinsey, A. (1953). *Sexual behavior in the human female.* Philadelphia, PA: Saunders.

Levinger, G. (1966). Sources of marital dissatisfaction among applicants for divorce. *American Journal of Orthopsychiatry, 36,* 803–807.

Lindeman, E. (1944). Symptomatology and management of acute grief. *American Journal of Psychiatry, 101,* 37–45.

Martin, D. (1976). *Battered wives.* San Francisco, CA: Glide.

Mrazek, P., & Kempe, C. (Eds). (1981). *Sexually abused children and their families.* Oxford, England: Pergamon Press.

Ochberg, F. (1980). Victims of terrorism. *Journal of Clinical Psychiatry, 41,* 73–74.

Peters, J. (1976). Children who are victims of sexual assault and the psychology of offenders. *American Journal of Psychotherapy, 30,* 398–421.

Pizzey, E. (1974). *Scream quietly or the neighbors will hear.* Essex, England: Anchorage.

Pizzey, E. (1975). Chiswick women's aid: A refuge from violence. *Review of Social Health Journal, 95,* 297–298, 308.

Ridington, J. (1977–78). The transition process: A feminist environment as reconstitutive milieu. *Victimology: An International Journal, 2*(3/4), 563–575.

Rosenfeld, A. (1979). Incidence of a history of incest among 18 female psychiatric patients. *American Journal of Psychiatry, 136,* 791–795.

Rounsaville, B. (1978). Theories in marital violence: Evidence from a study of battered women. *Victimology: An International Journal, 3*(112), 11–29.

Rounsaville, B., & Weissman, M. (1977–78). Battered women: A medical problem requiring detection. *International Journal of Psychiatry in Medicine, 8,* 191–202.

Scott, P. (1974). Battered wives. *British Journal of Psychiatry, 125,* 433–441.

Seligman, M. (1975). *Helplessness: On depression, development and death.* San Francisco, CA: W. H. Freeman.

Sgroi, S. (1982). *Handbook of clinical interventions in child sexual abuse.* Lexington, MA: Lexington Books.

Simrel, K., Berg, R., & Thomas, J. (1979). Crisis management of sexually abused children. *Pediatric Annals, 8,* 5–11.

Stark, E., Flitcraft, A., & Frazier, W. (1979). Medicine and patriarchal violence: The social construction of a "private" event. *International Journal of Health Service, 9,* 461–493.

Straus, M. (1974). Leveling, civility and violence in the family. *Journal of Marriage and the Family, 36,* 13–29.

Straus, M. (1977–78). Wifebeating: How common and why? *Victimology: An International Journal, 2*(3/4), 443–458.

Straus, M., Gelles, R., & Steinmetz, S. (1981). *Behind closed doors: Violence in the American family.* New York: Anchor Press/Doubleday.

Symonds, M. (1978). The psychodynamics of violence-prone marriages. *American Journal of Psychiatry, 38*(3), 213–222.

Tsai, M., Feldman-Summers, S., & Edgar, M. (1979). Childhood molestation: Variables related to differential impacts on psychosexual functioning in adult women. *Journal of Abnormal Psychology, 88*(4), 407–417.

Waites, E. (1977–78). Female masochism and the enforced restriction of choice. *Victimology: An International Journal, 2*(3/4), 525–534.

Walker, L. (1977–78). Battered women and learned helplessness. *Victimology: An International Journal, 2*(3/4), 535–544.

Walker, L. (1979). *The battered woman.* New York: Harper & Row.

Walker, L. (1984). *The battered woman syndrome.* New York: Harper & Row.

Washington, DC Police Foundation. (1983). *Police Foundation Report.* Washington, DC, Police Foundation.

# 8

# *Special Intervention Programs for Child Victims of Violence*

Howard B. Levy, Stephen H. Sheldon, and
Jon R. Conte

## INTRODUCTION

It appears that America has been having a love affair with violence. Indeed, concerned professionals and lay public alike have become increasingly frightened and disturbed by the magnitude of reports of violence in this country. Most distressing has been the disproportionate increase in cases of intrafamily violence, especially violence directed at children.

Straus, Gelles, and Steinmetz (1980) have reported that Americans are more likely to be murdered in their homes by members of their families than anywhere else or by anyone else. They have also reported that 1.4 to 1.9 million children between 3 and 17 years of age are vulnerable to physical injury by their parents (Gelles, 1982; Straus et al., 1980). These numbers are by no means inclusive and reflect only those cases that are identified and enter the "system."

Acts of force against children are not new. They have been recorded throughout history (DeMause, 1974). During this past century, organizations dedicated to the prevention of child abuse/neglect, in conjunction with specific government and private agencies, have developed and initiated efforts to provide protection for children. As we enter the mid 1980s, it is important that we recognize that child abuse and other child maltreatment issues have had the benefit of visibility, national recognition and prototypal legislation. Even so, adequate protection of children from acts of violence remains an unfulfilled promise. In spite of increasing involvement on the part of social service agencies, law enforcement and medical communities and our court systems, charges are frequently made that access to safeguards and services for children and their caretakers remain difficult and discouraging. Service provision often appears fragmented, poorly coordinated, and discontinuous. There remains a sense that individual children and their families become lost within a system that tends to shuffle people among separate service units.

This "system" is a composite of professional groups that include social service, medical, judicial, law enforcement, and mental health disciplines. Each discipline has a specific role in responding to violence and interacting with other members of the community. It is the availability and coordination of these independent systems, as they respond to victims and perpetrators of violence, that define the nature and parameters of a community response to violence.

This chapter first describes the roles, interrelationships, interdependencies, and foibles of various community agencies as they currently exist. A review of the inadequacies in each discipline that result in a potentially less than optimal response also is presented. A theoretical basis for community intervention utilizing known risk factors is suggested, stressing the proactive nonstatic nature of these "vulnerability" factors. Following this theoretical matrix, a coordinated community response is delineated. Last and most important in terms of long-range strategies for the future is a discussion of further policy development and research.

## THE SYSTEMS APPROACH TO INTERVENTION

### Identification and Reporting

Entry into the system of potential responses to family violence is dependent upon the identification of the child abuse victim and the subsequent report of that episode to the mandated state protection agency. The report is the trigger for the subsequent cascade of responses.

Each state has a child abuse reporting law which stipulates that certain professionals *must* report all cases of suspected child abuse and neglect to that state's child protection agency. Failure to report places the mandated professional at potential risk for civil liability. Those professionals designated as mandated reporters vary in each state but usually include physicians, teachers, social workers, and police officers. Child abuse reports are not limited to mandated reporters, however, and may be initiated by anyone who suspects that a child has been or is being abused. Once a report of abuse has been generated, an investigation is begun to determine whether the allegation of abuse is valid. Evidence is gathered from interviews with the child's caretakers, other family members, neighbors, and involved professionals. An appraisal of the child's home environment is also undertaken and assessed in terms of safety and adequate resources.

The report and subsequent investigation process are complex and their outcome can be affected by variations in the levels of knowledge, skill, and commitment of mandated reporters, nonmandated reporters and Child Protection Service (CPS) investigators. The child victim must therefore rely on the competence of the reporter and investigators. Adding to this potential confusion are the vastly different manifestations of child abuse and neglect. Signs and symptoms of abuse may relate to the specific area of the child's body that has been traumatized or may be symbolic. An example of the latter is the acute onset of bedwetting in a previously toilet-trained child who has sustained multiple inflicted bruises. Because children have a limited ability to defend or protect themselves against injuries, they may exhibit subtle personality or behavioral changes as sequelae to the violence they have sustained. A not infrequent example in this area is the deterioration in school performance of a child who has been sexually abused.

The investigation of a report of suspected child abuse usually involves interviews with the alleged victim and her or his family as well as the presumed abuser. Collateral interviews with neighbors or other professionals frequently occur simultaneously. As part of this information-gathering process, children are often interviewed and examined by physicians, although in many states this unfortunately is not a routine aspect of all child abuse investigations. Interviews typically occur in the child's and the family's environment (e.g., home, school, or neighborhood).

Training of investigators varies greatly between and even within states. Most states have deprofessionalized the CPS job classification so that prior social service or mental health education is not a requirement for job eligibility. Few states have developed detailed investigative guidelines or protocols, and policies vary greatly across states. This lack of standardized procedure appears to have resulted in a situation in which there is considerable individual CPS worker discretion in the handling of cases. More importantly, the accuracy of CPS decisions is an issue of considerable debate among professionals and one that suffers from a lack of empirical investigation.

Once a case of suspected abuse is founded or determined as having some validity by the investigation, a number of other systems are activated.

## Law Enforcement

The primary function of law enforcement is to investigate allegations of violations of the law and to gather evidence that may be used to prosecute those who break the law. This function is designed to protect society and the victim from additional illegal acts. The function of the police in gathering evidence includes interviewing crime victims and witnesses and collecting physical evidence. The different types of intrafamily violence result in significant variations in the extent to which victims are capable of providing a statement about their victimization, whether or not there are available witnesses who can corroborate what the victim has said and/or the presence of physical evidence. An example of the variation in victim capability is illustrated by the sexually abused two-year-old child who may not have the language skills to describe his or her abuse. In spite of these difficulties, increasing experience suggests that in the majority of reports of intrafamily violence police are able to obtain the information required to take further action.

Once a report is made to the police they initiate an investigation to determine whether there is credible evidence that a crime has been committed. This determination involves assessing victim and witness statements, collecting physical evidence and assuring that the chain of evidence remains intact. In cases of intrafamily violence police are allowed broad discretion about which steps to take immediately. Depending on the circumstances, they may arrest the offender, take temporary custody of child victims, or refer adult victims to temporary shelters. In some jurisdictions, perpetrators of intrafamily violence may be contacted by telephone and asked to come to the police station for booking. If victim advocates are available the police may be able to call upon them to help shepherd victims through the intervention process. These and other services help the police carry out their primary function of investigating crime while minimizing additional trauma to victims.

## Justice System

The justice system consists of the law enforcement and court subsystems (civil and criminal courts). Generally, each of the justice subsystems is charged with the broad mandate of protecting society from illegal acts. However, without an actual violation of the law, the justice system is prohibited from entering into the private lives of citizens. Interpersonal violence between strangers is almost universally regarded as an appropriate focus of justice system concern, but there is no such agreement about the role of the justice system in responding to the violent home: interpersonal violence between members of the same family is often regarded as a ''family matter'' in which the state should not intervene. The arguments for and against justice system involvement are often emotional and pragmatic (Conte, 1984).

Our assumption is that acts of interpersonal violence within a family must be responded to by all of the systems charged to deal with interpersonal violence. Failure to respond in a coordinated fashion places victims of intrafamily violence at a disadvantage relative to victims of extrafamily violence. Moreover, in dealing with violence committed within the family the justice system may respond, but in a different manner than it does in cases involving extrafamily violence. The manner and sensitivity with which the justice system responds to intrafamilial violence will determine the appropriateness of intervention by this discipline.

After a police report has been made and an investigation begun, two separate aspects of the justice system are often engaged.

*Criminal justice system.* The criminal justice system, which is responsible for *protecting society* through the prosecution and punishment of those who break the law, may be involved depending upon the type of crime and identity of the perpetrator. Criminal law stipulates that acts of sexual assault, battery, and physical assault are against the law, but the specifics of what constitutes criminal (in the family setting) rather than civil law violations, vary across jurisdictions.

In criminal law proceedings, although the victim is an interested party, his or her role is primarily that of a witness. Criminal justice proceedings are often criticized because of their apparent insensitivity to and lack of concern for the needs and rights of victims. Even though the primary function of the criminal justice system is the prosecution and punishment of offenders, there is an increasing awareness that the criminal justice system may also be used to encourage offenders to enter treatment.

The use of the criminal justice system as a means to encourage offenders to accept responsibility for their actions and to receive treatment that is aimed at reducing their potential for continued criminal behavior is hotly debated. Those who oppose the use of the justice system to force offenders into treatment argue that one cannot ''treat a crime,'' that it is impossible to coerce behavioral changes, and that forcing perpetrators into treatment denies them their rights to due process. Those who favor the use of the justice system to force offenders into treatment stress that many offenders have no insight into their behaviors and that they rationalize their acts of violence. For example, the sexual abuse of a child is explained as a means of teaching that child about sexuality. The psychological distortions associated with most acts of intrafamily violence require some mechanism to help the offender understand the illegal and harmful nature of his or her behavior. In many cases no alternative is available to replace the justice system as a mechanism for helping offenders accept responsibility for their behavior and enter treatment.

*Civil justice system*. Civil justice involvement in cases of intrafamily violence has the primary function of *protecting the victim*. Child protection investigations of reports of child abuse or neglect are mandated in every state. Although in some jurisdictions the police may be mandated to investigate reports, each state also has a child protection agency that must investigate all reports and take steps to protect the child. The mandated agency must also provide services to attenuate the conditions that were responsible for the child's injury. In many states a case of reported child abuse or neglect must be validated before any social service may be provided to the child or family. When a child is judged to be at serious risk, CPS may take temporary custody of the child and place him or her in a safe environment. This may involve placing the child with other relatives or in a foster home.

The civil justice system also includes the juvenile court, which has the long-term responsibility of protecting the child, and must often approve the plans formulated by the state social services department. Occasionally the juvenile court may also stipulate services designed to alter the conditions that required removal of the child from his or her home. This branch of the civil justice system is responsible for the legal termination of parental rights in those cases where it is determined that this action will be in the child's best interest. Civil justice action also may be helpful through the use of *no-contact orders*, by which perpetrators of violence are ordered out of the home and are not to have contact with other family members. Usually these orders stipulate a specific period of time.

Regardless of which aspect of the justice system is involved in intrafamily violence, there is increasing agreement that such involvement should be as sensitive and atraumatic as possible. Numerous innovations have been implemented to reduce the likelihood that this intervention will be a significant source of trauma in the lives of victims of intrafamily violence (Conte & Berliner, 1981). These innovations are diverse and include: teaching justice system personnel about the dynamics of interpersonal violence in order to lessen their misconceptions about family violence; training police and attorneys to be sensitive interviewers of victims of violence; reducing the number of times victims are required to repeat the story of their victimization; vertical prosecution, which allows the same prosecuting attorney to handle a case throughout its legal proceedings; whenever possible, removal of the offender rather than the victim(s) from the home; and pre-trial or post-conviction diversion programs that offer treatment as alternatives to incarceration.

## Social Services

The social services comprise a wide range of specific interventions that are designed to prevent or alleviate social problems or contribute to their solution. These services also are intended to improve the well-being of individuals, groups and communities. They may be provided by both private (voluntary) and government agencies. Although the scope of services varies in each community they usually include: financial supports such as food stamps and Aid to Families with Dependent Children; subsidized housing; homemaker and visiting nurse services; emergency food and clothing; temporary shelters; and job training.

These supports can provide essential ingredients in professional efforts to prevent and ameliorate the impact of intrafamily violence. An example of this is the use of homemakers as a means of keeping children safe, and at the same time avoiding the costs of out-of-home care in neglect cases. Income, housing, and food supports can significantly reduce the stress parents may be experiencing, and which also appears related to many acts of physical child abuse. The availability of temporary shelters supplemented by emergency food and other supports make it possible for women to protect themselves and their children from violence. These services offer women an option other than remaining in an abusive environment simply because they have no other means of financial survival. Job training and income supplements make it possible for mothers to support their families and improve their living conditions. These supplements may be pivotal factors in a process that reduces parent vulnerabilities associated with family violence. Although the availability of these services should reflect the measurement of user need, they are often available only to those cases identified as being at the most serious risk. Furthermore, various legislative changes have resulted in an absolute decrease in the availability of these services (L. Brown, personal communication, 1984).

## Mental Health

Mental health services encompass a continuum of specific interventions and also are designed to remediate specific behavioral aspects of individuals, families, or small groups that may be associated with intrafamily violence. Until recently there has been some distrust of mental health approaches since many mental health practitioners have tended to treat all intrafamily violence as an intrapsychic problem and the product of intra- or interpersonal variables. This view might dictate that the stress resulting from inadequate housing, food or other basic life-sustaining resources be treated with counseling rather than by helping the client obtain adequate support. The theoretical framework outlined in this chapter will suggest that violence may be the result of a number of vulnerabilities. Some of these vulnerabilities reside within individuals or families, while others reside in communities or are the result of state and federal policy decisions.

Recognition that intrafamily violence is the result of a number of interactive variables suggests that mental health services can be useful in many cases of interpersonal violence. These services often include: skill training such as parent training that teaches parents nonaversive child management techniques; parent education to increase parent knowledge of child development and nutrition; stress management classes; advocacy training/availability, in which therapists either advocate or teach clients those advocacy skills necessary to obtain their own goods and services; or individual, small group or family therapy.

## Medicine

It was not until the 1940s that physicians noted the specific association of healed fractures and chronic subdural hematomas in young children (Caffey, 1946). Less than a decade later, Silverman published an article recognizing that these injuries appeared to be the result of repeated nonaccidental traumas (Silverman, 1953). Although radiologists were at the forefront of medicine's involvement in the diagnosis of child abuse, it was not until Dr. C. Henry Kempe and his associates coined the term "battered child syndrome" that the medical profession became active in the area of child abuse and neglect intervention (Kempe, Silverman, Steele, et al., 1962). In spite of the medical community's late entry into the system of community response, it is often in a unique position to protect the child and maintain a therapeutic liaison with the family or caretakers. The physician reporter is unusual in the community system of interventions in that there is no burden placed upon him or her to validate a report or to win a case, to gain a conviction, or to obtain adequate information needed to incarcerate a perpetrator. The physician, by nature of his or her training, seeks only to be an advocate for the child and family. The doctor may therefore be able to avoid the pitfalls and handicaps of many of the other community intervention services.

The physician not only functions as a mandated reporter utilizing his or her diagnostic intervention skills, but can also provide acute treatment for any existing injuries. In addition, he or she may also be able to lay the foundation for any future rehabilitation of the child and his or her caretakers.

Unfortunately, in spite of their potential role as gatekeepers to the system, physicians are at times hesitant to report their suspicions of child maltreatment. They often lack adequate information related to child abuse and are inexperienced in handling these emotionally charged situations. These difficulties are frequently related to the inadequacy of preparatory curricula relating to family violence in medical schools. Inexperience and limited medical school coursework, however, are only two of the factors contributing to physicians' reluctance to report. Other issues that alter physician involvement are hesitancy to believe that violent acts against children can possibly be perpetrated by family members whom the physician has known over a period of years; hesitancy to become involved in judicial proceedings; disinclination to take time from a busy practice to provide court testimony; and fear of confronting the perpetrator (Helfer, 1975). Recent information suggests a continued belief of physicians that the "system" may be more disruptive than helpful, and emphasizes a perception by physicians that after they initiate a report they will be unable to obtain any follow-up (Sheldon & Levy, in preparation).

Nonetheless, the physician is often pivotal in gaining valuable information through the medical interview of the child and/or the caretaker, as well as from the subsequent examination and laboratory tests. The physician must ultimately be able to translate his or her knowledge of child development and the family as a unit with the physical examination and laboratory tests into a community treatment plan. The thoroughness and completeness of the interview, the examination, and the ability to collate this information may be exceedingly important to the outcome of the case. Unfortunately, the information needed to assess cases of intrafamily violence may be unfamiliar to the physician. This is especially true for those physicians involved in very technical or specialized areas of medicine. Lack of experience with the results of child abuse, other than those directly related to the injury, may result in the physician acting in a very pragmatic manner. Under such circumstances he or she may provide only acute treatment for the specific injury brought to his or her attention. In addition, confusion over certain aspects of reporting laws, exemplified by the word "suspicion" as it is used in child abuse reporting, may result in physician underreporting. These issues are exacerbated by the array of community services and networks that often confuse the physician. Many physicians are left with a sense of lack of accomplishment and are frustrated in attempts to shepherd their patients and their families through these systems.

## GAPS IN KNOWLEDGE

In spite of the vast number of research projects studying violence and its sequelae, several areas have not been adequately addressed. These gaps in our knowledge preclude any truly efficient or viable response to the problem of handling cases of violence and child abuse.

Although the more holistic interest in violence within the home is relatively new, there is an expanding research effort. This effort is likely to alter how professionals view the origins, effects, and ideal treatments of all types of family violence. Unfortunately, much of this research takes place within disciplines, and there is little cross-fertilization between professional disciplines. Overall, research and other activities focusing on any one type of violence have had little influence on other types of violence. Consequently, professionals concerned with physical child abuse are often not aware of developments in child sexual abuse. Neither group tends to be aware of the developments with children touched by domestic violence.

Several major gaps in current knowledge strike us as the most pressing in terms of community responses to the violent home.

### What Is the Etiology of Violence?

Most experts concur that exposure to discord, violence, and lack of resources are common elements in the background of individuals who become perpetrators of abuse/neglect. The exact etiology or imprinting pattern has remained elusive. It remains unclear if these factors must occur at a finite point in time, in a specific sequence or over a predetermined duration. Adding to this confusion is the question of why an individual perpetrates neglect (as opposed to sexual abuse or physical abuse) and not necessarily the same type of violence to which he or she had been exposed.

Much of the research on the origins of violence has tended to focus on a single type of violence (e.g., child abuse or sexual violence) and on a limited number of variables. We suggest that a multivariable approach may more profitably identify the set of variables associated with the various types of interpersonal violence. While it is likely to be some time before a single model of the genesis of violence is developed and validated, research that quantifies the variables will significantly contribute to understanding the occurrence of violence. Research directed at the correlations between various risk factors is likely to be of immediate utility in planning organized responses to violence.

## What Is the Prevalence of Child Abuse/Neglect?

There is still an uncertainty as to the actual incidence of violence directed at children and this reflects a lack of definition as well as the varying sensitivities and knowledge of reporters. Research thus far has led most investigators to believe that the abuse and neglect of children is underreported, but the magnitude of underreporting is still unknown. As eluded to earlier in this chapter, one of the major factors in underreporting rests with the lack of education and comprehension of abuse and neglect by both mandated and nonmandated reporters. A prime example is the lack of understanding by some physicians that failing to recognize and report abuse may lead to more serious harm of a child. A second example is the damage that comes from a CPS worker unfounding a case because it lacks sufficient evidence for legal action, when the "lack of evidence" is actually due to the worker's failing to understand another discipline's role or jargon. These disparities emphasize the need for a systems approach to child abuse and neglect reporting.

## What Are the Physical Findings in Child Sexual Abuse?

A previously underemphasized area has been the incidence of physical abnormalities present in victims of intrafamilial sexual abuse. Several investigators (Levy & Sheldon, 1985) have found a moderate degree of crossover abnormalities—physical injuries present in victims of sexual abuse that are distinctly different from the known sequelae of the sexual molestation. For example, it remains unclear as to the actual incidence of concomitant physical abnormalities occurring in cases of incest. The significance of sexually transmitted diseases in young children is only now becoming appreciated as they relate to the pervasiveness and varieties of transmittable illnesses. Only recently has Chlamydia trachomatis been recognized as an important disease of sexual origin in young children (Levy, Sheldon, & Ahart, in preparation). The extent of this entity's potential role in the subsequent infertility of infected children is unknown, as is the question of whether it is transmitted with any frequency by a nonsexual route in children beyond infancy. Furthermore, the potential ability of laboratories to provide information about Chlamydia, subtyped in a strain-specific fashion and cultured from the victim and the perpetrator, poses stimulating legal and medical issues. In addition, methods are now available to detect evidence of prior Chlamydia infection even after the host has been adequately treated.

In part, problems with sexually transmitted diseases in children are confusing and underrepresented because of state confidentiality laws. A requirement that these laws be qualified for young children is now more appreciated than previously.

*How Best to Treat Violence?*

Currently, there are few data that describe the effects of various services to either the victims of violence or the perpetrators. Decisions about which clients are best served and with which services are currently based on clinical experience or occasionally are based on the biases of individual social service workers. Perhaps more importantly, it is not clear that violent individuals who receive a package of services will benefit as measured by a reduction or elimination of their potential to commit further acts of violence. Concomitantly, while we know that physical wounds of violence do heal, it is not clear that the psychological consequences of interpersonal violence can be healed by any intervention without substantial scarring.

In an age of declining service dollars, knowledge about what types of services, for what types of clients, producing what kinds of effects, and how long these effects last strike us as fundamentally important. Society is no longer willing to "throw money" at problems. Therefore, any argument for spending money to reduce the problem of violence would be significantly strengthened if proponents were able to provide data supporting the assumption that intervention does produce a positive outcome.

*How Does a Community's Response to Violence Actually Operate?*

One of the most interesting issues surrounding a community's response to the violent home is the extent to which the response conforms to the ideal model that that community describes. We are unaware of any data describing how a community actually handles violence. Although community response involves interagency agreements designed to ensure coordination and integration across agencies, there is no evidence that these systems actually provide such responses. Similarly, we know of no data that describe a client's movement through the various systems or the consequences of the various systems' decisions about the client.

The latter is typified by our paucity of understanding as to what happens to abused children when police or CPS workers fail to take protective custody. How many of these children are ultimately reabused? How many are reabused in the time period shortly after the failure to take custody? Limited data, generated mainly by the medical community, are available but they show only that nonreporting statistically places these children at significant risk for further and more serious injury (Fontana & Besharov, 1979).

There are specific questions regarding how various subsystems operate and how the entire community response system actually functions. Although poorly handled cases are occasionally identified by one or another system in a community, it is not clear whether mishandling is an exception or a rule in most communities. Nor is it clear what happens to most cases of abused children who are identified. For example, in Cook County, Illinois, where a special sexual abuse unit has been formed to investigate cases of sexual abuse there has been an increase in the percentage of "founded" cases to over 70% of the more than 1,365 cases reported in 1983. However, the State of Illinois is able to provide financial support for the treatment of only a fraction of these cases. What happens to the remaining cases of sexually abused children identified by CPS is unknown at this time. Our knowledge base is in danger of remaining incomplete until some mechanism is developed to share information and improve communication among professionals.

## THEORETICAL BASIS FOR COMMUNITY INTERVENTION

The literature is replete with descriptions of risk factors for family violence and child abuse. Many cite the interplay between various factors including cyclical violence (children who grew up in a violent environment and experienced child abuse are more likely to grow up to be child or wife abusers), socioeconomic status, social stress within families, and social isolation (Gelles, 1982). Others have cited factors intrinsic to the child that are instrumental in child abuse including prematurity (Maden & Wrench, 1977), low birth weight (Park & Collmer, 1975), handicaps, retarded or delayed development (Steinmetz, 1978), congenital defects, psychomotor retardation, hyperactivity, chronic illness (Thompson, 1983), and children whose parents perceive them as different from other children (Steinmetz, 1978). Lastly, certain environmental factors are considered instrumental in the development of violence toward children such as large family size (Straus, Gelles, & Steinmetz, 1980), lack of parental attachment to child, low job satisfaction, alcohol abuse, and economic stresses (Gelles, 1982; Levy & Sheldon, 1984).

It must be noted, however, that none of the factors cited have been proven to be absolute predictors of child abuse or neglect. Child abuse is an interactional event (Kadushin & Martin, 1981) combining risks and vulnerabilities of the host, agent, and environment. Garbarino (1982) discusses the concept of vulnerabilities rather than risk as being an earlier determinant in child maltreatment. He states that "the vulnerable parent is one who need not become high risk unless conditions conspire to exploit or attack the parent. It is on the foundation of vulnerability that risk is built by environmental circumstances" (p. 45).

It is upon this foundation of vulnerabilities, as described by Garbarino, that we have developed a theoretical matrix to assess the likelihood of abuse in a given family over time. If proven functional, it will provide a practical basis for community intervention in the violent home.

Child abuse events do not appear to be isolated phenomena (Kadushin & Martin, 1981). They are stimulated by events which cascade into violent interactions. Most experts agree that there is a constant and varying interaction between the child, parents, and environment that may lead to abuse or neglect. Most descriptions of this dynamic milieu include only one or two dimensions. An ecological paradigm, however, requires a four dimensional analysis. The role of the child in the genesis of abuse is well supported in the literature. From the earliest parent-child interaction, the child is responsible for shaping and modifying parental behavior according to the child's behavioral, genetic and emotional makeup. Children (even the youngest infant) exhibit characteristics that are additive to the vulnerability of the situation. Some of these vulnerabilities include prematurity, behavior disorders, sleep disturbances, and congenital defects (see Table 1). Parental vulnerabilities might include a recent separation or divorce, economic hardship, aggressive personality, low self-esteem, and dependency (see Table 2). The child's vulnerabilities can exacerbate a parental vulnerability, increasing tension and interpersonal stress. Conversely, a lack of vulnerabilities may defuse a potentially violent interchange. The environment, comprised of the people, services, mores, values, and beliefs within the family's neighborhood, town/city, society, and culture, also has its vulnerabilities, which exist concomitantly with the parent's and the child's vulnerabilities. These include sanctioned corporal punishment, poverty, unemployment, lack of assistant housekeeping services, and lack of agency supports (see Table 3). In addition to the child's vulnerabilities, the concreteness of the parental strength, the presence or absence of a vulnerable environmental milieu, and time determine the degree of modification of the parent.

Our framework depicts the three interacting and overlapping spheres of parent, child, and environment existing within and being affected by a neighborhood, town, society, and culture—the ecological unit (see Figure 1). The spheres are constantly changing their characteristics and degree of influence resulting in a dynamic interaction of variables. The smaller

TABLE 1
Child's Vulnerability Factors

1. Hyperactivity
2. Prematurity
3. Low birth weight
4. Low I.Q.
5. Colic
6. Demanding
7. Withdrawn
8. Acquired defect
9. Congenital defect
10. Nonoptimal Brazelton score
11. Genetic abnormality
12. Chronic illness
13. Difficult, irritating behavior
14. Tense, high strung
15. Increased intensity of reactions
16. Irregularity of reactions and behavior
17. Indifferent
18. Adopted
19. Dependent
20. Emotional unresponsiveness
21. Habits which get on parent's nerves
22. Separation
23. Tantrums
24. Nightmares
25. Sleep disturbances
26. Child seen as worse than others

spheres revolve within two larger ones: the society and the culture in which the family exists.

Characteristics of the child, the parents, and the environment may be placed on separate axes of a three dimensional model (see Figure 2). A matrix may then be established containing eight separate cells in three dimensions. The spheres of family, individuals within the family, environment, culture, and society reside within the matrix. Environmental vulnerability factors are placed on the x axis, child vulnerabilities on the y axis, and parental vulnerabilities on the z axis. Therefore, environmental factors move the ecologic unit from right to left within the matrix; child factors move the unit from top to bottom and parental factors move the unit from front to back. The construct assumes a dynamic nature of interrelationships. Constantly the ecological unit is changing and segments

TABLE 2
Parental Vulnerability Factors

---

 1. Anxiousness
 2. Aggressiveness
 3. Suspicious of others
 4. Dependent
 5. Less able to seek support from others
 6. Less nurtured as children
 7. Poor understanding of parenting
 8. Do not encourage reciprocity with child
 9. Frustration of dependency needs
10. Psychopathology
11. Low self-esteem
12. Low satisfaction with family life
13. Depression
14. Impulsiveness
15. Identity problems
16. Low intelligence
17. Self-centered
18. Marital strife
19. Frequent job changes
20. Alcoholism
21. Abused or neglected as child
22. Look to children to satisfy own needs
23. Jealousy
24. Inability to deal with child's needs
25. Inappropriate demands on child
26. Lack of knowledge of child development
27. Expectations too high for developmental level of child
28. Lack of consistent positive reinforcement
29. Use of extremes of physical punishment
30. Easily upset or angry
31. Use of threats and complaints
32. Use of broad range of discipline techniques
33. Single parent
34. Young parent
35. Less frequent interactions with child
36. More negative interactions with child
37. Separation of parent and child
38. Poor health
39. Recent separation or divorce
40. Economic hardship

---

TABLE 3
Environmental Vulnerability Factors

1. Sanctioned use of force in society
2. Separation
3. Unstable marriage
4. Divorce
5. Unemployment
6. Poverty
7. Lack of agency supports
8. Inability to seek supports
9. Child labor
10. Young marriage
11. Children thought of as property
12. Sanctioned corporal punishment
13. Social isolation
14. Absent extended family
15. Cultural practices of brutality as initiation rites
16. Lack of assistant housekeeping services

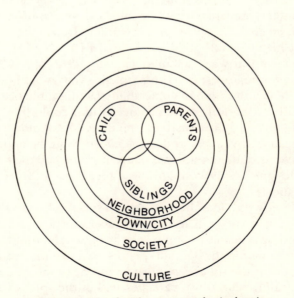

*Figure 1.* The family as an ecological unit

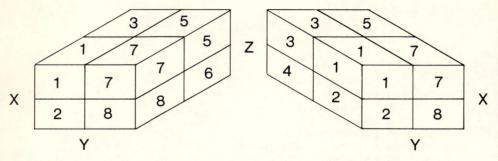

*Figure 2*. Environmental (x), child (y) and parent (z) vulnerabilities to child abuse

are influencing each other. These interactions vary from time to time, resulting in fluid movement between cells. At an isolated point in time, the position within the cells might be identified. With the addition of the variable of time, the direction of movement might be approximated. When vulnerability factors are qualitatively added to the construct (" + " meaning the presence of vulnerability factors and " – " meaning the absence of vulnerability factors), the cells may be defined as in Table 4.

Situational analysis may then predict that a violent act against the child would most likely occur when the ecological unit approaches or lies within cell number six in which all vulnerability factors are present. The risk would be high when the unit lies within cells 4, 5, or 8, and the direction of movement is toward cell number six. Cells 2, 3, and 7 represent lower risk while the lowest risk for a violent event would occur in cell number one. If quantification of vulnerability factors could be established, the mathematical location of the ecological unit could be determined. When time is added to the construct, the direction of movement might also be elucidated. If velocity and acceleration could be approximated, a mechanism for quantitative analysis of a family unit and their vulnerability could be designed. This would provide a reproducible mechanism for accurate diagnosis.

The community provides the cultural and social spheres within which the ecological unit revolves. If accurate diagnosis can be made, community resources must be available to impact on the vulnerabilities. Intervention must come from within the defined spheres; external interventions, that is, those outside of the spheres requiring modification, are generally ineffective in dealing with those variables within the spheres.

## IMPLICATIONS FOR RESEARCH,
## SERVICE AND SOCIAL POLICY

This chapter has suggested a number of points relative to how communities do and should respond to violence against children. Some of these points have their origins in empirical work; others are an outgrowth

TABLE 4

| Cell | Definition | Analysis |
|------|-----------|----------|
| 1 | child (c) – parent (p) – environment (e) – | *Lowest Risk Cell:* absence of all vulnerabilities. |
| 2 | c + p – e – | *Low Risk Cell:* the vulnerable child is in a nurturant, low-risk environment with strong parents exhibiting minimal vulnerabilities. |
| 3 | c – p + e – | *Low Risk Cell:* the vulnerable parent is in a supportive environment and the child manifests minimal vulnerabilities. |
| 4 | c + p + e – | *High Risk Cell:* the vulnerable parent is faced with a difficult child who manifests his or her own significant vulnerabilities. However, the environment is supportive. With minimal change in environmental factors, an abusive or neglectful event may occur. |
| 5 | c – p + e + | *High Risk Cell:* parental vulnerabilities are high and the environment is not supportive. However, the child is *not* manifesting behavior or characteristics that might precipitate an abusive event. |
| 6 | c + p + e + | *Highest Risk Cell:* parental vulnerabilities are high as are the child's. The environment is not supportive and the risk of a violent act occurring is great. |
| 7 | c – p – e + | *Low Risk Cell:* parent's and child's vulnerabilities are minimal. Though the environment is not supportive, parent's and child's strengths reduce the risk of a violent event. |
| 8 | c + p – e + | *High Risk Cell:* The child manifests significant vulnerabilities and the environment is not supportive. The absence of violent acts relate to the concreteness of parental strengths. Minimal changes in the vulnerability of the parents might precipitate a violent act. |

of direct practice in community settings, responding to the victims and the perpetrators of violence. As we review this chapter several major areas stand out as the most important in thinking *how things might be different for children*.

## Multivariable Matrix

Considerable empirical work to date suggests that there are a number of factors associated with violence within the home. These variables have been identified in a host of research studies addressing the specific aspects of violence in individual family members and communities. Much additional empirical work is still needed to understand the specific combination of intraindividual, interpersonal, and community variables associated with the various types of violence. Current knowledge supports the matrix suggested previously in this chapter as an organizing framework.

## Service Implications

Preliminary as it may be, the matrix suggests a number of specific service interventions that can potentially reduce the vulnerabilities associated with violence within the home. While many of these interventions are of unproven significance, there is sufficient reason to assume that some are in fact change producing enough to warrant further investigation.

## Violence is the Problem of the 1980s

Every statistic supports the belief that interpersonal violence is the problem of the 1980s. The direct cost of violence in terms of individual and social responses to injury, and the disruption of individual and family life, combined with the costs of intervention by various professionals, has not been calculated. It is likely that it may be beyond meaningful comprehension. The indirect costs in terms of suffering, lost potential, decrease in productivity and allocation of some of the assumed costs of violence (e.g., juvenile delinquency) is likely to be incalculable.

## Implications

In this final section of the chapter, we would like to discuss some of the implications of the issues we have raised. We have attempted to focus on those issues that can be responded to in the immediate future. Our intent is to discuss those issues that can potentially result in practical actions to reduce violence against children.

## Research

The call for more research is almost obligatory in a chapter such as this. As pressure for available funds has significantly increased in the last five years, federal and state funding for research has dramatically decreased. This has resulted in a situation in which the very real needs of abused children and their families must be weighted against the need to understand more about the causative factors. The battle this creates between service providers and researchers is unfortunate. It strikes us as an indication that the survival of individual groups and the preservation of turf may be more important than the desire to reduce violence. Although we are mindful of competition for funding those activities that impact on the suffering of children and their families versus the longer range research activities useful in preventing future suffering, we believe there are a number of research activities of immediate concern:

*Cost of violence.* Calculating the cost of violence in terms of the direct and indirect consequences is likely to require considerable creativity. Nevertheless, if reasonable cost-estimating procedures can be developed, the forthcoming information will be extremely helpful in making future social-policy decisions concerning the reduction of family violence.

*Empirical description of the community's response.* As we described previously in this chapter, there are clear ideas about how community systems should respond to the violent home. What remains unclear is whether present community responses conform to the existing models for coordinated interagency actions. It is also unclear whether the systems actually perform their roles as described in these models. Practical research is needed that describes the manner and consequences of the way communities actually handle cases of violence against children. This research should identify those factors that support and those that impede the operation of a coordinated, victim-sensitive community.

*Outcome studies.* Little data are available concerning the power of individual or aggregate interventions to actually reduce the incidence of violence against children. Although there are a number of potentially effective intervention strategies, little available data support the actual effectiveness of these interventions. As the pressure for existing funds increases, it is likely that available research monies will be diverted to interventions that have demonstrated effectiveness.

*Etiological research.* In terms of developing long-range strategies directed at decreasing violence against children, additional research on the causes and factors associated with the development and maintenance of violence is essential. Much of the research to date has focused on a limited set of variables, which often reflect only individual or intrafamily variables. The matrix outlined earlier in this chapter suggests that etiological research addressing a wider range of individual, familial, and community variables may be more successful in identifying factors associated with the development of violence.

## Services

A need for more services to violent homes is apparent, but may remain unavailable for the foreseeable future, in light of the present budgetary constraints and priorities. Decisions about which services should be offered to violent homes is hampered by the lack of data describing the effects of those various services. Equally problematic is the general lack of understanding about how the current social service and mental health service delivery systems actually operate. It is imperative that as we are faced with fewer available services, we develop an efficient and compassionate method of selecting clients and assuring access. Presently, access to services appears to be based more on the individual discretion of social service workers than on any organized plan within the social service departments of most states. This state of affairs suggests a number of implications:

*Investigative protocols.* Most state social service departments limit their policies and procedures to investigative formats (e.g., how soon after a report is filed must an investigation be concluded or what specific forms must be completed by what date). A more productive approach might be to determine which factors should be considered in investigating a report of violence against a child. Most notably missing in many CPS investigations is a systematic assessment of psychosocial variables (e.g., vulnerabilities thought to be associated with the risk for violence). The development of assessment strategies that incorporate these risk factors and the subsequent training of CPS workers to conduct such assessments are likely to be quite helpful in the early identification of cases at risk for more serious violence.

*Decision-making criteria.* Although there are few data describing the operation of the multidisciplinary community response system, experience suggests that this system often operates in a capricious manner. Variations in individual case decisions are determined more by which worker has the case than by any internal aspects of the case itself. It appears that cases are often handled in a manner that violates good case management principles and community-developed models. This state of affairs suggests that detailed decision-making criteria should be developed and employed by each system. These criteria should assist each system in making appropriate decisions and ensure that cooperation and coordination across systems actually occurs.

Many communities have also found that the establishment of multidisciplinary review teams, which periodically review case decisions, can be helpful in improving the operation and efficiency of the community's response to these cases. This concept should be expanded to allow individual workers to request consultation from these review teams and external experts, as well as to periodically identify difficult cases for review.

## Policy

The implementation of any policy intended to reduce the incidence of violence against children will require substantial efforts to alter the present trends of our federal and state policymakers. It is mandatory that our legislators understand that further reductions in social and economic supports for children and their families are counterproductive and possibly catastrophic. The recognition that violence against children is the result of a number of factors is implicit in developing a compassionate and practical solution. The vulnerabilities that appear to be related to violence against children cannot be resolved by establishing computerized central registries. These registries identify cases of abuse but are unable to provide the necessary services needed to reduce or eliminate the risk to children and their families.

Perhaps more fundamentally, society must make essential decisions about whether it is willing to carry out those activities that are likely to reduce the vulnerabilities associated with abuse. Recent history suggests that society may not be willing to make that commitment.

# REFERENCES

Caffey, J. (1946). Multiple fractures in the long bones of infants suffering from chronic subdural hematomas. *American Journal of Roentgenology, 56*, 163–173.
Conte, J. R. (1984). The justice system and sexual abuse of children. Social Service Review, University of Chicago, Dec., 556–568.
Conte, J. R., & Berliner, L. (1981). Prosecution of the offender in cases of sexual assault against children. *Victimology, 6*, 102–109.
DeMause, L. (1974). *The history of childhood*. New York: Harper & Row.
Fontana, V. J., & Besharov, D. J. (1979). *The maltreated child*. Springfield: Charles C Thomas.
Garbarino, J. (1982). Healing the social wounds of isolation. In E. H. Newberger (Ed.), *Child abuse* (pp. 43–55). Boston: Little, Brown, & Co.
Gelles, R. J. (1982). Child abuse and family violence: Implications for medical professionals. In E. H. Newberger (Ed.), *Child abuse* (pp. 25–41). Boston: Little, Brown & Company.
Helfer, R. E. (1975). Why most physicians don't get involved in child abuse cases and what to do about it. *Children Today, 4*, 28–32.
Kadushin, A., & Martin, J. (1981). Child abuse as an interactional event. In A. Kadushin & J. Martin (Eds.), *Child abuse: An interactional event* (pp. 47–89). New York: Columbia University Press.
Kempe, C. H., Silverman, F. N., Steele, B. F., et al. (1962). The battered child syndrome. *Journal of the American Medical Association, 181*, 17–24.
Levy, H. B., & Sheldon, S. H. (1984). A hospital's response to the increasing incidence of child abuse and neglect in an inner-city population. *The Mount Sinai Journal of Medicine, 51*(2), 161–165.
Levy, H. B., & Sheldon, S. H. (1985). *Prepubescent sexual abuse*. Submitted for publication.
Levy, H. B., Sheldon, S. H., & Ahart, S. L. (In preparation). *Chlamydia trachomatis infections in sexually abused children*.
Maden, M. F., & Wrench, D. F. (1977). Significant findings in child abuse research. *Victimology, 2*(2), 196–224.
Park, R. D., & Collmer, C. W. (1975). Child abuse: An interdisciplinary analysis. In M. Heatherington (Ed.), *Review of child development research* (Vol. 5). Chicago: University of Chicago Press.
Sheldon, S. H., & Levy, H. B. (In preparation). *Physician resistance to child abuse reporting*.
Silverman, F. N. (1953). The roentgen manifestations of unrecognized skeletal trauma in infants. *American Journal of Roentgenology, 69*, 413–427.
Steinmetz, S. K. (1978). Violence between family members. *Marriage Fam. Rev., 1*(3), 1–16.
Straus, M. A., Gelles, R. J., & Steinmetz, S. K. (1980). *Behind closed doors: Violence in the American family*. New York: Anchor Press.
Thompson, M. (1983). Organizing a human service network for primary and secondary prevention of the emotional and physical neglect and abuse of children. In J. E. Leavitt (Ed.), *Child abuse and neglect: Research and innovation* (pp. 49–73). The Hague, The Netherlands, Martinus Nijhoff Publishers.

# 9

# *Special Intervention Programs for Child Witnesses to Violence*

## Robert S. Pynoos and Spencer Eth

( Children who witness extreme acts of violence represent a population at significant risk of developing anxiety, depressive, phobic, conduct, and post-traumatic stress disorders.)Consequently, there is a need to investigate the nature and the course of children's reactions and to develop methods of early preventive interventions.

During the past four years, we have completed pilot investigations of the traumatic consequences for children who witness any of three types of violence likely to have the greatest personal impact on a child: 1) the murder of a parent; 2) the rape of a mother; and 3) the suicidal act of a parent. Witnessing such events resulted in signs and symptoms of post-traumatic stress in nearly 80% of some 100 uninjured child witnesses we have studied. Recent findings suggest that these psychological consequences for traumatized children may persist for years (Terr, 1984). The post-traumatic stress disorder (PTSD) symptoms in child witnesses can also become chronic, and the children can benefit from prompt psychological assistance. Work with this group of children is of special importance because the psychological needs of child witnesses are commonly neglected by the family, school, law enforcement agencies and mental health professionals.

In this chapter is presented an overall plan of how to assist these children. Different therapeutic approaches are discussed including direct work with the child, working therapeutically through family members, interventions at school, and mental health consultation with law enforce-

This chapter was supported by funds provided by the Robert E. Simon Foundation. Editorial assistance was provided by Margaret Kelly.

ment agencies. General principles are outlined that underlie work with the child in any of these settings, and issues specific to each therapeutic avenue are addressed.

## EXPOSURE TO VIOLENCE

In discussions of violence in the home, the primary attention has been on spouse beating and child abuse. As evidenced by other contributions to this volume, the extent of domestic violence in our society has been unappreciated and the psychological consequences for the victim too often ignored. It should also be recognized that these violent acts also result in an even larger number of child witnesses (Pfouts, Schopler, & Henley, 1982) and that other violent acts in the home—for example, parental suicidal behavior—are often overlooked completely as a source of emotional trauma to the child. Furthermore, children are also exposed to many violent crimes in their homes and neighborhood (i.e., armed robbery, homicide, or rape) that do not necessarily prompt any social service or mental health intervention.

Within the past 20 years, the rate of violent crime in the United States has increased dramatically in relationship to other Western countries, reaching what may be deemed as "an epidemic of violence" (West, 1984). As of 1980, the estimated homicides per year exceeded 24,000 (Center for Disease Control, 1984). Of these, at least 40% were the result of domestic violence. The Sheriff's Homicide Division of Los Angeles County (personal communication, 1984) estimates that dependent children witness between 10% and 20% of the approximately 2,000 annual homicides in their jurisdiction. If a similar exposure rate applies to other urban areas, then several thousand children per year witness a murder and, commonly, the victim is one of their parents.

In 1980, there were over 77,000 reported rapes outside of marriage in the United States (Center for Disease Control, 1984). In contrast to homicide, rape is seriously underreported. Recent household surveys indicate that, at a minimum, there is a 10 : 1 ratio of unreported to reported rapes, with an estimated annual incidence of approximately 800,000 rapes. Forty percent of all rape victims are in the 20- to 39-year old, child-bearing age group, and over 40% of all rapes occur in the home. Thousands of children each year may therefore be exposed to the rape of their mother. In Los Angeles County alone, Sergeant Beth Dickerson (Chair, California Association of Sexual Assault Investigators) estimates that children are in the home when a rape occurs as much as 50% of the time, and that children directly view the assault in approximately 10% of the cases reported to the Sheriff's office (B. Dickerson, personal communication, 1984).

Suicide and suicidal behavior are violent acts, and as such, present a major source of childhood exposure to violence. There is evidence of an epidemic increase in the prevalence of suicide attempts in the United States and other Western countries during the past several decades, although the rate of actual suicides has remained stationary (Weissman, 1974). Although this increase in suicide attempts is most notable in married women (Aitkens, Buglass, & Kreitman, 1969), studies using general population comparisons (Weissman, 1974) reveal a statistical excess also of separated and divorced persons of both sexes among those who attempt suicide. Given the increase in parental suicide behavior, the likelihood of a child witnessing some portion of this form of violence has itself increased dramatically in recent years, so that many thousands of children each year are directly or indirectly exposed to the suicidal behavior of a parent.

### POST-TRAUMATIC STRESS DISORDER (PTSD): A DEVELOPMENTAL MODEL

It is important to adopt a four-category approach to childhood trauma in designing a therapeutic plan of intervention with a child exposed to a violent act (see Table 1). First, one must recognize the phenomenology of violence-related PTSD, that is, those symptoms that unavoidably result from a traumatic state. Second, one must delineate those early efforts by the child to master the anxiety or avoid its renewal, including efforts to assure him- or herself that the violence will not recur. Third, one must examine the possible mediating influences that enhance or adversely affect trauma resolution. These include a number of child-intrinsic factors as well as additional environmental stresses. And last, one must anticipate that the demands of trauma mastery will have an impact on the child. One must monitor that impact to determine whether trauma resolution significantly influences current childhood tasks and future development by hindering normal progression or prematurely propelling the child into more mature roles.

*Phenomenology*

Child witnesses to a parent's homicide, rape, or suicidal behavior frequently demonstrate symptomatology fulfilling the four major DSM-III (American Psychiatric Association, 1980) criteria for PTSD: 1) the per-

Table 1

Goals of Evaluation and Treatment Planning

1. Recognize phenomenology of violence-related PTSD
2. Elucidate methods employed to contend with traumatic anxiety
3. Enumerate factors that enhance or adversely affect trauma resolution
4. Explore influence of trauma resolution on childhood tasks

ceived presence of a distressing, traumatic event: children will often describe the event as so upsetting as never to be forgotten; 2) reexperiencing of the occurrence: in young children this frequently takes the form of traumatic play and dreams as well as intrusive images or sounds; 3) psychic numbing or affective constriction: children may exhibit subdued or mute behavior, or commonly adopt an unemotional or third-person, nearly journalistic attitude toward the event; 4) incident-specific phenomena that were previously not present. Children are as likely as adults to suffer from startle reactions and avoidant behavior linked to trauma-specific reminders and they may be especially susceptible to sleep disturbances (Frederick, 1983). Distinct phase-specific features of PTSD in children affect the clinical presentation and course of recovery. These developmental factors influence the child's capacity to cope with the distress and to contend with traumatic anxiety (Eth & Pynoos, 1984).

One important goal of any therapeutic work with a victim or witness of violence is to help identify those traumatic reminders that elicit psychophysiologic reactions and intense perceptual or affective responses. Fear and avoidance of renewed traumatic anxiety associated with these environmental or ideational stimuli are related to the appearance and chronicity of incident-specific symptoms. Therefore, generalities about the violent event cannot substitute for a full exploration of the violent occurrence and the surrounding circumstances.

### Mastery/Management of Traumatic Anxiety

Mastery/management is an area of special interest in our research. There are as yet no taxonomies of coping for children comparable to those available for adults (Garmezy, 1983). We have been interested in both the child's cognitive and emotional efforts to cope with traumatic anxiety and helplessness. Insights into these processes have contributed significantly to our understanding of how to conduct therapeutic interviews with children traumatized by acts of violence.

We have found four common psychological methods employed by school-age children for limiting traumatic anxiety in the immediate weeks or months after a violent occurrence:

1) By denial-in-fantasy the child tries to mitigate painful reality by imaginatively reversing the injurious outcome.
2) By the inhibition of spontaneous thought the child works to avoid reminders of the violent actions.
3) In "fixation to the trauma," evidenced by incomplete, journalistic recountings of the event, the child hopes to make the harmful occurrence more tolerable through reiteration.
4) In his or her preoccupation with fantasies of future harm, the child avoids directly addressing the initial violence by supplanting the memories of the occurrence with new fears.

These strategies of emotional coping may persist or remit, only to reappear with traumatic reminders.

The child witness may be mentally involved with continued cognitive reappraisals of the actions of all participants and witnesses to the violent act. To offset his or her traumatic helplessness, the child must consider, if only in fantasy, alternate actions that could have prevented the occurrence, interrupted the violence before harm was done, reversed the physical harm, or gained safe retaliation. What is remarkable about the "inner plans of action" (Lifton, 1979) of the child witness is the dominance of fantasies of third-part intervention, either directly by the child or by another person. Intervention fantasies may also serve as a continuing source of self-blame for not having done more and result in post-traumatic guilt. Developmental considerations are important determinants of these cognitive efforts (Eth & Pynoos, 1984) and familiarity with the phase-specific cognitive capacities is essential to effective therapeutic interventions.

As has been pointed out in various discussions of adult coping, generalities across different types of stressful events may prove inadequate because of the importance of situational influences (Abramson, Garber, & Seligman, 1980). Particular tasks of mastery may be associated with the psychological challenge presented by each specific type of violence. For instance, in cases of mutilating injury to the parent, the child witness may engage in efforts to restore an image of the parent as physically intact in his or her efforts to contend with the memories of the visual horror.

## Mediating Influences

Many previous discussions of childhood trauma have placed too much emphasis on whether premorbid factors put a child at greater risk of being traumatized. We would rather place the emphasis on uncovering those factors that enhance or impede the recovery phase. In our clinical appraisal of the child in the immediate aftermath of a violent trauma we recognize the influence of each of the following post-trauma influences:

1) Preexisting psychopathology
2) Preexisting stress or conflict
3) Recovery from physical injury
4) Family circumstances and adequacy of social support
5) Available emotional assistance to child
6) Parental or guardian psychopathology
7) New stresses secondary to traumatic event
8) Issues of assigning human accountability
9) Conflict of loyalty involving significant others
10) Previous experience with violent trauma
11) Demands of criminal or civil proceedings

The task of trauma mastery is extremely demanding and requires considerable psychological effort and attention of the child. Therefore, any factor that reduces the child's capacity or opportunity to focus on this all-important task may lead to maladaptive resolution or prolongation of symptomatology. Child-intrinsic factors—for instance, the presence of an attention-deficit disorder—may interfere by distracting the child from being able to maintain the needed sustained attention even within the therapeutic consultation.

As recognized with adults, post-traumatic stress disorders are apparently more severe and longer lasting when a stressor is of "human design" (American Psychiatric Association, 1980), especially in the case of human-induced violence (Frederick, 1980). As we have observed, struggles over assigning human accountability may add considerably to the child's traumatic burden after witnessing an extreme act of violence. Blame may be easy to assign, as in the case of a stranger-assailant; but the effort may cause an intense conflict of loyalty if a parent is to be held at fault. The violence may prompt fantasies of revenge or an identification with the aggressor that can seriously jeopardize the child's confidence in his or her own impulse control and create fears of counter-retaliations.

The presence of significant psychopathology in the child's guardian or caretaker can jeopardize the child's own efforts to achieve an adaptive resolution of the trauma. For example, in one case, the psychotic delusions of the grandmother-guardian of a four-year-old girl seriously interfered with the child's efforts to maintain reality testing about her mother's murder. Furthermore, the anxieties or fears of the parent or guardian can easily be communicated to the child and the child's course of recovery may depend on that of the parent or guardian (Mercier & Despert, 1943; Silber, Perry, & Bloch, 1958).

Extrinsic factors may require the child to turn his or her attention elsewhere in the acute aftermath or may interfere with spontaneous efforts to achieve some psychological closure. Many violent events cause an immediate upheaval in the child's life: unexpected separation from parents, dislocation of family residence, change of schools, increased family discord, and required participation in criminal proceedings. These additional stresses can deplete the child's inner resources.

### Impact on the Child

Finally, there is need to monitor the following important interactions between the task of trauma mastery and the ongoing developmental processes:

1) immediate developmental issues
2) effect on cognition and learning
3) effect on affective life—the child's view of the stability or nature of human relationships
4) developmental progression—accentuation, premature closure or regression
5) interaction of trauma and grief in cases of lethal violence
6) future orientation—change of life attitude, selection or restriction of life choices

Young children are likely to demonstrate an increase in anxious attachment behavior and other regressive symptomatology (Bowlby, 1977; Elizur & Kaufman, 1982; Thomas & Chess, 1977). School-age children are more likely to react to traumatic violence with aggressive or inhibited behavior and with psychosomatic complaints. Adolescents may embark upon a period of post-traumatic acting-out behavior expressed by school truancy, precocious sexual activity, substance abuse and delinquency.

Exposure to violence can cause deleterious effects on cognition, including memory, school performance and learning (Bowlby, 1979; Cain

& Fast, 1972; Gardner, 1971). Significant alterations in personality after traumatic childhood events have also been reported (Gislason & Call, 1982). These alterations can include both counterphobic and inhibitory features. Further, children may develop radically new views about the safety and security of human relations as well as their own future. Children may envision a foreshortened future adult life as Terr (1979) reported or, as we have found, a need to live in a fortressed environment and avoid intimate interpersonal relationships, including marriage. This change in future orientation may be one of the most significant markers of childhood trauma.

If the violence results in the death of the parent then the child is faced with the dual task of trauma mastery and bereavement. As we have observed, there is an important interplay between these two psychological demands on the child. Traumatic issues related to the violence commonly interfere with the mourning process and, therefore, increase the risk of pathological or aborted grief (Eth & Pynoos, 1985).

## ANALOGOUS MODEL

In searching for an analogous model of therapeutic trauma consultation, we have been impressed with the resemblance between our technique and that adopted by military psychiatrists for the treatment of soldiers who have viewed a buddy killed or maimed in combat (Fox, 1974; Glass, 1947, 1954; Grinker & Spiegel, 1943; Kardiner, 1941; Lifton, 1979). The common principles include:

1) the finding that the witnessing of extreme violence constitutes a unique, severe psychic trauma;
2) the importance of "front-line" intervention before maladaptive ego resolution is organized;
3) since "ego constriction" is a primary consequence of the trauma, the direction of major efforts at ego restitution and coping enhancement;
4) the understanding that mastery requires an affectively experienced "reliving," including a comprehensive review of the traumatic event;
5) full exploration of aggressive themes, especially retaliation fantasies which threaten ego restoration;
6) relieving the demands of an "outraged superego" which responds to the passivity of the trauma experience by insisting that more should have been done to save the victim;

7) appreciation that absent or pathological grief results from efforts to avoid reevoking traumatic anxiety; and

8) recognition that sustained mastery can be achieved only through reintegration into the group, family or community.

### EARLY ACCESS

Children have been a forgotten lot in our expanding knowledge of the aftereffects of severe trauma and the need for early intervention. Adult clinical experience as well as current theories of post-traumatic stress reveal an urgent need to intervene at the earliest occasion possible. Only during the acute phase after the traumatic event can one observe the manifest appearance of the traumatic anxiety and easily identify the incident-specific traumatic reminders from which the individual seeks psychological protection.

With the passage of time the two most important psychological consequences, the contraction of ego functioning and the dulling of one's emotional life, result in maladaptive trauma resolution. Consistent with the clinical findings of Grinker and Spiegel (1943) in their work with traumatized soldiers, we have observed, for example, that when we have consulted with a child some years after witnessing his or her parent's murder, the traumatic references are much more disguised in their projective drawing and story-telling. Attention can still be directed toward the traumatic references, but even when we are as thorough in our exploration of the traumatic experience, the emotional release or restoration of spontaneous affect so observable during the acute phase is often not nearly so apparent.

Soon after we began our studies we discovered that children exposed to extreme acts of violence rarely receive any prompt psychological help. Our interest in homicide began after one child was referred for treatment some months after his mother had been murdered. When we contacted the investigating officers, we discovered that there were several more children in their active homicide files who had witnessed a parent's killing. We also learned that the homicide detectives in such cases often acted as reluctant family advisors with family members asking the assigned police officer, for instance, if a child should attend the funeral. The officers themselves, fully aware of the horror and mutilation of a murder scene, expressed their concern for the psychological welfare of the child witnesses. We were able to see these other affected children without encountering significant resistance from the officers, the families or the children themselves.

Since all homicides are reported to law enforcement we began to contact the police and sheriff's departments. The officers and detectives specializing in homicide were receptive to our overtures and several meetings were scheduled. Eventually, we were invited to lecture at the police academy about the importance of our work and the critical role the police play for the child exposed to violence. We also obtained the interest of the Sheriff of the County of Los Angeles, Sherwood Bloch, who sent a memorandum to his Homicide Division supporting our work and inviting the officers to have families contact us.

We then approached the District Attorney's Office. Prosecutors tended to be cautious about psychiatric involvement, in part because of their fear that we might unduly influence and thereby contaminate criminal witnesses. However, they soon came to recognize that therapeutic interventions produced a less traumatized, more verbal and, therefore, potentially more effective child witness. We also presented our work to a meeting of all of the assistant district attorneys. In the end we were able to follow the referred children throughout subsequent criminal proceedings without objection from the prosecutors, who allowed us not only to help prepare children for courtroom testimony but also to conduct post-testimony follow-ups.

We were most successful in gaining a cooperative alliance with the Victim-Witness Assistance Programs operated from the City and County District Attorneys Offices. The Victim-Witness Assistance counselors were active in notifying us of appropriate children, securing parental consent, and bringing the children to sessions. These programs can also fund treatment of eligible children. In addition, we worked closely with the county child protective service. Child victims of violence frequently require immediate placement and other concrete services, and the child's case-worker remains a critical person in arranging for care.

School psychological counseling services serve as another important source of referral. Since a change in school behavior and performance may be one of the earliest observed effects of acute trauma, these school psychologists have an important role to play in early case detection and in liaison with classroom teachers, school administration, and the children's families. Nevertheless, school personnel often overlook the link between the emergence of acute conduct disturbances or school failure and some violent disturbance at home or in the community. School psychologists welcomed special training in recognizing the signs and symptoms of trauma in children exposed to violence, and in the availability of experts for consultation. Our work with individual schools led to a meeting of school psychologists within the Los Angeles Unified School

District and we hope to develop means to monitor children in school for signs of an acute exposure so that prompt assistance or consultation can be implemented.

More recently, we have expanded our contacts with the Los Angeles rape-response network. As the data presented earlier in this paper suggest, many children are exposed to sexual assaults of their mother. Although the rape victim herself often receives counseling, no inquiry is made routinely about whether any children were present during the attack. An important opportunity for intervention with the victim's children is therefore lost. However, as attention is brought within this network to these overlooked children, we have slowly begun to receive referrals.

Our work with children exposed to parental suicide behavior has primarily been hospital-based. The original study involved consulting with the families and direct interviews with children whenever a parent was hospitalized for a first-known suicide attempt. Most of the attempts may well have been lethal if not for fortunate intervention. In more than half of these cases, a child was involved in discovering the suicidal parent. To our surprise, even though the hospital units placed a major emphasis on family therapy, rarely was any attention placed on the aftereffects on the child members of the family. The study found a great degree of apprehension and overidentification with the child among mental health professionals; they did not wish to become aware of the traumatic consequences for the children.

As a result of our work to establish prompt referrals from all of the agencies mentioned, we have been able to see some children as early as the first day of a parental murder, and in most cases, within the first few weeks after the violent occurrence. The opportunity to conduct a therapeutic consultation with children and their families necessitated the development of an interview format designed to meet the special needs of these acutely traumatized children. The format had to have generic application and address those issues common to exposure to violent events. The interview we devised has undergone a series of revisions as our experience has grown, and particularly as we have learned from the children's own comments in review of the consultation.

### Child Interview Techniques

Anyone who has attempted to assist a child recently exposed to an extreme act of violence will understand the difficulty in knowing how to proceed. Direct inquiry about the traumatic event may be unproductive, leaving the interviewer feeling stymied and the child further entrenched in detachment. Family members as well as professional colleagues may fear that direct intervention with the child will only exacerbate the trauma. Our extensive experience, however, supported by the work of several other investigators (Ayalon, 1983; Frederick, in press) confirms that open discussion of the trauma offers immediate relief, not further distress, to the child.

The initial consultation with the child offers a unique opportunity to provide significant assistance to the child, and in many cases, may be the only such occasion in the acute aftermath of the traumatic event. There have been many anecdotal clinical descriptions of trauma work with children. Each demonstrates special considerations in this type of work. From our review of these reports, as well as from more than one hundred interviews we have conducted, we have arrived at some general interview principles that all effective techniques share. Special interview techniques, similar to the one we have developed (Pynoos & Eth, in press), are necessary to permit the child spontaneously and fully to describe his subjective experience and to catalyze constructive efforts to offset the residue of the traumatic helplessness.

In the opening phase, the interviewer allows the child to express the impact of the trauma in play and fantasy and through metaphor—in our version by use of a projective, free drawing and storytelling task. This opening enables the consultant to identify the child's preliminary means of coping and defensive maneuvers and the most likely means to emotionally engage the child in approaching the traumatic experience.

In the trauma phase, the interviewer shifts attention to the actual traumatic episode. In order to foster mastery of the traumatic anxiety, he overcomes the child's efforts to avoid and deny and supports a thorough exploration of the child's experience. Frederick (in press) has suggested that trauma mastery based on the incident-specific experience of the child is the sine qua non of successful resolution of post-traumatic stress symptoms.

In the third and final phase, the consultant can then assist the child in addressing his current life concerns with an increased sense of security, competence and mastery. The consultant is careful to permit closure to the trauma exploration phase and to achieve a proper leavetaking.

*First stage: Opening*
    Establish the focus
    Free drawing and storytelling
    Traumatic reference

*Second stage: Trauma*
A. Reliving the experience
   Emotional release
   Reconstruction
   Perceptual experience
   Special detailing
   Worst moment
   Violence/physical mutilation
B. Coping with the experience
   Issues of human accountability
   Inner plans of action
   Punishment or retaliation
   Fears of counter-retaliation
   Challenge to child's impulse control
   Influence of previous trauma
   Traumatic dreams
   Future orientation
   Current stresses
*Third stage: Closure*
   Recapitulation
   Underscore realistic fears
   Universalize the child's responses
   Describe expectable course
   Acknowledge child's courage in undertaking the interview
   Invite child critique of consultation
   Proper leave-taking

The explicit goal of the therapeutic consultation is to identify the immediate effects of the trauma, with the child's attention and energy reserved exclusively for this role. Sharing the traumatic memories with the consultant begins the process of mastering the experience. By speaking and playing, the child can partially compensate for the passive helplessness of the witness. In addition, the session bolsters the child's observing ego and reality-testing functions, which in turn tend to dispel cognitive confusion and encourage active coping. Rather than dampen all of his or her feelings, the child must regain confidence that he or she is not helpless in the face of his emotions and need not fear either a destructive loss of impulse control or a flood of unbearable emotion.

The key concept in the opening stage is that elements of the violent event remain intrusive and will inevitably appear somewhere in the drawing or story. This traumatic reference must be identified by the interviewer, even though the child may seek to suppress associations to the violence. This projective task provides the interviewer with clues to the sources of the child's anxiety and current means of coping.

The second or trauma stage is marked by the transition from the child's drawing and story to an explicit discussion of the actual event and is a critical moment for both the clinician and child. David Levy (1938) provided the first description of how an "emotional release" occurs when the therapist addresses the child's efforts to cope with recent trauma as exhibited in his imaginative play. Catharsis does not adequately describe the goal of the emotional release. Before the child proceeds to "relive the experience," first he or she must no longer feel as threatened by his or her emotional responses and gain hope that he or she can begin to cope with them.

As the reconstruction continues, the child is directed to maintain a focus on the central action of the violence when physical harm was inflicted. Although a marked increase in anxiety may proceed the child's doing so, afterwards the child appears strengthened in his or her mastery of the trauma. During the exploration, the child will frequently be noted to invest a particular detail with special traumatic meaning. This detail is psychodynamically helpful in pointing toward the child's initial identification. The interviewer also should ask at some point what the worst moment was for the child. Even young children are able to articulate a uniquely painful moment, and will feel especially close to and understood by the therapist. Finally, the impact of the violence can be approached. The child is helped to describe and even draw the actual physical injuries witnessed that may serve as the source of recurrent, intrusive memories which seem difficult to unburden.

After this thorough exploration of the event, the interviewer can discuss with the child a number of issues that relate to the child's coping process. Although the child may refer to the event as an accident, the child nevertheless will struggle with issues of human accountability. The interviewer may wonder aloud, "How come it happened?" or "What would make someone do something like that?" One can then explore the child's immediate efforts to reverse his or her helplessness at the time of the event by later cognitive reappraisals. The child is invited to offer his or her imaginative plans of action that seek to alter the precipitating events, undo the violent act, reverse the lethal or injurious consequences or gain safe retaliation. These cognitive reappraisals often provide important clues to the presence of any post-traumatic guilt experienced by the child.

Many children express particular relief at drawing or acting out their fantasy of punishment or revenge. The child is helped to understand that these fantasies serve to counter the helplessness felt at the time of the event, and express the wish to put to rest any thoughts of further threat. Viewing an open display of aggression may erode the child's trust in adult restraint and cause him or her to fear his or her own ability to handle angry feelings. The child is assisted to distinguish his or her own aggressive impulses from those of the assailant.

Probably the best gauge of the effectiveness of the trauma exploration is that the child will now openly discuss a number of life stresses brought on by the event and display the wish to be an active participant in the decisions being made about his or her care. The interviewer offers to be a child advocate with his or her parents, guardian or social service agency to accomplish some of these goals—for instance, being allowed to have friends from his or her old school visit.

During the closure stage of the interview we underscore the realistic fears associated with danger and normalize the anxiety in reexperiencing the event in the session. In cases of traumatic death, relieving the burden of the intrusive recollections can allow the mourning process to be resumed (Eth & Pynoos, 1985). Because of the precarious position of the traumatized child, the gains accrued during the interview can easily be jeopardized. However, children seem noticeably less alienated after the session, and the human relatedness established with the interviewer can often be transferred to the child's immediate family.

Properly conducted therapeutic consultation can facilitate the child's acceptance of continued or future psychotherapy. The child must not fear his or her capacity to tolerate the occurrence of traumatic anxiety and helplessness in the course of any further psychotherapy, or need for avoidance will prevent him or her from being willing to participate. Follow-up meetings or referrals for formal psychiatric treatment are arranged as indicated.

It should be understood that the interview is designed for use within weeks of the violent act. With the passage of time the method becomes problematic as the traumatic reference grows obscure, memories are repressed and the child becomes increasingly reluctant to face renewed traumatic anxiety. However, even years later a child may be relieved to have a chance to unburden him- or herself, and the therapist may find these interview principles helpful.

In cases of parental death, early therapeutic attention to the trauma of being witness to the violence or its injurious aftermath can have a beneficial effect on the child's mourning and overall outcome. Similar to Lindy et al. (1983), we, too, have been impressed that after proper attention is paid to the traumatic elements, many children will then exhibit a spontaneous progression to open expressions of grief. Children who had previously shown no signs of grief will suddenly begin to cry over the loss, to reminisce with warmth and sadness over memories of the deceased, and to directly seek comfort and aid in addressing the reality of the death and the life changes that have resulted.

*Family Work*

Treatment of young children through the therapeutic assistance of the parents has been an established practice whenever a child develops acute symptomatology after a stressful occurrence. In the case of Little Hans, Freud (1909/1953) described how he conducted the treatment of an acute phobia in a young boy by instructing his parents as to appropriate serial therapeutic interventions. More recently, Schetky (1973) and Pruett et al. (1979) both have reported case examples of the use of parents or guardians to treat children whose parent was murdered. Furman (1981) has fully described the technique of working therapeutically through the family members whenever a child is grieving over the loss of a parent.

All the recommended procedures entail having the parents or guardians give careful reports of the child's behavior and words to the therapist who then advises the family members: first, of ways to elicit more verbal meaning from the child about his responses, and then of any needed steps they can take to ameliorate the continued conflict or stress. Furman describes most clearly how the family member must engage in important affective exchanges with the child to legitimize the child's feelings and to correct cognitive confusions. We have also found this method to be of special importance. However, the clinician has to be especially alert to certain therapeutic issues resulting from violent traumatic experiences that can hinder successful use of family members.

After a violent trauma, family and friends may undergo a period of distress and suffering. During this interval, the child's caretaker may be in a traumatized and, perhaps, grief-stricken state, and may be unable emotionally to meet the challenge of providing the needed emotional support to the child. The child's family may be so preoccupied with personal reactions to the violence that they overlook the special needs of the child, or well-intended family members may seek to shield the child from any potentially upsetting reference to the violence (Schetky, 1973). Furthermore, the stigma attached to the violence may result in family members providing misleading explanations or prohibiting the child's making any mention of the incident.

Prior to our individual interview with the child, we meet with the parent or guardian and discuss the nature of his or her own and the extended family's response. Preparation of the family member often first requires providing some temporary relief to them as well. Their distress may come from unexpected sources. In a number of instances after a parental murder, for example, we have found that the grandparent, who is acting as guardian, is contending with earlier memories of traumatic and violent losses brought back to mind by this incident. One grandmother brought to the first meeting a poem that she'd written years before in memory of a son killed in combat during World War II. Before approaching the more recent violence, she required an opportunity to talk of this earlier violent death.

In studies of children who lived through natural disasters, more resilience was apparently exhibited in children whose families tolerated temporary behavioral regressions and invited verbal discussions of the event and its aftermath (Bloch, Silber, & Perry, 1956). In cases of family trauma, other investigators (Cain & Fast, 1972; Bowlby, 1979) have reported that misleading explanations, conspiracies of silence, and prohibitions against the child mentioning details of the event can all contribute to chronic difficulties in learning and cognition or to an inability to identify accurately one's emotional responses.

Family members may be very unfamiliar with the nature of post-traumatic symptomatology, its appearance, course, and meaning. We have worked with a colleague, Kathy Nader, M.S.W., to devise a questionnaire that allows us to review with the child's caretaker the common behavior alterations that may be observed in the post-trauma period, and in doing so, to provide the caretaker with some immediate clinical education.

One goal of this work with the family is to enhance their willingness and toleration of the child's discussion of the occurrence, not simply in the immediate aftermath, but in the months ahead when anniversary or other traumatic reminders may stimulate renewed recollections. One means we employ is to request the child's permission after the initial individual interview to have the parent or guardian join us, and share with them the disturbing aspects of the event that have remained with the child. In fact, the ego restitution initiated during our therapeutic consultation with the child can be consolidated, expanded and offered as a model for other family members (Polak, Egan, Vandenbergh, & Williams, 1975).

*Liaison with the School*

Liaison with the child's school is essential to any successful intervention program for children exposed to violent acts. Children commonly exhibit changes in school behavior and cognitive performance that serve as key indicators of the traumatic course and recovery. Many of the children we have studied demonstrated the immediate onset of learning disorders related to an inability to concentrate on academic tasks. The cognitive performance difficulties result from the intrusive recollections of and associations to the violent event, the interference of depressive affect, and the evolution of a cognitive style of "forgetting." The behavioral change most noticed by teachers is the unexpected appearance of aggressive behavior that may progress to a conduct disorder. Although less often noticed, nonparticipation and inhibited behavior may also occur. If such changes begin to appear it is important to correctly attribute them to the traumatic consequences and to institute adequate psychological interventions. Although the child's teachers are not likely to be familiar with the signs to look for in the classroom, in our experience they are very interested in gaining the understanding needed to assist the child during the course of acute trauma resolution and to cooperate with the consultant in monitoring the adequacy of recovery.

In addition, when the violent occurrence is public, as in cases of homicide, awareness of the event can precipitate anxiety in other students and teachers, prompt more general classroom changes in behavior, and disrupt the educational process. Fortunately, the structure of a school renders it highly susceptible to outside therapeutic influence. Over the past several years we and our colleagues have developed a group consultation technique for use in elementary and preschool classrooms touched by violence (Eth, Silverstein, & Pynoos, 1984). It is well documented that children will respond symptomatically to a violent tragedy involving a person known to them, from a president to a classmate's parent (Harrison, Davenport, & McDermott, 1967; McDonald, 1964). When that happens, the classroom may be the ideal locus for a group consultation. It has been noted that since children can readily discuss their feelings during structured school activities, this setting offers an opportunity for enhancing coping skills (Bloch, Silber, & Perry, 1956). The group consultation economically addresses both the primary symptom of any anxiety in the children and the secondary loss of school function. The breakdown of classroom cohesion exacerbates stress and, in another context, has been termed a loss of communality (Erikson, 1976). For the directly affected child, the existence of a cohesive, secure and less anxious classroom environment can be of great importance in providing the proper opportunity during the school day for recovery while home life remains unsettled or under severe stress.

## Liaison with the Judicial System

Children who are victims or witnesses of crimes routinely become involved with the judicial system. We have found that there is a continuing interaction between the course of a child's response to a violent crime and the subsequent criminal proceedings (Pynoos & Eth, 1984). The child's efforts at mastering the trauma of being a witness to violent acts can either be enhanced or impeded by required judicial participation. As part of our consultation service, we therefore will follow children from the initial police investigation through testimony in open court and defendent sentencing.

Previous clinical reports (Terr, 1981) have neglected to consider correlations between children's symptoms and ongoing criminal proceedings. For example, prompt arrest can alleviate the initial fear, while trial postponement may result in prolonged anxiety. We have observed a number of cases in which specific symptoms, such as unconscious reenactment behavior or traumatic dreams, have reappeared at critical junctures during the procedures. Our present legal system is often insensitive to, and ill-prepared to deal with, the special needs of the child witness. However, it is possible for the child to view his or her involvement in legal activities as a challenge rather than a threat (Folkman & Lazarus, in press). Since the judicial proceedings adjudicate blame, there is a necessary link between judicial outcome and trauma resolution. For example, by the time of sentencing, children who are preoccupied with fantasies of revenge will seem to welcome being unburdened of the responsibility for obtaining justice. We have observed examples where a child's aggressive traumatic play and dangerous reenactment behavior abated in the weeks after a murderer's conviction and incarceration.

Although it is a difficult position to achieve, we have sought to become recognized as experts in childhood trauma who, while declining assignment to any specific adversarial judicial agent, still serve a special role in assisting the child. We think it is of critical importance to keep separate the therapeutic role of assisting the child to address the trauma and the questioning of the child for legal purposes. We do not act as agents of the police and interview children in order to establish criminal evidence. Rather, we have been able to educate police officers to the prospect that a less traumatized child is likely as a result to be a more effective legal witness. Similar to what occurs in family courts, perhaps it would be best if the juvenile or criminal court judge assigned a child trauma consultant to assist the child through the criminal proceedings.

Unlike the clinical interview, testifying on the witness stand may lead to further distress rather than relief. If court appearances are required, we retain the role of child consultant. This role differs from that of the traditional expert witness who offers testimony or advice on the verification of the child's evidence. We will not only help prepare the child for the stress of testifying but will provide post-testimony support to the child so that his or her subjective experience on the stand can be therapeutically reviewed. Witnessing a violent act of high personal impact, such as the homicide or rape of a parent, is so important a core memory that to have it challenged under cross-examination could cause the child to question his or her own sense of reality. After the child testifies, reconfirmation may, therefore, be of significant value.

Similar issues arise when civil proceedings are initiated. Temporary placement may need to be decided because of an emergency situation. However, one must be cautious in rendering an opinion about custody preference prior to addressing the acute trauma sequelae. We think questions of custody should not be addressed before the child receives adequate early trauma treatment so that the child can be a more active participant in discussion of alternatives. We have observed that therapists too often become involved in evaluating the child to render an opinion for one side in a custody hearing while the child remains untreated for prominent signs of severe post-traumatic stress.

## FUTURE RESEARCH

Research efforts are needed to investigate all four previously outlined categories of traumatic consequences (see p. 195). Psychophysiological investigations may provide needed information about the onset and course of sleep disturbances, startle reactions and gastrointestinal disturbances that are so often associated with traumatic anxiety. The use of EEG recordings could help to determine the nature of the sleep disorder and the importance of stage four sleep phenomena as reported by Fisher (1965). Investigation of the acoustic startle reaction in children (Ornitz, personal communication, 1985) after exposure to gunfire could help delineate the location and permanence of any neurophysiological changes. Constitutional factors may play a key role in the intensity and direction of these psychophysiological reactions (Weiner, 1982).

Insight into these mechanisms may lead to rational psychopharmacological or behavioral interventions to treat these symptoms if they persist or become debilitating. Preliminary reports (Burstein, 1984) of such interventions in adult victims have been promising, although sufficient physiological understanding is not yet available to justify similar research with children.

Investigations into children's coping processes and their developmental and environmental determinants will be essential in furthering our understanding of the vulnerable and resilient child. However, as Folkman and Lazarus (in press) have argued for adults, one must avoid the pitfall of overgeneralizations that lead to the unlinking of the coping process from the situational influences. The use of reliable inventories of coping processes in children would allow us to compare the responses to different forms of violence, and to document over the course of recovery the changing pattern of cognitive and emotional coping that appears most efficacious.

Although our single session technique has proven helpful, these children often require further treatment. There is an immediate need for investigation of brief, focal psychotherapy for use with children traumatized by exposure to violence. Examples are available from adult studies to suggest that this form of therapy may be especially important in the treatment of post-traumatic stress disorders (Horowitz & Kaltreider, 1979). These methods will need modification to take into account developmental considerations that will influence symptom course and the maturity of cognitive and emotional means of coping.

Group therapy and self-help groups for victims of many types of natural and human-induced disasters have proved valuable in the recovery of adults. They often permit destigmatization and universalizing of one's personal responses, as well as a shared understanding of the expected course of recovery (Parson, 1984). The appropriate use of similar groups in attending to the child exposed to extreme acts of violence offers another channel needful of careful implementation and clinical review.

Education of professional groups, parents, and communities can serve several purposes. Demystification and destigmatization of the course of symptomatology after violent events can both provide a more supportive environment for recovery and enhance efforts to implement programs for early detection and treatment. We are presently completing separate pamphlets explaining childhood post-traumatic stress disorders, one directed at professionals including pediatricians, school psychologists, and mental health practitioners, and another for distribution to parents and community groups, especially in the aftermath of some violent or other traumatic occurrence. However, there has been little research into the best methods of public education in this field, and programs to evaluate this important area are needed.

## REFERENCES

Abramson, L., Garber, J., & Seligman, M. (1980). Learned helplessness in humans. An attributional analysis. In J. Garber & M. Seligman (Eds.), *Human helplessness*. New York: Academic Press.

Aitkens, R., Buglass, D., & Kreitman, N. (1969). The changing pattern of attempted suicide in Edinburgh, 1962–67. *British Journal of Preventive Social Medicine, 23*, 111–115.

American Psychiatric Association. (1980). *Diagnostic and statistical manual of mental disorders* (3rd ed.). Washington, DC: Author.

Ayalon, O. (1983). Coping with terrorism. In D. Meichenbaum & M. Jaremko (Eds.), *Stress reduction and prevention*. New York: Plenum.

Bloch, D. A., Silber, E., & Perry, S. E. (1956). Some factors in the emotional reactions of children to disaster. *American Journal of Psychiatry, 113*, 416–422.

Bowlby, J. (1977). The making and breaking of affectional bond, Part I. Aetiology and psychopathology in the light of attachment theory. (50th Maudsley lecture). *British Journal of Psychiatry, 130*, 201–210.

Bowlby, J. (1979). On knowing what you aren't supposed to know and feeling what you are not supposed to feel. *Canadian Journal of Psychiatry, 24*, 403–408.

Burstein, A. (1984). Treatment of post-traumatic stress disorder with imipramine. *Psychosomatics, 25*, 681–687.

Cain, A., & Fast, I. (1972). Children's disturbed reactions to parent suicide: Distortion and guilt, communication and identification. In A. Cain (Ed.), *Survivors of suicide*. Springfield, IL: Charles C Thomas.

Center for Disease Control (1984). *Violent crime summary of morbidity*. Violence Epidemiology Branch.

Elizur, E., & Kaufman, M. (1982). Children's bereavement reactions following death of the father: II. *Journal of the American Academy of Child Psychiatry, 21*, 474–480.

Erikson, K. T. (1976). Loss of communality at Buffalo Creek. *American Journal of Psychiatry, 133*, 302–305.

Eth, S., & Pynoos, R. (1984). Developmental perspectives on psychic trauma in children. In C. Figley (Ed.), *Trauma and its wake*. New York: Brunner/Mazel.

Eth, S., & Pynoos, R. (1985). Interaction of trauma and grief in childhood. In S. Eth & R. Pynoos (Eds.), *Posttraumatic stress in children*. American Psychiatric Press.

Eth, S., Silverstein, S., & Pynoos, R. (1984). Mental health consultation to a preschool following the murder of a mother and child. *Hospital and Community Psychiatry, 36*, 73–76.

Fisher, C. (1965). Psychoanalytic implications of recent research on sleep and dreaming. *Journal of the American Psychoanalytic Association, 13*, 197–303.

Folkman, S., & Lazarus, R. (in press). Personal control and stress and coping processes. *Journal of Personality and Social Psychology*.

Fox, R. P. (1974). Narcissistic rage and the problem of combat aggression. *Archives of General Psychiatry, 31*, 807–811.

Frederick, C. (1980). Effects of natural v. human induced violence upon victims. *Evaluation and Change*, Special Issue, 71–75.

Frederick, C. (1983). Violence and disasters: Immediate and long-term consequences. In *Helping victims of violence*. Ministry of welfare and cultural affairs. The Hague: Government Printing Office.

Frederick, C. (in press). Children traumatized by catastrophic situations. In S. Eth & R. Pynoos (Eds.), *Posttraumatic stress in children*. Washington, DC: American Psychiatric Association Press.

Freud, S. (1953). Analysis of a phobia in a five-year-old boy. In J. Strachey (Ed. and Trans.),

*The standard edition of the complete psychological works of Sigmund Freud* (Vol. 10). London: Hogarth Press. (Original work published 1909)

Furman, E. (1974). *A child's parent dies*. New Haven: Yale University Press.

Furman, E. (1981). Treatment-via-the-parent: A case of bereavement. *Journal of Child Psychotherapy, 7*, 89–101.

Gardner, G. E. (1971). Aggression and violence—the enemies of precision learning in children. *American Journal of Psychiatry, 128*, 445–450.

Garmezy, N. (1983). Stressors of childhood. In N. Garmezy & M. Rutter (Eds.), *Stress, coping and development in children*. New York: McGraw-Hill.

Gislason, I. L., & Call, J. (1982). Dog bite in infancy: Trauma and personality development. *Journal of the American Academy of Child Psychiatry, 21*, 203–207.

Glass, A. J. (1947). Effectiveness of forward treatment. *Bulletin of the U.S. Army Medical Department, 7*, 1034–1041.

Glass, A. J. (1954). Psychotherapy in the combat zone. *American Journal of Psychiatry, 110*, 725–731.

Grinker, R. R., & Spiegel, J. P. (1943). *War neuroses in North Africa: The Tunisian campaign*. The Air Surgeon, Army Air Forces. New York: Josiah Macy, Jr. Foundation.

Harrison, S. I., Davenport, C. W., & McDermott, J. F. (1967). Children's reactions to bereavement. *Archives of General Psychiatry, 17*, 593–597.

Horowitz, M. J., & Kaltreider, N. B. (1979). Brief therapy of the stress response syndrome. *Psychiatric Clinics of North America, 2*, 365–377.

Kardiner, A. (1941). The traumatic neuroses of war. *Psychosomatic Medical Monograph*. New York: Paul Hoeber.

Levy, D. M. (1938). Release therapy in young children. *Psychiatry, 1*(3), August, 387–390.

Lifton, R. J. (1979). The psychology of the survivor and the death imprint. *Psychiatric Annals, 12*, 1011–1020.

Lindy, J. D., Green, B. L., Grace, M., & Titchener, J. (1983). Psychotherapy with survivors of the Beverly Hills Supper Club fire. *American Journal of Psychotherapy, 37*, 593–610.

McDonald, M. (1964). Children's reactions to the death of a mother. *Psychoanalytic Study of the Child, 19*, 358–376.

Mercier, M., & Despert, J. (1943). Effects of war on French children. *Psychosomatic Medicine, 5*, 266–272.

Parson, E. R. (1984). The role of psychodynamic group therapy in the treatment of the combat veteran. In H. Schwartz (Ed.), *Psychotherapy of the combat victim*. New York: Spectrum.

Pfouts, J., Schopler, J., & Henley, H. C. (1982). Forgotten victims of family violence. *Social Work, 27*, 367–368.

Polak, P. R., Egan, D., Vandenbergh, R., & Williams, W. V. (1975). Prevention in mental health: A controlled study. *American Journal of Psychiatry, 132*, 146–149.

Pruett, P. R., et al. (1979). Home treatment for two infants who witnessed their mother's murder. *American Journal of Psychiatry, 132*, 647–657.

Pynoos, R., & Eth, S. (1984). The child as witness to homicide. *Journal of Social Issues, 40*, 87–108.

Pynoos, R., & Eth, S. (in press). Witness to violence: The child interview. *Journal of the American Academy of Child Psychiatry*.

Pynoos, R., Gilmore, K., & Shapiro, T. (1983). *The response of children to parental suicidal acts*. Paper presented at the Annual Meeting of the Academy of Child Psychiatry, San Francisco, October 1983.

Schetky, D. H. (1973). Preschooler's response to murder of their mothers by their fathers: A study of four cases. *Bulletin of the American Academy of Psychiatric Law, 6*, 45–57.

Silber, E., Perry, S., & Bloch, D. (1958). Patterns of parent-child interaction in a disaster. *Psychiatry, 21*(2), 159–167.

Terr, L. (1979). Children of Chowchilla: A study of psychic trauma. *Psychoanalytic Study of the Child, 34*, 547–623.

Terr, L. (1981). Psychic trauma in children. *American Journal of Psychiatry, 138*, 14–19.

Terr, L. (1983). Chowchilla revisited: The effects of psychic trauma four years after a school bus kidnapping. *American Journal of Psychiatry, 140,* 1543–1550.

Terr, L. (1984). Children at acute risk: Psychic trauma. In L. Grinspoon (Ed.), *Psychiatry update*, Vol. III. Washington, DC: American Psychiatric Press.

Thomas, A., & Chess, S. (1977). *Temperament and development.* New York: Brunner/Mazel.

Weiner, H. (1982). The prospects for psychosomatic medicine: Selected topics. *Psychosomatic Medicine, 40,* 491–517.

Weissman, M. (1974). The epidemiology of suicide attempts. *Archives of General Psychiatry, 30,* 737–745.

West, L. J. (1984). *The epidemic of violence.* Paper presented at the Annual Meeting of the American Psychiatric Association.

# Part IV

# COMMUNITY INTERVENTION PROGRAMS

# 10

# *Preventing Family Violence: Family-Focused Programs*

## Carolyn Swift

### INTRODUCTION

Family violence and prevention, as fields of study in the social sciences, have developed along parallel tracks. Both look at practices that are centuries old, but neither can claim a knowledge base of more than a decade or so. In both fields, initial theories have been simplistic, while today, both benefit from a systems approach. The most powerful prevention programs take place at the macrocosmic level, where interventions are designed to change societal institutions and practices. It is at this level that the issues of inequitable distribution of power and resources are most effectively addressed. However, individual human service workers and their agencies have limited resources to devote to systems change. In addition, the realities of their funding bases and community supports rarely permit them to commit resources to institutional change. For these reasons, much of the preventive work of social service agencies and their staffs is with the individuals and families they serve. In support of their work, this chapter explores efforts to prevent family violence at the microcosmic level. Prevention strategies focused at the macrocosmic level are addressed in detail elsewhere in this volume (Lerman, Chapter 11). This chapter begins by tracing the commonalities shared by the fields of family violence and prevention. A generic model for preventing dysfunctional behavior is then presented. Current beliefs about the causes of family violence are reviewed, and specific programs are discussed as applications of the prevention model.

The idea of prevention is not new. It is embedded in folklore: "A stitch in time saves nine." It is reflected in the wisdom of the sage: "An ounce of prevention is worth a pound of cure." Family violence is not new

219

either. Biblical references, ancient myths, and fairy tales describe violence between husband and wife, parents and children, and siblings. Folktales are compelling because they embody the collective experience of the human condition. Wicked stepmothers, jealous husbands, and cruel and heartless fathers know no country or tongue. As characters they crop up in the folktales of countries around the globe. Their actions speak to the fragility of human relationships and the need to find ways of ensuring personal health and safety within intimate family bonds.

Theories have only recently begun to emerge to explain the causes of family violence. The serious study of this subject is less than 25 years old, dating from Henry Kempe's identification of the battered child syndrome (Kempe et al., 1962). As Gelles (1980) points out, there were no articles on family violence in the *Journal of Marriage and the Family* during its first 30 years of publication, nor did the journal review the subject in its decade review of family research and action in the sixties. One of the consequences of the emergent state of scholarship on family violence is the simplicity of initial attempts to explain it. Early investigators tended to identify a single event or condition as the "cause." They then located this cause in the individual—either the abuser or the victim—and labeled it a defect in personality or adjustment. Both child abuse and spouse abuse were initially explained as a function of the personalities of the participants (Keller & Erne, 1983; Newberger & Newberger, 1982).

Current etiologies of family violence reflect a systems approach. A variety of integrative models have been suggested. Each assumes that abuse is multidetermined. The imbalance of power between the sexes and sex-role stereotypes are seen as major determinants of abuse, particularly spouse abuse (Breines & Gordon, 1983; Dobash & Dobash, 1979; Straus, 1980b). For both child abuse and spouse abuse the critical variables include environmental stressors such as life-change events, social isolation, poverty and cultural norms, and variables associated with individual family members that may increase the risk of family violence—such as anger proneness and nonnormative status (Gelles, 1973; Justice & Justice, 1976; Keller & Erne, 1983; Young, 1976). More recently, sociopsychological models have looked at repetitive patterns of abuse across generations. In the case of spouse abuse, repetitive cycles of abuse and reconciliation within such relationships are also seen as helping maintain the abuse (Hilberman, 1980; Walker, 1984).

As a behavioral science, the field of prevention has undergone a similar process of theoretical development. Preventive health strategies are part of our everyday lives. Most of us know that exercise, good nutrition, weight control and stress reduction, for example, can prevent the development of some physical and mental illnesses. However, prevention has become a bona fide field of study only within the last decade. Scholarly journals and texts devoted to prevention have been in existence less than five years.

The classic prevention model comes from the field of public health, where the condition to be prevented is physical illness. This classic model casts health outcomes in terms resulting from the interactions of persons with their environments: In public health language, disease is caused by the impact of environmental stress on a host population. Given this simple formula, the solution to preventing disease is straightforward—preventionists intervene to change either the environment, the host population or both. Environmental interventions are usually aimed at eliminating the noxious stressor or reducing its intensity. Host-focused interventions concentrate on strengthening the defenses of the host population to resist the impact of stress.

Examples illustrate these two classic prevention strategies. Confronted with the problem of preventing malaria, public health officials chose the first option—eliminating the noxious stressor. They destroyed the breeding ground of malaria-carrying mosquitoes by spraying the swamps that served as the insects' habitat. The second strategy, strengthening the host population, is seen in the conquest of polio. Instead of ridding the environment of the noxious stressor—the polio virus—health authorities found it more practical to strengthen the defenses of the host population, primarily children, through inoculation. Both of these examples, each using a different method, achieved the same results: the negative health outcome—disease—was prevented.

Note that the choice between the two prevention strategies in these examples is ethically value-free. Whether to target the stressor or host is a practical issue. Answers to questions such as, which is more accessible? which strategy is less costly? or which is more effective? determine the selection. It is ethically irrelevant—of interest primarily to cost accountants—whether the stressor is eliminated or the host population strengthened. Either way, the prevention mission is accomplished. Ecologists are not alarmed at the prospect of mosquitoless swamps, and ethicists are not concerned that children are forced into a defensive posture vis-à-vis the polio virus. In the case of physical disease, potential victims are generally at liberty to pursue victim-free status by the most expeditious means available, whether this be by eliminating the stressor or strengthening the host.

The public health prevention model had its major application in preventing the impact of nonhuman stressors on human hosts. Applying this model becomes awkward in situations in which both the stressor and the host are human beings. The discovery that the behavior of other human beings is a source of environmental stress has enormous significance for prevention theory (Cassel, 1974). Once social behavior is seen as a source of psychosocial stress, the dichotomous simplicity of the classic prevention model breaks down.

Family violence is a case in point. If the behavior of one human being or group causes the physical or mental victimization of another human being or group, then prevention strategists are confronted with a dilemma. Their choice of either of the two classic strategies has ethical—and perhaps ecological—implications. Stressor-focused interventions become more complicated, since battering husbands and abusing mothers cannot be targeted for eradication in the same way that mosquitoes or viruses can. Adding humans to the list of environmental stressors complicates prevention analysis because human stressors are, in reality, "double agents." They function both as *sources* of stress for others, and as *targets* of stress themselves, from both human and nonhuman sources.

The dilemma is not avoided by choosing the second classic strategy. Strengthening the host population in family violence situations means teaching wives and children at risk for abuse how to negotiate, fight, escape, or mobilize law enforcement or other institutional alternatives. The ethical problem here is that this is a blame-the-victim approach. The responsibility is placed on the potential victim to avoid being criminally attacked by a family member. The solution to the preventionist's dilemma goes beyond the classic simplicity of the public health model. Effective prevention programs must incorporate the complexity of the multiple forces which determine behavior.

## PREVENTION MODEL

George Albee (1981) has developed an equation that incorporates a systems approach into the strategy for prevention of mental and emotional illness. The equation has broad applicability for projecting prevention programs across a variety of behavioral and social problems, including family violence. It provides a useful conceptual schema for organizing the major factors associated with health and behavior, and for suggesting ways in which these factors interact to produce health and behavioral outcomes.* The formula can be applied individually to either the stressor or

---

*The equation is not intended, nor does it lend itself easily, to being operationalized in any literal mathematical sense. Conceptual issues (e.g., overlapping variables) and logistical issues (e.g., valid and reliable instruments are not available to measure the variables) are barriers to attempts at mathematical translation.

the host, to the family as a system, or to an entire population at risk.

Adapted here for family violence, the equation draws together critical variables, and outlines their general relationship to each other:

$$\text{Incidence of Dysfunction} = \frac{\text{Stress} + \text{Risk Factors}}{\text{Social Supports} + \text{Coping Skills} + \text{Self-Esteem}}$$

Primary-prevention activities are those that reduce the incidence of dysfunctional health or behavioral outcomes in targeted populations. A glance at the equation immediately suggests two prevention strategies. In order to reduce the incidence of family violence, either the value of the numerator must be decreased or the value of the denominator increased. Note that the top line of the equation contains the factors in the environment and in the person that contribute to the dysfunctional outcome, while the bottom line contains the factors that operate to prevent the unwanted outcome. Since human service workers generally have little control over the life stresses to which their clients are exposed, their efforts are usually focused on ''bottom line'' activities; that is, increasing the social supports, coping skills, and self-esteem of the people they serve. What follows is an exercise in applying Albee's formula to family violence. The exercise is intended to illustrate the model, not serve as an exhaustive analysis.

Incidence refers to new cases of disorder that occur within a specified time period in a population. A critical issue in designing interventions to prevent family violence is the selection of the specific health or behavioral outcome to be prevented. Is the goal to reduce the incidence of new victims each year or to reduce the incidence of new abusers? The first goal is directed to preventing victimization, the second to preventing the development of abusive behavior. The choice of outcome determines which populations are identified as at risk and whether stressor or host-focused strategies are used. While it is logical that for abuse to end, abusive behavior must be stopped, until the very recent past, the victim (host) has borne the major responsibility for prevention efforts. Societal institutions have traditionally sanctioned, in custom and law, the abuse of wife by husband and child by parent. Increasingly, the professional community has begun to focus on the abusive behavior itself (the stressor) as the appropriate target for prevention efforts. Since the state of the prevention art is imperfect, stressor-focused interventions cannot be guaranteed to eliminate all violence from the home. Therefore, it is appropriate to develop host-focused interventions as well, to protect the safety of potential victims. The assumption here, then, is that both strategies are needed.

Stress is used in the equation to refer to 1) the life change events associated with family violence, such as unemployment, pregnancy and the onset of parenting, and 2) chronic systemic stressors such as poverty and sexist cultural norms. Risk factors refer to constitutional character-istics of the person or population targeted for prevention efforts. Persons are considered to be at risk if they are members of a group for which the incidence of a specified disorder is above the base rate for that disorder in a population (Vance, 1977). In the case of family violence, sex, age, and nonnormative parental or child status are risk factors. Males are at risk for developing abusive behavior toward other family members. Fe-males and children are at risk for victimization by family violence.

Social supports refer to social networks and resources such as immedi-ate family members, relatives, friends, neighbors, and co-workers. Pro-fessionals such as physicians, clergy, counselors, and other human service workers augment natural supportive networks. Coping skills refer both to broad levels of competence as well as to specific skills related to the behavior targeted. For example, parenting skills and those involved in negotiating and defusing anger are linked to outcome in situations of fami-ly conflict. Self-esteem carries the same meaning here as in the general psychological literature: In general, it refers to the image or assessment of one's own personal resources and capacities.

## PROGRAMS TO PREVENT FAMILY VIOLENCE

Projecting strategies to prevent family violence, using Albee's formula, involves two basic tasks. The first task is to identify the specific stresses and risks associated with family violence and develop interventions to eliminate or reduce these in targeted families. The second task is to iden-tify the characteristics of supportive networks, the specific coping skills and the level of self-esteem or combinations of these factors associated with healthy family functioning, and develop interventions to increase these in targeted families. In practice, many prevention programs incor-porate elements of both tasks.

### Reducing Stress

Stress is a major contributor to family violence. Sources of stress in-clude life change events (e.g., unemployment and the onset of parenting) and chronic or systemic conditions (e.g., social isolation, low socioeco-nomic status, and certain cultural norms). This section reviews the rela-tionship between these sources of stress and family violence, and suggests prevention programs consistent with the prevention model presented.

*Unemployment*. Marital violence has been found to increase directly with the increase of stressful events experienced by families (Straus, Gelles, & Steinmetz, 1980). A single stressful event does not usually cause breakdown. It is the piling up of stressful events over a short period of time that is damaging. Suddenly losing a job is a major shock. In our country in the last few years, unemployment has affected as many people as the death of a loved one, major illness and divorce (Buss, Redburn, & Waldron, 1983). The devastating impact of involuntary layoff or termination results from the many changes it brings. Loss of income directly affects the family's capacity to provide for basic human needs such as shelter, food, clothing and transportation. For many males, unemployment also threatens the ability to fulfill the perceived male role of breadwinner. Anxiety, depression, loss of self-esteem, and alcoholism are commonly found in unemployed males (Buss et al., 1983). Increased levels of both spouse abuse and child abuse have also been found in families in which the male is unemployed (Gil, 1970; Prescott & Letko, 1977; Straus et al., 1980). Inability to provide for his family's needs, together with his reduced social status and the frustrations of constant exposure to the round-the-clock pressures of parenting, are believed to contribute to abusive behavior.

The most direct and effective interventions to prevent violence resulting from unemployment are those that eliminate this stressor by returning these men to the work force. While local and federal government agencies are assigned this task, a variety of other institutions and human service organizations have entered the field in the last few years. Community job fairs match employers with job seekers and create an arena in which unemployed peers can exchange information and tips in their search. In some of the communities hardest hit by unemployment, loosely organized barter groups have formed, generally within neighborhoods (R. Schelkun, personal communication, Jan. 1981). Typically, members of these groups exchange services such as child care, house and car repair or items such as home-baked or canned goods and used clothing. In one community, a drop-in center located in a union hall served a coordination, education and referral function (Buss et al., 1983).

These community activities, especially barter groups, serve several preventive functions. They fill the time of the unemployed family member in productive pursuits, provide for some of the basic needs of the affected families, maintain the dignity of family members by valuing reciprocal contributions, and focus the time and energies of family members on events outside the family itself, thus providing a respite from the unaccustomed, constant presence resulting from sudden unemployment. Widespread integrated social networks in some communities, like Youngstown, Ohio, provide ready self-help groups in times of crisis: "These networks may assist in fulfilling the financial needs of workers, may provide therapy for problems, and may be instrumental in locating and obtaining jobs" (Buss et al., p. 88).

The Employment Transition Program (ETP) of the University of Michigan's Industrial Development Division is a model prevention program for the unemployed (Hess, 1983). This five-day training program attempts to provide unemployed participants with the skills to control their own careers. The goal is reentry into the labor force. To this end, the classic prevention strategies of stress reduction and skill building are used. By analyzing economic and labor market information, participants come to an understanding of the societal forces underlying their unemployment. This learning is designed to reduce their self-blaming behavior and help restore their self-esteem. It also provides them with information needed to consider options for redirecting their careers. The practical skills of job searching, resume writing and interviewing are also taught. This program combines the three "bottom line" prevention resources: It provides the added social support of a group of unemployed peers along with expert program staff; it increases the specific coping skills needed to obtain jobs; and it aims at restoring self-esteem by reducing self-blaming behavior. A profile of average ETP participants shows them to be middle-aged (49 years), with limited education (11 years) and substantial seniority in previous jobs (19 years). A manual, pre- and post-tests and an experimental design spanning four years permits the program to train trainers and to follow up their participants' subsequent attempts to reenter the work force.

*Onset of parenting.* The onset of parenting marks one of life's major transitions. It signals passage to a generative stage of life. It also brings substantial changes in the economic and social life of the family. Pregnancy is associated with increased levels of spouse abuse (Eisenberg & Micklow, 1977; Gelles, 1975). A recent study of women seeking emergency room treatment found that battered women were twice as likely to be injured during pregnancy as nonbattered women (Kahn, 1984). Their pregnancies were significantly more likely to terminate in abortion or miscarriage. If the pregnancy is unplanned and unwanted, the baby is at high risk for child abuse.

The most practical prevention strategies to reduce unwanted pregnancies are sex education and birth control. In prevention terms, both are effective coping skills. However, less than 10% of the children in this country receive any kind of sex education (Dunwoody, 1982b). The continuing opposition of many segments of our society to these prevention strategies means that pregnant women and children will continue to suffer from family violence.

The onset of parenting demands resources and skills that many adults do not have. Alpert and her associates (1983) have developed a scale to assess the stresses associated with becoming a parent. Of 21 events, the most stressful was the major illness of a child. The second most stressful event was frequent conflicting demands for time by the spouse and the child. Also ranked as highly stressful were decisions about which one of the parents was responsible for child-care tasks, conflicting demands between the needs of the self and the child, and loss of sleep in the months following childbirth.

Preventive interventions to reduce the stress of pregnancy and the onset of parenting include prenatal classes, early intervention programs and parent education. While these programs all involve the strategy of building supportive networks—through classes or home visits—the major prevention strategy employed is an increase in parents' skills in coping with the responsibilities of parenthood.

Comprehensive prevention programs for expectant families include three components. The first two are classic examples of teaching coping skills through anticipatory guidance, a process in which persons about to experience a stressful situation rehearse the anticipated sequence of events and plan coping strategies to meet the crisis (Bloom, 1971). These skills prepare parents for the experiences of birth and child care. First, the prospective parents are recruited for classes covering the stages of pregnancy and the birth experience itself—classes on natural childbirth are among the most popular. Second, child development and parenting skills are taught. Skills such as feeding and bathing the baby are often included in the prenatal curriculum, since capturing the parents' time after the baby is born is difficult.

The third component deals with the practices and procedures of the hospital's maternity unit. Under optimum conditions the mother participates actively—this means with little or no anesthesia, and with the option to view the delivery (e.g., through overhead mirrors), hold the baby immediately after birth, and breast-feed if she wishes. It is important that the father be included in the birth process as well. This accomplishes two preventive aims: It provides for mutual support between the parents, and it ensures the father's participation in the bonding process. The family should be encouraged to spend time alone with the baby within the first few hours of birth. There should be rooming-in arrangements that include the mother's option to assume major care of the infant as well as extended visiting privileges for the father. Ideally, the hospital or related agency maintains a schedule of follow-up visits to the family to answer questions about child care and put the family in touch with community resources. Gray (1982) describes three current models of perinatal positive parenting programs: The Institute for Family and Child Study at Michigan State University, Vanderbilt University School of Medicine and the Rural Family Support Project in Indiana.

Parent education takes many forms, ranging from formal curricula in secondary schools and college-level courses in child development to short courses offered by mental health centers or other community agencies and brief pamphlets distributed by mail, such as the Pierre the Pelican series (Roland, 1978) of the State of Louisiana. Parenting classes are generally targeted to mothers or couples. In increasing recognition of the importance of the father's role in parenting, some 100 U.S. firms are providing parent education programs at the work site (Klinman & Kohl, 1984). Two models of parent education programs are described here. One is a grass-roots program (USEP) and the other (PET) was developed by a professional.

United Services for Effective Parenting (USEP) is an organization of over 170 parenting programs in Ohio (Badger & Burns, 1982). USEP began in 1974 as an advocacy organization for birth-to-three programs and the families they serve. Almost 16,000 children under three and their families are served annually in the state. A third of the staff members are volunteers, mostly parents. Program activities include short courses on Infant Enrichment Through Mother Training, newsletters, surveys, resource and referral directories and annual conferences. USEP has developed an effective model for organizing parents and professionals into a delivery system for parent education and early intervention services.

Thomas Gordon (1983) believes that it is not the earliest years, but the 10 years following infancy that are most critical for parenting. He believes that parents go through a behavioral shift—from responder to controller —in experiencing their child's transition from infancy to childhood. He argues that the conventional role of parent as disciplinarian assumes a hierarchy of power in the family and a system of rewards and punishments that lead to inevitable parent-child conflicts. To prevent such conflicts and their potential for abuse Gordon teaches a simple model of parenting that shares many components with accepted prevention strategies. First, he teaches parents that the child's behavior is motivated to meet physical and psychological needs, not to annoy or challenge parents. By emphasizing communication skills he helps parents accept responsibility for their own reactions, while teaching children the consequences of their behavior.

A basic part of Gordon's course is his concept that both parent and child can interact to fulfill the needs of each—his "No-Lose," "Win-Win" method. PET eliminates punishment of children. It is designed to raise their self-esteem and advocates their involvement in family problem-solving. The model is one of participatory democracy. Over half a million parents in the U.S. and 15 foreign countries have been exposed to PET. Gordon (1977) cites ten research studies documenting changes in parents resulting from their exposure to the course. Changes mentioned include significant increases in 1) parents' confidence and self-esteem in their role, 2) mutual acceptance, understanding and trust between parent and child, and 3) democratic parental attitudes toward the family as a unit. Significant decreases were found in authoritarian attitudes and behavior on the part of parents. Changes cited in the children of PET graduates include higher self-esteem and improved school performance.

*Social isolation*. Other major sources of stress for families, in addition to life change events, are chronic deficits in social or material resources. It is generally believed that socially isolated families—those with minimal ties to relatives, neighbors and the surrounding community—show higher rates of both spouse abuse and child abuse than less isolated families (Gelles, 1974; Gil, 1970). Preventive interventions for these families include early intervention programs and supportive group experiences. In general, close ties with relatives, friends and neighbors supply a continuing stream of support to family members. Supportive behaviors include listening to problems, giving advice and material supplies, exchanging favors such as child care, and seeking these same behaviors in return. This reciprocal aspect of the relationship makes social network support different from—and in this way superior to—professional therapeutic services (Mitchell & Trickett, 1980). By asking for and receiving help in return, relatives and friends of family members confirm that person's skills as a problem solver and value as a significant other. The positive consequences of reciprocity in personal relationships are reported in many studies (Cohen & Sokolovsky, 1978; Mitchell & Trickett, 1980; Tolsdorf, 1976) and form the basis of Riessman's Helper Therapy (Riessman, 1965).

Early intervention programs offer a variety of supports for isolated families with children (Bond & Joffe, 1982; Heber et al., 1972; Moss, Hess, & Swift, 1982). Programs are usually targeted to pregnant women and mothers of newborn babies who are considered to be at risk for the development of a range of negative outcomes, including child abuse, retardation, developmental delay and school behavior problems. Most programs use paraprofessional staff made up of parent aides as the primary service deliverers. They make regular—usually weekly—home visits to targeted families, from the time of the mother's pregnancy through the infant's first year. Visits generally continue with reduced frequency until the child enters school. Parent aides are trained to listen to the mother's concerns and assist her in problem solving around the family's physical and psychological needs. In addition, they demonstrate parenting skills and specific infant stimulation techniques. The aides are trained to link families to the community's resource and referral networks.

The Optimum Growth Project (South County Mental Health Center, 1980), a model early intervention program, won the National Mental Health Association's first Lela Rowland Prevention Award. This is one of the few relatively low-cost preventive programs for families that provide experimental evidence of a direct impact on reducing family violence. An evaluation during the third year of the program showed that mothers receiving home visits improved significantly compared to control group mothers in caring for their children's physical needs and interacting with them. "Less than one percent of test group mothers had been reported for child abuse and neglect as compared with 7.7% of comparison group mothers" (p. 7).

Early intervention programs provide one-on-one support for isolated mothers through the use of parent aides. Another way to build the mother's social supports is by expanding her social networks. This has been done by linking her to a variety of peer groups. Mutual support groups are a relatively recent, but extremely important, source of social resources for parents. In an age of increasingly transient and mobile families, many parents find themselves uprooted from home communities, faced with raising children in unfamiliar neighborhoods, separated from their customary network of relatives and friends. The trauma of divorce adds to the alienation of many of today's parents. Parents Without Partners is organized to provide both social support and resources to divorced and widowed parents. Compassionate Friends provides support for parents who have lost a child through death (Videka-Sherman, 1982). Parents United is directed to families in which incest has occurred (Giarretto, 1981). Parents Anonymous is a self-help group for abusing parents (Comstock, 1982). The preventive value of the latter two groups is twofold: First, they actively help members to stop abusing their children; second, their educational outreach programs educate the general public to the problem of child abuse, and through this activity may influence high risk families to seek help prior to the occurrence of abuse. These self-help groups have chapters nationwide.

Local communities have developed a variety of other supportive groups to reduce the isolation of families in their midst. One of the most promising and creative is the approach of the Children's Aid Society of Metropolitan Toronto (Breton, Welbourn, & Watters, 1981). While this group pioneered their model with abuse-prone mothers, their methods are appropriate for use with nonabusing, socially isolated and other high-risk mothers as well. Agency staff began with the assumption that abusive mothers are unable to nurture their children because they have not received adequate nurturing themselves. Program strategy was also influenced by findings of a general lack of verbal communication coupled with a reliance on physical contact in abuse-prone families (Elmer, 1967). In an attempt to remediate the mothers' early failure experiences, a group model was developed that included socially sanctioned touching and non-threatening conversation. Since hairdressing combines both of these behaviors, a hairdresser was added to project staff and this activity became the focus of the group.

The group's format evolved over several replications. For example, the first group was successful in maintaining volunteer attendance and active participation until the staff decided to drop nurturance and initiate a problem-solving format. This led to the breakup of the group. Staff learned from this experience that the mothers found the leap from nurturance to exposure of personal problems too threatening. Even though the group broke up, the experience proved to be a positive one, since the mothers reportedly stopped abusing their children. Later groups accomplished the shift in format more gradually, focusing on nonpersonal, nonthreatening problem solving and generic coping skills. The model is reported to be successful in helping the mothers achieve a series of positive outcomes—e.g., to gain social skills, find employment, accept parent aides in their homes, send children to nursery schools, and separate from abusive partners.

Social isolation is also a major issue in elder care. In a recent survey of persons caring for an elderly family member, the average age of the elderly was 82 (Steinmetz, 1982). The caretakers did not report being burdened by performing personal or household services for the elder, but major conflict arose around social activities. Elders were often cut off by death or major illness from significant family members or friends of long standing, and were not interested in developing new social contacts. This insistence on fulfilling all their social needs within the family places immense strain on caretakers. Programs that take the elder out of the home for part of the day—senior citizens' centers, golden age groups—or those that provide respite care in the home appear most promising in their potential to prevent abuse.

Gender issues have often been overlooked in the literature on family violence. The mother has been delegated the role of primary parent and the father relegated to the background in terms of child care responsibilities. Sexist biases assume that mothers have an exclusive role in bonding at birth (Arney, 1980), and that her care and supervision continue to be primary through childhood and adolescence. Increasingly in recent years, scientists and practitioners have begun to examine the role of the father and to restructure that role as a more active, influential one (Pleck, 1984; Baruch & Barnett, 1983, 1984).

The work place is beginning to recognize the importance, for their employees, of supporting fathers' roles. A fourth of this nation's large firms grant fathers one or more days of paid leave at the time of childbirth (Kamerman, Kahn, & Kingston, 1983). Other innovative benefits related to fathering that are occurring with increasing frequency include part-time work schedules and days off for child care (Putnam, 1984). It is in the context of new recognition of the importance of fathering that we consider the role of social networks for men and their potential for preventing family violence.

Straus (1980a) found that men who did not belong to any organizations, such as clubs, business or professional groups, unions, or lodges, assaulted their wives at a much higher rate than men who were actively involved. The same study showed that men who rarely attended religious services also had a higher rate of spouse abuse than men who attended weekly. These results confirm the supportive effects of social networks. However, these networks can also have negative effects. When the norms of the network support the abusing behavior, then close network ties can maintain rather than reduce family violence:

> . . . the assumption that the kin network will be opposed to violence is not necessarily correct. For example, a number of women indicated that when they left their husbands because of a violent attack, their mothers responded with urgings for the wife to deal with the situation by being a better housekeeper, by being a better sex partner, or just by avoiding him, etc. In some cases, the advice was "you just have to put up with it for the sake of the kids—that's what I did!" (Straus, 1980a, p. 246)

*Low socioeconomic status.* Early investigators believed that family violence was classless. While it is true that such violence occurs across all socioeconomic classes, it is now clear that it occurs most often in the lower socioeconomic class (Gelles, 1980; Straus et al., 1980). This finding makes sense, since poverty is a source of severe, chronic stress. Prevention programs addressing the broader social issue of poverty are dealt with elsewhere in this volume (Gil, Chapter 6). This chapter suggests approaches for those working with poor families.

Most of the preventive approaches described—family planning programs, those focusing on unemployment, early intervention, parent education, and building social networks—are useful in working with families across the socioeconomic spectrum, including poor families. A pattern that emerges clearly in working with poor battered women or those whose husbands abuse their children is that many stay in the abusing situation out of economic necessity. Women with higher educations, those who have jobs outside the home, and those with higher paying jobs tend not to put up with the abuse (Okun, 1983; Semmelman, 1982; Walker, 1984). It follows that interventions supporting the employment of both husband and wife have preventive potential. The unemployed husband, as noted earlier, is at risk for developing abusing behavior and the unemployed wife is without resources or options to escape if abuse develops. For these reasons, the strategy of supporting education or training, for either or both marital partners, may be effective in preventing family violence.

*Cultural norms.* Certain cultural norms are a source of systemic stress in families. Two norms that have been linked to family violence are the power imbalance between female and male heads of house and the use of physical force to discipline or control family members. Both sexes are burdened by discriminatory traditions and practices that dictate the "appropriate" role of each in family life and in the world outside the family. In each case, role restrictions and prescriptions set up situations that increase the likelihood of abuse. Sex-role socialization sets up a power imbalance within families with the male in the dominant role and the female in a subordinate role. This imbalance leads to abuse of power as expressed in economic, social and, in the case of family violence, physical ways. Television and movies glamorize violent acts, mirroring the norm that assigns the victim role to women and the aggressor role to men (Greenberg, 1982). Physical abuse of wives by their husbands has a long history of acceptance in Western custom and law.

Our culture also has a long tradition of physical discipline and punishment of children. Such punishment has been shown to lead to a variety of negative outcomes: low self-esteem (Coopersmith, 1967), aggression and violence toward siblings (Straus et al., 1980), and delinquency and criminality (McCord & McCord, 1958). In the extreme, physical punishment perpetuates the cycle of abuse that erupts in succeeding generations of families. Parent education courses that teach alternatives to physical punishment are effective preventive interventions for individual families (Gordon, 1977).

What sorts of prevention programs are there to help individual families combat the norms that feed family violence? Programs that support more balanced roles for both sexes within the family as well as in the world of work, programs that support the role of fathers in nurturing and caring for their children, parent education courses that reinforce these responsibilities, and job sharing for couples all contribute to equalizing parental responsibilities between mother and father. The more time fathers spend with their children and in the routine responsibility of child care and household tasks, the greater their self-esteem and sense of competence as fathers (Baruch & Barnett, 1983). Programs supporting women's options for careers outside the home, those promoting equal pay for equal work and programs devoted to eliminating sex discrimination in the work place should ultimately contribute to equalizing the power balance and reducing the likelihood of abuse between marital partners. Widely available, high quality day care should be within the means of every family so that both working and nonworking parents could have needed respite from the intense, continuous task of child care (Levine, 1982). Child care has become a concern of both the public and private sectors. For example, in a recent five-year period (1978–1983), employer-supported child care programs increased significantly, from 105 to 600 (President's Advisory Council, 1984).

## Reducing Risk Status for Family Violence

*Sex and age.* Males are at risk for becoming abusers,* and women and children are at risk for becoming victims. Explanations for these relative risks are widely reported in the literature and will not be repeated here. Interventions at the macrocosmic level are needed to change the cultural norms and practices that maintain these differential risks through sex-role conditioning. Those working with individual families may find it useful to attempt to reduce the risk status of particular family members through skill-building techniques, discussed later in this chapter.

---

*While both mothers and fathers abuse their children, mothers are reported slightly more frequently as abusers. This appears to reflect not so much a sex difference as the relative exposure of each parent to the experience of child care—often unrelieved child care. Studies demonstrating an increase in child abuse by unemployed fathers underscore this point.

*Nonnormative status.* Nonnormative status also appears to increase the risk of abuse. There is evidence that stepchildren suffer higher rates of abuse (Daly & Wilson, 1980; Hunter, Kilstrom, Kraybill, & Loda, 1978), particularly sexual abuse (Finkelhor & Hotaling, 1984; Swift, in press). Premarital counseling for parents contemplating second marriages would provide anticipatory guidance and coping skills for problems commonly found in stepfamilies (Anderson, Larson, & Morgan, 1981). Educational interventions in elementary school teaching children escape and avoidance behaviors would be helpful to all children (Cooper, Lutter, & Phelps, 1983). Such training would have the added advantage of providing stepchildren with protective skills without singling them out as a high risk population. Premature or low birth weight children are at higher risk for abuse (Parke & Collmer, 1975). Children perceived to be "different" by their parents, as well as handicapped, developmentally delayed or retarded also appear to be at higher risk than other children (Gelles, 1980; Gil, 1970). Early intervention programs, mutual support groups, respite care and provision of specific training in the skills needed to care for such children are all sound preventive measures.

*Status incompatibilities.* The cultural norms that identify the husband as the head of house are challenged when the wife has a higher educational or occupational status. Status inconsistencies and incompatibilities have been found to be risk factors associated with abuse between couples (Hornung, McCullough, & Sugimoto, 1981; Walker, 1984). The highest risk, including life-threatening violence, is associated with asymmetric status pairs, such as a wife whose occupational status is high relative to her husband or a husband who is an occupational underachiever. One approach to preventing violence in asymmetric status pairs would be to educate the husband to understand that his wife's career achievements do not reduce his own. Utilization of resources such as counseling or male support groups might reduce the husband's feelings of personal threat. In extreme cases, separation or divorce may be necessary to avoid violence.

*Intergenerational cycle of abuse.* Another risk factor is exposure to abuse in childhood. Family violence cycles through generations, repeating patterns of abuse in succeeding cohorts of victims. The repetitive cycle seems to be associated both with childhood victimization and with exposure to the victimization of other family members. Many studies report that parents who abuse their children are more likely to have suffered abuse as children than other parents (Conger, Burgess, & Barrett, 1979;

Gelles, 1980; Hunter & Kilstrom, 1979; Hunter et al., 1978; Lystad, 1975; Melnick & Hurley, 1969; Schneider, Hoffmeister, & Helfer, 1976). Men who batter their wives or female partners are over three times as likely to have grown up in a battering home than nonbatterers and to have suffered abuse as children (Walker, 1984).

It is not only the child victims of abuse that are at risk for developing later abusive behavior. Simply observing family violence appears to teach the child violent solutions to interpersonal problems. According to a national survey, those who observed their parents hitting each other were more likely to be abusive toward their own children (Gelles, 1980). Battered women tend to abuse their children at a higher rate than nonbattered women (Walker, 1984). When these women leave their battering partners and enter relationships with nonbattering men, abuse of their children tends to drop (Walker, 1984). Modeling, then, is a significant teacher of violent behavior.

The two classic prevention strategies—reducing stress and strengthening coping skills and resources—are both relevant to breaking the intergenerational cycle of abuse. To reduce the abused child's experience of stress, the abuse must be stopped and the child's safety guaranteed. Once this is done, there must be careful management of how and what the child is told about the parents' behavior, court decisions and actions of service agency staff (Aber, 1980). Since many abused children are either aggressive or socially withdrawn (Martin, 1976), training in social skills and anger control may strengthen them against the development of later abusive behavior (Keller & Erne, 1983). Strengthening supportive networks for abused children and for their families in the next generation is a promising prevention approach. Hunter and Kilstrom (1979) found that parents with access to more supportive resources did not repeat the abuse of the earlier generation. Strengthening parent-infant bonding may also be effective in breaking the cycle. Parents of newborns who do not repeat abuse were found to visit their infants in the hospital more often than abuse-repeating families (Hunter & Kilstrom, 1979).

*Increasing Social Supports*

The value of supportive relationships for healthy functioning and their role in buffering the destructive effects of stress has been extensively documented (Gottlieb, 1981, 1983; Mitchell & Trickett, 1980). The self-help groups and early intervention programs described above exemplify this strategy. Educational interventions such as parenting courses or workshops for the unemployed also serve this purpose, since they usually involve meetings with groups of peers and professionals in leadership roles. In addition to these standard sources of social support, two supportive processes, each involving families in different ways, have important consequences for healthy family functioning. The first is the process of parent-infant bonding. The second is the legislative process and related enforcement practices.

*Parent-infant bonding.* The amount of time parents and infants spend together in the first few days of life has important consequences for their later relationship. Mothers who are permitted to hold their infants for several hours immediately after birth and to assume major responsibility for their care are found to show more attachment behavior in later months and years than mothers who experience the conventional routine of most hospital maternity wards (Kennell, Jerauld, Wolfe et al., 1974; Kennell, Voos, & Klaus, 1976; Klaus, Jerauld, Kreger et al., 1972). Restricted family-infant contact at birth has been associated with later child abuse (Hunter et al., 1978; Hunter & Kilstrom, 1979). In a recent control-group study, six extra hours of mother-infant contact in the first two days after birth reportedly led to a dramatic difference in the frequency of child abuse two years later (Daly & Wilson, 1980). Separation of infants and mothers during the first 48 hours after birth puts the child at high risk for later abuse. Lynch (1975) found that 40% of a sample of severely abused children had experienced such separations compared with only 6% of their nonabused siblings.

The positive value of bonding is enhanced by recent research showing that newborns have a much greater capacity to see, hear and respond to human faces and voices than was previously thought possible (Brazelton, 1973; Eisenberg, 1976; Fantz, Fagan, & Miranda, 1975). Infants are born ready to interact with their caretakers (Emde, Swedberg, & Suzuki, 1975; Gregg, Haffner & Korner, 1976). While the beneficial effects of bonding have been documented, most hospitals in this country continue to follow procedures designed for the convenience of the hospital staff rather than for the benefit of the infant and his or her parents. There is currently an active movement to change hospital routines to reflect the knowledge gained from bonding studies.

*Family violence legislation and enforcement.* Social supports are usually thought of as rooted in the family, the neighborhood (with its churches and schools) and the work site. The community at large, through its institutions and practices, is a major source of support for its members. Communities' attitudes about family violence reflect today's changing mores. This shift is apparent in the expansion of social services and options for victims (e.g., foster homes and safe houses). These options have become available in most communities only within the last decade. In prevention terms, these services are host-focused interventions that treat the problem rather than prevent it. A signal of increasing community support for preventing family violence is seen in recent legislative changes and enforcement of laws related to this problem.

The law is a powerful force in controlling behavior. The last half of this century has witnessed a parade of causes seeking social justice through legislative change. However, passing laws to prohibit discriminatory practices does not guarantee these practices will end. Attitudes, as expressed in norms and customs, may take generations to change. Victims of family violence have suffered a history of benign neglect at best, and abandonment at worst, by this nation's legal system. One problem has been the lack of adequate legislation to protect victims of family violence. A second problem has to do with enforcement. Even in situations in which the law provides clear protection to victims, police have traditionally declined to arrest offenders. When police have made arrests, the courts have traditionally failed to convict. Over the last decade, discriminatory laws have been changed and new laws passed that create legal remedies for victims. These changes include eviction of the abuser from the home, mandatory arrest of batterers who violate protection orders and warrantless arrests for misdemeanor offenders involving domestic abuse (Lerman, 1982, this volume, Chapter 11). Enforcement practices have also begun to reflect increasing societal support for the rights of persons to be safe from attack by family members. A number of police departments have been sued because of the failure of police officers to make appropriate arrests or to enforce laws ensuring the safety of family members.

These changes have major significance for prevention. First, legislation codifies societal norms, even if attitudinal change comes slowly: "The legislation of one generation may become the morality of the next" (Walker, 1964). In discussing rape reform legislation, Loh (1981) echoes this point:

> The role of rape law as catalyst for attitude change may be greater than any immediate impact on the criminal justice system. The criminal law serves not only a general deterrent function. It also has a "moral or sociopedagogic" purpose to reflect and shape moral values and beliefs of society . . . The new rape law symbolizes and reinforces newly emerging conceptions about the status of women and the right of self-determination in sexual conduct . . . Conviction of rape, rather than of some surrogate defense, is a dramatic lesson

about society's disapprobation of the act, and helps to strengthen the public code. (p. 50)

The second preventive effect of legislation is in its power to deter the act prohibited. Research has demonstrated that it is the *certainty* of punishment (not its severity) that is effective in deterring crime (Andenaes, 1975; Erickson & Gibbs, 1973; Tittle, 1969). Unfortunately, the certainty factor has historically operated in reverse in the case of family violence. Abusers have traditionally been able to count on avoiding prosecution. It has been estimated that out of 10,000 men who assault their wives annually, only 800 are arrested, and only two end up going to jail (Dunwoody, 1982a).

Now studies are emerging that demonstrate effectiveness of the certainty principle in preventing crimes of domestic violence. A majority of domestic assault victims who seek prosecution find the action effective in stopping the violence, according to a Justice Department study in four major U.S. cities (Smith, 1981). The study focused on misdemeanor assaults among family members and friends in Charlotte, North Carolina, Los Angeles, Minneapolis, and Brooklyn. Victims expressed the most satisfaction with outcome in court systems in which judges lectured the defendants on the gravity of the crime and warned them of the legal consequences of continued battering.

One of the most frustrating outcomes of domestic disputes for law enforcement personnel—and a reason often given for failure to arrest—is the frequency with which victims bring charges and then drop them. The results of the Justice Department study refute the conventional wisdom that sees the time spent processing these cases as wasted. Even cases that ended up being dismissed were found to be effective in stopping violence:

> The informal resolutions that may have been reached outside the courtroom and the cessation of the violence may have been possible *because* the victim communicated the message to the abuser that "things have gone too far." Especially for the first time offender, the prospect of prosecution may be sufficiently frightening to alter his conduct toward the victim. (Smith, 1981)

In summary, changes in domestic violence legislation and enforcement are slowly beginning to change society's norms about what is and is not acceptable behavior in families. The hard-won victories of individuals in challenging specific discriminatory laws or enforcement practices serve preventive goals, since these victories set the standards by which subsequent behavior is judged.

*Increasing Coping Skills*

Most prevention programs for families include some sort of skill component. It should be understood that the incidence of family violence in society at large will be little affected by skill-building programs targeted to specific families, since sex-role stereotyping and discriminatory laws and customs, if unchanged, will continue to contribute to intrafamilial violence. However, skill building with individual family members may reduce their personal risk for victimization. The workshops, parenting courses, and other interventions described above are designed to increase the capacity of family members to resolve stressful situations (e.g., unemployment and parenting problems). Skill-building interventions are useful in facilitating normal developmental passages from one life stage to another. Such interventions may also reduce risk status in individual situations. Arming individual women and children with escape, avoidance or physical defense techniques, for example, may reduce the risk status they occupy because of their sex or age (Bart, 1981; Cooper, Lutter, & Phelps, 1983; McIntyre, 1981).

This section focuses on another skill that is critical to the prevention of family violence in individual situations: the control of anger and aggressive behavior. There is substantial evidence that men who are violent at home are also likely to be violent outside the home (Walker, 1984; Fagan, Stewart, & Hansen, 1983). Walker (1984) found that the rates of arrest and convictions for violent crimes were twice as high for batterers as nonbatterers. Animals, children, and people encountered in public places, such as streets, parks, and bars, are targets for such men. A study of rearrests of batterers in Brooklyn two and one-half years after conviction "suggests that a sizeable minority of defendants develop patterns of violence which are vented both within their homes and among their families and friends and outside their homes among strangers in society" (Smith, 1981). Approximately 10% of the defendants were rearrested for new crimes committed against the original victim. Over 30% were arrested for new crimes that did not involve the original victim—approximately half of these crimes were violent.

Anger has received comparatively little attention from researchers and scholars. While anger and aggression are not the same, the arousal of anger increases the probability of aggression. A prevention approach applicable to individuals at risk for developing physically abusive behavior is training in anger and conflict management. Novaco's (1977) three-phase model for high risk populations includes cognitive preparation, skill acquisition and application practice.

In the cognitive preparation phase, participants begin by learning to identify the situational cues that arouse their anger. These cues include perceptions of others' intentions, imminent pain, or personal injury or loss. They then learn to analyze their own feelings in response to the perceived threat. The self-assessment includes such questions as "Will I be able to block the threat, or stop it from happening?" "What will happen if I attack?" "Will I be attacked in return?" What people tell themselves when they start to get angry, their "self-talk," is a key determinant of their subsequent actions. The labeling involved in the self-talk process influences the way the person sizes up the situation. Rationalizations and justifications ("I'm right and she's wrong"), as well as calculations of the likelihood that planned actions will succeed ("I'm stronger than she is"), influence behavior in interpersonal situations.

Novaco's approach is similar to the preventive technique in anticipatory guidance. Both are based on the assumption that a large part of behavior is controlled cognitively—by the person's perceptions, interpretations, and self-talk in the situation. The second phase of Novaco's anger-control model involves skill acquisition and rehearsal. In this phase, participants become experts about their own anger patterns. They learn to become aware of the feelings and thoughts that signal anger arousal. A particularly important skill involves the ability to reinterpret the anger-arousing situation in ways that reduce or eliminate the angry response. Applied to family violence, this skill means, for example, that parents learn to hold in check their anger responses long enough to realize that their child's misbehavior may be accidental, due to hunger, fatigue or some other cause over which the child has little control. The "ability to alternatively construe provocation," as Novaco describes it, requires both impulse control and self-talk to supply neutral or nonprovocative reasons for the behavior of others.

The third phase of training involves application and practice. The procedures here are essentially desensitization techniques. The learner is exposed to situations that have aroused anger in the past. Beginning with mildly arousing real-life situations, the newly learned skills and self-talk are tested. If the learner manages well, provocations are escalated. Ideally, mastery of anger control occurs across the continuum of provocative situations.

Novaco (in press) cites a series of studies demonstrating that stress-inoculation approaches to anger management are effective. The technique has been applied to child-abusive parents (cited in Nomelini & Katz, in press). Adolescent anger has also been successfully defused and controlled through stress inoculation (Feindler & Fremouw, 1983). A "think aloud" program has successfully taught aggressive young boys to modify their responses in social situations (Camp, 1977; Camp, Blom, Herbert, & van Doorninck, 1977). The finding that these boys, before intervention, were not using verbal mediation techniques to manage their own behavior suggests that communication skills should be a major component of any preventive strategy directed to individual families.

## Increasing Self-Esteem

Self-esteem refers in general to the way one feels about oneself—how one values oneself in various life roles. There are few experimental studies in the field of family violence which address self-esteem apart from other measures of subject functioning. Many of the studies cited earlier as demonstrating reductions in stress and increases in social supports and/or coping skills also demonstrate increases in self-esteem in subject populations (Breton, Welbourn & Watters, 1981; Gordon, 1977; Hess, 1983; Mitchell & Trickett, 1980; South County Mental Health Center, 1980).

Current literature reflects conflicting findings related to levels of self-esteem in battered women. The traditional view is that these women suffer from low self-esteem (Carlson, 1977; Duncan, 1982; Hilberman, 1978; Mills, 1984). Their low self-regard is one of the factors that keeps them in the relationship according to this view. Wardell and her colleagues (1982) suggest that what appears to observers to be passivity, dependence and a low self-image may in fact be a normal response to situations of severe threat to health and life in which victims have few options for avoidance or escape: "In such situations, to notice that one lacks alternatives signifies rationality, not a poor self-image" (Wardell, Gillespie, & Leffler, 1982, p. 76). The finding of low self-esteem in battered or sexually abused women is usually interpreted as resulting from the abuse situation (Goldstein, 1983; Shields & Hanneke, 1982).

Several recent studies (Feldman, 1983; Walker, 1984) report finding no differences in self-esteem between battered and nonbattered women. "It was predicted that battered women's self-esteem would be quite low and our results, surprisingly, show the opposite. They perceived themselves as stronger, more independent, and more sensitive than other women or men. It is possible that battered women develop a positive sense of self from having survived in a violent relationship which causes them to believe they are equal to or better than others" (Walker, 1984, p. 100). Walker notes that these findings appear to be incompatible with the victims' reports of depression and other measures she interprets as demonstrating learned helplessness.

Two studies shed light on this apparent contradiction. Thome (1982) found that battered women felt adequate self-esteem when they dealt with the world outside the home, but felt less self-esteem when they dealt with their mates. This finding suggests that investigators of family violence should assess self-esteem separately in these two arenas of functioning. While Feldman (1983) found no differences in self-esteem between battered and nonbattered women, she found significant differences in self-esteem between battered women who stayed in the battering situation and those who left it (the latter had higher scores). As is often the case with research in a relatively young field, conflicting results may be symptomatic of a too simple formulation of the research issues.

Low self-esteem has also been found in males who abuse partners and/or children (Davidson, 1978; Doherty, 1983). A finding with major implications for prevention is that the self-esteem of children in homes where the mother is physically abused is adversely affected (Lombardi, 1982).

It is clear from this overview that the relationship between self-esteem and family violence is a complicated one. The relationship should be investigated for all family members, not just the abuse victim or the abuser. In addition, the investigator should examine self-esteem 1) both within and outside the abusive situation, and 2) for those who stay in and those who leave the situation. Finally, standard definitions of abuse and measures of self-esteem should be used so as to facilitate comparison of the results of multiple studies.

Until such refinements are incorporated into the methodology of family violence research, it is premature to draw definitive conclusions about the relationship between self-esteem and family violence. However, interventions with populations at risk in which either coping skills or social supports or both are increased suggest that these variables contribute to elevating self-esteem and, cumulatively, to creating preventive outcomes.

## SUMMARY

This chapter begins by tracing the development of family violence and prevention as fields of study. A model for preventing family violence is then presented. The model links stress and risk factors as major contributors to family violence and identifies social supports, coping skills and self-esteem as factors that contribute to healthy family functioning. Specific programs are presented as examples of preventive approaches consistent with the model.

Increasingly, major institutions in our society are advocating develop-

ing resources to prevent family violence rather than continuing to treat
its victims. This philosophy is put succinctly in the Report of the Attorney
General's Task Force on Family Violence (1984):

> The best of all strategies for dealing with family violence is to pre-
> vent it from occurring in the first place. A major part of the battle
> in preventing family violence is to spread knowledge. Potential vic-
> tims and abusers must know that family violence is not sanctioned,
> and is not a private matter, but instead comprises criminal offenses
> that will be vigorously prosecuted. Potential victims particularly
> young children must be told of ways to protect themselves; poten-
> tial abusers must learn how to deal constructively with the problems
> common in relationships and the difficult task of raising children.
> The public at large must be aware of the magnitude and urgency of
> the problems represented by family violence and the costs to socie-
> ty if prevention is not given high priority, for many of today's abused
> children will be tomorrow's abusers, runaways, and delinquents. (At-
> torney General, 1984, p. 64)

## REFERENCES

Aber, J. (1980). The involuntary child placement decision: Solomon's dilemma revisited.
   In G. Gerbner, C. Ross & E. Zigler (Eds.), *Child abuse: An agenda for action*. New York:
   Oxford University Press.
Albee, G. (1981). Preventing prevention in the community mental health centers. In *The
   Health Care System and Drug Abuse Prevention: Toward Cooperation and Health Pro-
   motion*. Washington, DC: U.S. Government Printing Office, DHHS Pub. No. (ADM)
   81-1105, 38–44.
Alpert, J., Richardson, M., & Fodaski, L. (1983). Onset of parenting and stressful events.
   *The Journal of Primary Prevention, 3*, 149–159.
Andenaes, J. (1975). General prevention revisited: Research and policy implications. *Jour-
   nal of Criminal Law and Criminology, 66*, 338–365.
Anderson, J., Larson, J., & Morgan, A. (1981). PPSF/Parenting Program for Stepparent
   Families: A new approach for strengthening families. In N. Stinnett, J. DeFrain, K. King,
   P. Knaub & G. Rowe (Eds.), *Family strengths: Roots of well-being* (Vol. 3, pp. 351–363).
   Lincoln, NE: University of Nebraska Press.
Arney, W. (1980). Maternal-infant bonding: The politics of falling in love with your child.
   *Feminist Studies, 6*(3), 547–570.
Attorney General. (1984). *Report of the Attorney General's Task Force on Family Violence*.
   Washington, DC: U.S. Dept. of Justice.
Badger, E., & Burns, D. (1982). A model for coalescing birth-to-3 programs. In L. Bond &
   J. Joffee (Eds.), *Facilitating infant and early childhood development* (pp. 513–537).
   Hanover, NH: University Press of New England.
Bart, P. (1981). A study of women who both were raped and avoided rape. *The Journal
   of Social Issues, 37*, 123–137.
Baruch, G., & Barnett, R. (1983). Correlates of father's participation in family work. *Working
   papers* (No. 106). Wellesley, MA: Center for Research on Women.
Baruch, G., & Barnett, R. (1984). Father's participation in family work: Effects on children's
   sex role attitudes. *Working papers* (No. 126). Wellesley, MA: Center for Research on
   Women.

Bloom, B. (1971). A university freshman preventive intervention program: Report of a pilot project. *Journal of Consulting and Clinical Psychology, 37*, 235–242.

Bond, L., & Joffe, J. (Eds.). (1982). *Facilitating infant and early childhood development.* Hanover, NH: University Press of New England.

Brazelton, T. (1973). Neonatal behavioral assessment scale. *Clinics in developmental medicine.* No. 51. Philadelphia: J. B. Lippincott Co.

Breines, W., & Gordon, L. (1983). The new scholarship on family violence. *SIGNS, 8,* 490–531.

Breton, J., Welbourn, A., & Watters, J. (1981). A nurturing and problem-solving approach for abuse-prone mothers. *Child Abuse and Neglect, 5,* 475–480.

Buss, T., Redburn, F., & Waldron, J. (1983). *Mass unemployment: Plant closings and community mental health.* Beverly Hills: Sage.

Camp, B. (1977). Verbal mediation in young aggressive boys. *Journal of Abnormal Child Psychology, 86,* 145–153.

Camp, B., Blom, G., Herbert, F., & van Doorninck, W. (1977). "Think aloud": A program for developing self-control in young aggressive boys. *Journal of Abnormal Child Psychology, 5,* 157–169.

Carlson, B. (1977). Battered women and their assailants. *Social Work, 2,* 455–460.

Cassel, J. (1974). Psychosocial processes and "stress": Theoretical formulation. *International Journal of Health Services, 4,* 3, 471–482.

Cohen, C., & Sokolovsky, J. (1978). Schizophrenia and social networks: Ex-patients in the inner city. *Schizophrenia Bulletin, 4*(4), 546–560.

Comstock, G. (1982). Preventive processes in self-help groups: Parents anonymous. *Prevention in Human Services, 1*(3), 47–53.

Conger, R., Burgess, R., & Barrett, C. (1979). Child abuse related to life change and perceptions of illness: Some preliminary findings. *Family Coordinator, 28,* 73–78.

Cooper, S., Lutter, Y., & Phelps, C. (1983). *Strategies for free children: A leader's guide to child assault prevention.* Youngstown, Ohio: Ink Well Press.

Coopersmith, S. (1967). *The antecedents of self-esteem.* San Francisco: Freeman.

Daly, M., & Wilson, J. (1980). Discriminative parental solicitude: A biographic perspective. *Journal of Marriage and the Family, 42,* 277–288.

Davidson, T. (1978). *Conjugal crime.* New York: Hawthorne Books.

Dobash, R. E., & Dobash, R. (1979). *Violence against wives.* New York: Free Press.

Doherty, S. (1983). Self-esteem, anxiety and dependency in men who batter women. *Dissertation Abstracts International, 44/05-A,* 1384.

Duncan, D. (1982). Cognitive perceptions of battered women. *Dissertation Abstracts International, 43/01-B,* 245.

Dunwoody, E. (1982a). Canadian National Clearinghouse on Family Violence. Canada holds hearings on family violence. *Response, 5*(2), 8–9.

Dunwoody, E. (1982b). Sexual abuse of children: A serious, widespread problem. *Response, 5*(4), 1–2, 13–14.

Eisenberg, R. (1976). *Auditory competence in early life: The roots of communicative behavior.* Baltimore, MD: University Park Press.

Eisenberg, S., & Micklow, P. (1977). The assaulted wife: "Catch 22" revisited. *Women's Rights Law Reporter, 3–4,* 138–161.

Elmer, E. (1967). *Children in jeopardy.* Pittsburgh: University of Pittsburgh Press.

Emde, R., Swedberg, J., & Suzuki, B. (1975). Human wakefulness and biological rhythms after birth. *Archives of General Psychology, 32,* 780–783.

Erickson, M., & Gibbs, J. (1973). The deterrence question: Some alternative methods of analysis. *Social Science Quarterly, 54,* 534–551.

Fagan, F., Stewart, D., & Hansen, K. (1983). Violent men or violent husbands. In D. Finkelhor, R. Gelles, G. Hotaling & M. Straus (Eds.), *The dark side of families* (pp. 49–67). Beverly Hills: Sage Publications.

Fantz, R., Fagan, J., & Miranda, S. (1975). Early visual selectivity as a function of pattern variables, previous exposure, age from birth and conception, and expected cognitive deficit. In L. B. Cohen & P. Salapatek (Eds.), *Infant perception: From sensation to cogni-*

*tion*. New York: Academic Press.

Feindler, E., & Fremouw, W. (1983). Stress inoculation training for adolescent anger problems. In D. Merchenbaus & M. Jarenko (Eds.), *Stress reduction and prevention*. New York: Plenum Press.

Feldman, S. (1983). Battered women: Psychological correlates of the victimization process. *Dissertation Abstracts International, 44/04-B*, 1221.

Finkelhor, D., & Hotaling, G. (1984). Sexual abuse in the national incidence study of child abuse and neglect: An appraisal. *Child Abuse and Neglect, 8*, 23–33.

Gelles, R. (1973). Child abuse as psychopathology: A sociological critique and reformation. *American Journal of Orthopsychiatry, 43*, 611–621.

Gelles, R. (1974). *The violent home*. Beverly Hills: Sage Publications.

Gelles, R. (1975). Violence and pregnancy: A note on the extent of the problem and needed services. *Family Coordinator, 24*, 81–86.

Gelles, R. (1980). Violence in the family: A review of research in the seventies. *Journal of Marriage and the Family, 42*, 873–885.

Giarretto, H. (1981). A comprehensive child sexual abuse treatment program. In. P. Mrazek & H. Kempe (Eds.), *Sexually abused children and their families*. New York: Pergamon Press.

Gil, D. (1970). *Violence against children: Physical child abuse in the United States*. Cambridge: Harvard University Press.

Goldstein, D. (1983). Spouse abuse. In A. Goldstein (Ed.), *Prevention and control of aggression* (pp. 37–65). New York: Pergamon Press.

Gordon, T. (1977). Parent effectiveness training: A preventive program and its delivery system. In G. Albee & J. Joffee (Eds.), *Primary prevention of psychopathology: The issues* (pp. 175–186). Hanover, NH: University Press of New England.

Gordon, T. (1983). Transforming early parenthood to promote family wellness. In D. Mace (Ed.), *Prevention in family services: Approaches to family wellness* (pp. 133–147). Beverly Hills, CA: Sage.

Gottlieb, B. (Ed.). (1981). *Social networks and social support*. Sage Studies in Community Mental Health, 4. Beverly Hills: Sage.

Gottlieb, B. (1983). Opportunities for collaboration with informal support systems. In S. Cooper & W. Hodges (Eds.), *The mental health consultation field* (pp. 181–203). New York: Human Sciences Press.

Gray, E. (1982). Perinatal support programs: A strategy for the primary prevention of child abuse. *Journal of Primary Prevention, 2*, 138–152.

Greenberg, B. (1982). Television and role socialization: An overview. In D. Pearl, L. Bouthilet, & J. Lazar, *Television and behavior: Ten years of scientific progress and implications for the eighties, Vol. 1*. DHHS Pub. No. (ADM) 82-1195. Washington, DC: U.S. Government Printing Office.

Gregg, C., Haffner, M., & Korner, A. (1976). The relative efficacy of vestibular-proprioceptive stimulation and the upright position in enhancing visual pursuit in neonates. *Child Development, 47*, 309–314.

Heber, R., Garber, H., Harrington, S., Hoffman, C. & Falender, C. (1972). *Rehabilitation of families at risk for mental retardation*. Madison, WI: University of Wisconsin.

Hess, R. (1983). Early intervention with the unemployed: Employment Transition Program of the University of Michigan. *Journal of Primary Prevention, 4*, 129–131.

Hilberman, E. (1978). *Battered women: Issues of public policy*. A consultation sponsored by the U.S. Commission on Civil Rights, January 30–31.

Hilberman, E. (1980). Overview: "The wife-beater's wife" reconsidered. *American Journal of Psychiatry, 137*, 1336–1347.

Hornung, C., McCullough, B., & Sugimoto, T. (1981). Status relationships in marriage: Risk factors in spouse abuse. *Journal of Marriage and the Family, 43*, 675–92.

Hunter, R., & Kilstrom, N. (1979). Breaking the cycle in abusive families. *American Journal of Psychiatry, 136*, 1320–1322.

Hunter, R., Kilstrom, N., Kraybill, E., & Loda, F. (1978). Antecedents of child abuse and neglect in premature infants: A prospective study in a newborn intensive care unit. *Pediatrics, 61*, 629–635.

Justice, C., & Justice, R. (1976). *The abusing family*. New York: Human Sciences Press.

Kahn, M. (1984). Battered women: A five-year study. *ADAMHA News, 10*, 6.

Kamerman, S., Kahn, A., & Kingston, P. (1983). *Maternity policies and working women*. New York: Columbia University Press.

Keller, H. R., & Erne, D. (1983). Child abuse: Toward a comprehensive mode. In A. P. Goldstein (Ed.), *Prevention and control of aggression* (pp. 1–36). New York: Pergamon Press.

Kempe, H., Silverman, F., Steele, B., Droegemueller, W., & Silver, H. (1962). The battered child syndrome. *Journal of the American Medical Association, 181*, 107–112.

Kennell, J., Jerauld, R., Wolfe, H., Chester, D., Kreger, N., Alpine, W., Steffa, M., & Klaus, M. (1974). Maternal behavior one year after early and extended post-partum contact. *Developmental Medicine and Child Neurology, 16*, 172–179.

Kennell, J., Voos, D., & Klaus, M. (1976). Parent-infant bonding. In *Child abuse and neglect: The family and the community*. Cambridge, MA: Ballinger.

Klaus, M., Jerauld, R., Kreger, N., McAlpine, W., Steffa, M., & Kennell, J. (1972). Maternal attachment: Importance of the first post-partum days. *New England Journal of Medicine, 286*, 460.

Klinman, D., & Kohl, R. The Fatherhood Project. (1984). *Fatherhood USA: The first national guide to programs, services, and resources for and about fathers*. New York: Garland.

Lerman, L. (1982). Court decisions on wife abuse laws: Recent developments. *Response, 5*(3), 3–4, 21–22.

Levine, J. (1982). Day care challenges and opportunities in the 1980s. In N. Stinnett, J. DeFrain, K. King, H. Lingren, G. Rowe, S. Van Zandt & R. Williams (Eds.), *Family strengths: Positive support systems* (Vol. 4, pp. 15–31). Lincoln, NE: Nebraska University Press.

Loh, W. D. (1981). What has reform of rape legislation wrought? *The Journal of Social Issues, 37*, 28–52.

Lombardi, J. (1982). Growing up with violence: An analysis of retrospective accounts of female offspring. *Dissertation Abstracts International, 43/06-A*, 2118.

Lynch, M. (1975). Ill health and child abuse. *The Lancet, 2*, 317–319.

Lystad, M. (1975). Violence at home: A review of the literature. *American Journal of Orthopsychiatry, 45*, 328–345.

Martin, H. (Ed.). (1976). *The abused child: A multidisciplinary approach to developmental issues and treatment*. Cambridge, MA: Ballinger.

McCord, J., & McCord, W. (1958). The effects of parental modes on criminality. *Journal of Social Issues, 14*, 66–75.

McIntyre, J. M. (1981). *Victim response to rape: Alternative outcomes* (Final Report). National Center for the Prevention and Control of Rape, National Institute of Mental Health.

Melnick, B., & Hurley, H. (1969). Distinctive personality attributes of child-abusing mothers. *Journal of Consulting and Clinical Psychology, 33*, 746–749.

Mills, T. (1984). Victimization and self-esteem: On equating "husband abuse" and "wife abuse." *Victimology, 9*(2), 254–261.

Mitchell, R., & Trickett, E. (1980). Social network research and psychosocial adaptations: Implications for community mental health practice. In P. Insel (Ed.), *Environmental variables and the prevention of mental illness*. Lexington, MA: D. C. Heath & Company.

Moss, J., Hess, R., & Swift, C. (Eds.). (1982). *Early intervention programs for infants*. New York: The Haworth Press.

Newberger, C. M., & Newberger, E. H. (1982). Prevention of child abuse: Theory, myth, practice. *Journal of Preventive Psychiatry, 4*, 443–451.

Nomelini, S., & Katz, R. (in press). Effects of anger control training on abusive parents. *Cognitive therapy and research*.

Novaco, R. (1977). A stress inoculation approach to anger management in the training of law enforcement officers. *American Journal of Community Psychology, 5*(3), 327–346.

Novaco, R. (in press). Anger and its therapeutic regulation. In M. Chesney, S. Goldston, & R. Roseman (Eds.), *Anger and hostility in behavioral and cardiovascular disorders.* New York: McGraw-Hill.

Okun, L. (1983). *A study of woman abuse: 300 battered women taking shelter, 119 women-batterers in counseling.* University of Michigan, *Dissertation Abstracts, 44/06-B,* 1972.

Parke, R., & Collmer, C. (1975). Child abuse: An interdisciplinary analysis. In M. Hetherington (Ed.), *Review of child development research* (Vol. V, pp. 1–102). Chicago: University of Chicago Press.

Pleck, J. (1984). Men at work: A new focus on fatherhood activists. *Research Report, 4*(1), 1–2.

Prescott, S., & Letko, C. (1977). Battered women: A social psychosocial perspective. In M. Roy (Ed.), *Battered women: A psychosociological study of domestic violence* (pp. 72–96). New York: Van Nostrand Reinhold.

President's Advisory Council on Private Sector Initiatives. (1984). *Employer options to support working families.* Unpublished executive summary. Available from The White House, Washington, DC.

Putnam, J. (1984). *Men's lives: Changes and choices* (Vol. 4, No. 1, pp. 1–2). Research Report, Wellesley College Center for Research on Women.

Riessman, F. (1965). The "helper" therapy principle. *Social Work, 10,* 27–32.

Roland, L. (1978). *Pierre the pelican series of the state of Louisiana: Post-natal series.* New Orleans: Family Publication Center.

Schneider, C., Hoffmeister, J., & Helfer, R. (1976). A predictive screen questionnaire for potential problems in mother-child interaction. In R. Helfer & H. Kempe (Eds.), *Child abuse and neglect: The family and the community.* Cambridge, MA: Ballinger.

Semmelman, P. (1982). *Battered and nonbattered women: A comparison.* Ohio State University, *Dissertation Abstracts, 43/08-B,* 2716.

Shields, N., & Hanneke, C. (1982). Battered wives' reactions to marital rape. In D. Finkelhor, R. Gelles, G. Hotaling & M. Straus (Eds.), *The dark side of families* (pp. 132–148). Beverly Hills: Sage.

Smith, B. (1981). *Non-stranger violence: The criminal court's response.* Washington, D.C.: National Institute of Justice, U. S. Department of Justice.

South County Mental Health Center. (1980). A nomination of the Lela Rowland Prevention Award 1980: The Optimum Growth Project.

Steinmetz, S. (1982). Family care of elders: Myths and realities. In N. Stinnett, J. DeFrain, K. King, H. Lingren, G. Rowe, S. Van Zandt, & R. Williams (Eds.), *Family strengths: Positive support systems* (Vol. 4, pp. 213–233). Lincoln, NE: University of Nebraska Press.

Straus, M. (1980a). Social stress and marital violence in a national sample of American families. *Annals New York Academy of Sciences, 347,* 229–250.

Straus, M. A. (1980b). The marriage license as a hitting license: Evidence from popular culture, law and social science. In M. Straus & G. Hotaling (Eds.), *The social causes of husband-wife violence.* Minneapolis, MN: University of Minnesota.

Straus, M., Gelles, R. & Steinmetz, S. (1980). *Behind closed doors: Violence in the American family.* New York: Anchor Books.

Swift, C. (in press). Community intervention in sexual child abuse. In S. Auerbach & A. Stolberg (Eds.), *Crisis intervention with children and families.* New York: Hemisphere.

Thome, M. (1982). An analysis of differences between battered and nonbattered women with respect to sex role acceptance, life histories and personal adjustment. *Dissertation Abstracts International, 43/09-B,* 3047.

Tittle, C. (1969). Crime rates and legal sanction. *Social Problems, 16,* 409–423.

Tolsdorf, C. (1976). Social networks support and coping: An exploratory study. *Family Process, 15*(4), 407–417.

Vance, E. (1977). A typology of risks and the disabilities of low status. In G. Albee & J. Joffee (Eds.), *Primary prevention of psychopathology: The issues* (Vol. 1, pp. 207–237). The University Press of New England.

Videka-Sherman, L. (1982). Effects of participation in a self-help group for bereaved parents: Compassionate friends. *Prevention in Human Services, 1*(3), 69–77.

Walker, L. E. (1984). *The battered woman syndrome.* New York: Springer.

Walker, N. (1964). Morality and the criminal law. As cited in J. Andenaes, General prevention revisited: Research and policy implications. *Journal of Criminal Law and Criminology, 66,* 339–365.

Wardell, L., Gillespie, D., & Leffler, A. (1982). Science and violence against wives. In D. Finkelhor, R. Gelles, G. Hotaling & M. Straus (Eds.), *The dark side of families* (pp. 69–84). Beverly Hills: Sage.

Young, M. (1976). Multiple correlates of abuse: A systems approach to the etiology of child abuse. *Journal of Pediatric Psychology, 1,* 57–61.

# 11

# *Prosecution of Wife Beaters: Institutional Obstacles and Innovations*

## Lisa G. Lerman

## INTRODUCTION

At least one-fifth of the homicides and perhaps an even larger proportion of the assaults, batteries, and burglaries in the United States are committed within families or within intimate relationships. Forty percent of female homicide victims are killed by family members (FBI, 1980). For decades, these crimes have posed a major problem for police, prosecutors, and courts. Many criminal justice officials argue that prosecuting intrafamily crimes is inappropriate because it is disruptive to family life, that it is frustrating because victims often drop charges, and that it is a waste of resources needed for "real crime." During the last decade, as public awareness of the seriousness and pervasiveness of spouse abuse* has grown, new legal remedies for battering have been examined and developed to improve the justice system's response to people in chronic violent relationships.

Recent efforts on behalf of battered women have focused on setting up shelters and hotlines, improving the police response to domestic disturbance calls, and developing legislation providing civil injunctive relief for battered women. Experience with civil legal remedies has led many peo-

---

This chapter is a revision of L. G. Lerman, *Prosecution of Spouse Abuse: Innovations in Criminal Justice Response*, 1980, Washington, DC, Center for Women Policy Studies. Reproduced with permission.

*Spouse abuse* is used here to refer to violence between adults who are intimates regardless of their marital status or living arrangements.

 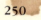

ple who work with violent families to turn to the criminal courts to obtain leverage over batterers and court orders enforceable by criminal penalties. Criminal law is increasingly used both to punish violators of protection orders and as an independent legal option that may be initiated instead of or in addition to a protection order. Much recent attention has focused, therefore, on identifying and eliminating obstacles to criminal prosecution of wife beaters.

This chapter describes the experiences of those who have solved some of the problems which plague prosecutors who handle spouse abuse cases. It sets out practical options by which prosecutors can successfully pursue family violence cases and can effectively reduce domestic violence in their communities. Changes are suggested in policies on screening, charging, and dismissal of charges, and in procedure for protecting victims of abuse and preparing them to participate as complaining witnesses. The report also recommends dispositions aimed at rehabilitating batterers and strategies for improving police reporting and investigation of domestic cases.* The research for this report was conducted during 1979 and 1980. The purpose of the study was to identify innovations within prosecutors' offices in the handling of spouse abuse cases, to examine the effectiveness of those innovations, and to explore the possible transferability of the changes in procedure to other prosecutors' offices. The goal was to find the prosecutors who were very concerned, active, and successful in using law enforcement to stop family violence and to share their experience and their ideas with other prosecutors.

First examined were the efforts being made by the 29 demonstration projects that were funded by the Law Enforcement Assistance Administration (LEAA) in 1978. The first stage was a review of extensive files maintained on these projects at the Center for Women Policy Studies, whose Family Violence Project provided technical assistance to the demonstration projects. From these files, including grant proposals, materials generated by the programs, quarterly reports, and evaluations, an initial determination of which projects were based in or had close ties with prosecutors' offices was made. Site visits to 11 of these projects, both to collect information for this report and to help the project staff with program

---

*The research for this chapter was conducted as part of the Center for Women Policy Studies' (CWPS) Family Violence Project. Under grants from the Law Enforcement Assistance Administration, U.S. Department of Justice, and the Administration for Children, Youth, and Families, U.S. Department of Health and Human Services, the CWPS Family Violence Project has provided technical assistance to federally funded demonstration projects on family violence and disseminated information to service providers nationwide since 1976.

development issues, were conducted, with lengthy interviews with most project staff and relevant law enforcement officials.*

In some instances, there were opportunities to talk with victims of abuse or abusers who were served by the projects; in other instances there were opportunities to sit in on interviews, staff meetings, court proceedings, and other events that occurred in the work of the projects. Each site visit usually ended with a meeting with the project director to discuss the researcher's observations and to talk about possibilities for further improvements of law enforcement response to battered women. After the site visit, frequent telephone contact occurred with each program.

As research progressed, two other prosecutors' offices, one in Los Angeles and one in Seattle, were identified as having taken significant initiatives on spouse abuse without LEAA funds. Site visits were made to both of these programs.

Telephone and in-person interviews were conducted with numerous other prosecutors from towns and cities across the United States, with some of these conversations occurring at conferences of law enforcement officials. Many in-person and telephone interviews with advocates for abused women also were conducted. Several programs provided materials used in processing domestic violence cases for prosecution. Others sought the researcher out for consultation on problems arising in their law enforcement system.

All of the interviews were unstructured; the goal in talking with people was to find out what the prosecutors' offices did or did not do in each community, identify the causes of obstacles or inaction, identify strategies that had been adopted to overcome those obstacles, and get any available information about the effectiveness of the innovations in stopping violence.

This report represents a synthesis of what was learned from 13 site visits, 20 conferences, and hundreds of informal conversations. In addition to gathering information from the field, all of the published articles that discuss the prosecution of spouse abuse were reviewed. The methodology used in conducting this study was closer to that used by an investigative reporter than that used by a social scientist. All of the data that had been compiled by the programs about their case loads were collected; the researcher did not collect additional data.

---

*The projects visited were located in Philadelphia, Pennsylvania; Portland, Oregon; White Plains, New York; New York City; Miami, Florida; Cleveland, Ohio; Salem and Milford, Massachusetts; Faribault, Minnesota, Santa Barbara, California, and Wilmington, Delaware.

This chapter will first offer a brief survey of the literature on these issues, followed by an analysis of what obstacles exist within the criminal justice system to prosecution of spouse abuse. Following that is a description of methods for reducing case attrition, and finally, a discussion of some sentencing options in dealing with men convicted of spouse abuse.

One of the most important of recent studies is "Prosecutorial and Judicial Handling of Family Violence" by Raymond Parnas (1973). Parnas examined projects which had developed new ways of processing domestic cases. The projects concentrated on using informal prosecutor hearings, information and referral programs, arbitration, peace bonds, and family courts in order to avoid prosecution of family violence cases and to channel such cases to social service personnel and psychologists. Parnas pointed out that prosecutors are ill-equipped to perform psychoanalysis and cannot deliver the primary counseling services needed by violent families. His conclusion, succinctly stated, is that "effective diversion requires problem-solving techniques rather than simple problem-controlling hardware" (Parnas, 1973, p. 759).

A similar view is articulated by Martha and Henry Field (1973). Examining criminal justice intervention in domestic violence cases, the Fields suggest that the criminal justice system is ineffective in achieving "deterrence, incapacitation, prevention, retribution, or rehabilitation." They assert that the dynamics of violent intimate relationships "place them more appropriately within the bailiwick of the helping professions" (Field & Field, 1977, p. 160). The authors suggest several alternatives, including improved reporting of domestic violence calls to identify serious cases, seling services.

Sue Eisenberg and Patricia Micklow (1977) take a different approach in examining prosecution as a remedy for domestic abuse. They criticize crisis intervention and arbitration as relying excessively on mediation or conciliation, with "the effect of deprecating the severity of the complaints" and translating "patterns of repetitive, serious, violent behavior into social disturbances, family spats, or quarrels" (Eisenberg & Micklow, 1977, p. 160). The authors suggest several alternatives, including improved reporting of domestic violence calls to identify serious cases, limited use of pretrial detention, clear prosecutor guidelines on the exercise of discretion in filing charges, and judicial insistence on complete records in spouse abuse cases.

Legal Services Attorney Marjory Fields (1978) describes in detail the failure of prosecutors to treat battering cases seriously, and suggests that prosecution is useful because it "restores some of the power balance that the husband has destroyed by his violence" (p. 252) and encourages improved police response. Fields criticizes remedies focused on mediation as ineffective in resolving serious disputes, particularly in a situation in which one party dominates the other. Fields encourages prosecutors to protect battered wives while criminal charges are pending by requesting conditions on pretrial release, and to understand the positive reasons why battered women often drop charges, which include cessation of violence after charges are filed, or departure to a safer residence and more secure environment while the batterer is in custody.

⏚ In 1978, prosecutors from around the country attended a conference on prosecution of spouse abuse cosponsored by the National District Attorneys Association and the Center for Women Policy Studies. According to the conference report by attorney Terry Fromson (1980), conference participants agreed that spouse assault is just as criminal as violent conduct between other people, and thus should not be treated less seriously by the criminal justice system. The report suggests that problems with victim noncooperation might be reduced through increased services to battered women who become complaining witnesses. It also discusses the use of civil injunctive relief and mediation in cases in which prosecution is deemed inappropriate.

Since 1980 a number of books and articles have been published in this area: a report by the U.S. Commission on Civil Rights (1982) titled ''Under the Rule of Thumb: Battered Women and the Administration of Justice''; Susan Schecter's (1982) *Women and Male Violence: The Visions and Struggles of the Battered Women's Movement*; an important study of the deterrent effect of arrest of wife beaters sponsored by the Police Foundation and conducted by Larry Sherman and Richard Berk (1983); two articles by Lerman entitled ''Mediation of Wife Abuse: The Adverse Impact of Alternative Dispute Resolution on Women'' (1984a) and ''A Model State Act: Remedies for Domestic Abuse'' (1984b).

⏚ In the last several years, there has been a trend away from mediation, crisis intervention, and similar informal procedures that were used in family violence cases in the early 1970s. Recent experimental programs and demonstration projects have increased the use of formal criminal charges in domestic assault cases. Through close coordination with mental health agencies, and through the development of extensive victim services, prosecution has become an appropriate and a desirable legal remedy for many battered women. Innovative programs emphasize the importance of enforcement of court orders, penalties, and rehabilitative measures.

Between 1978 and 1980 the Law Enforcement Assistance Administration funded 29 demonstration projects on criminal justice response to domestic violence around the country. Their mandate was to encourage and coordinate efforts of police, prosecutors, hospitals, and mental health and social service agencies.

Many of these demonstration projects had several components that provided services to violent families including shelters, prosecution units, mental health facilities, protection-order clinics, and public education and training facilities. Some of the projects which were based in or closely linked with prosecutors' offices have had remarkable success in prosecuting spouse abuse cases. Police referrals to prosecutors increased, the rate of case attrition due to victim noncooperation was reduced (in some cases to below 10%), the rate of convictions or guilty pleas rose, and recidivism rates dropped. In some cities, assistance for victims and court-mandated treatment for abusers are now established practices.

The projects funded by the LEAA Family Violence Program were only a small part of the wider grass-roots movement focused on reducing violence within families. Some have continued their work despite termination of federal funds, while other projects have been developed independent of the LEAA Program. All of these have made significant contributions to the improvement of criminal justice handling of family violence.

Although all of the options presented in this report are replicable, the changes that ought to be implemented in any given community depend on the structure of its criminal justice system, on what programs already exist, and on which agencies are most likely to provide financial and political support for an effort to upgrade prosecution of spouse abuse. For example, if pretrial diversion is unknown to the community, implementation of a diversion program might be more difficult than encouraging more aggressive prosecution. If mental health facilities already receive referrals from the criminal courts, advocacy of court-mandated treatment for abusers might be productive.

Prosecution is not presented as the best or the only legal option that should be available to violent families, but as the most serious and sometimes the only effective action that can be taken to stop violence within a family. At present most battered women do not, in fact, have the option to file charges because the obstacles posed by the system are so great.

## OBSTACLES TO SUCCESSFUL PROSECUTION

Many prosecutors believe that family violence is better handled by social service agencies or domestic relations courts than by criminal courts. They believe that most domestic cases are trivial crimes, and that the more serious cases are impossible to prosecute. From the prosecutor's perspective, the primary problem with prosecution of spouse abuse is that it is time wasted, since most victims request that charges be dropped before dispositions are reached. Given the enormous caseloads of most prosecutors, the result is that domestic violence cases are assigned lower priority than robbery, arson, and other crimes between strangers.

Sometimes victims of abuse request that charges be dropped because of fear of reprisal if charges are pursued or because of mistrust of or lack of information about the criminal justice system. In some cases, requests for dismissal are based on the victim's emotional attachment to the abuser, in others simply to the time which would be lost from work by participating as a complaining witness.

There are, nevertheless, reasons why prosecution may be the most appropriate course in domestic abuse cases. First, the failure of the criminal justice system to enforce the law against abusers contributes to the perpetuation of violence within families. It is well-established that spouse abuse is epidemic in the United States, pervading every race and ethnic group, every economic class, every geographic area (Schulman, 1979; Straus, 1977–1978). Battering can no longer be regarded as merely an "individual" problem or a "relationship" problem but must be viewed as perpetuated, at least in part, by inadequate or inappropriate responses by the institutions from which violent families seek help. A poignant example of the role of institutions in perpetuating family violence is that of hospitals that routinely distribute sedatives to women who complain of abuse. The sedation makes it less likely that the victim will take any action to protect herself from subsequent abuse (Stark, Flitcraft, et al., 1981).

Police who refuse to make an arrest because injuries are not visible and prosecutors who refuse to file charges because they believe victims will not testify communicate to victims and batterers that family violence is not a serious crime. This gives batterers tacit permission to continue their violent behavior. Efforts to improve prosecutorial policy on family violence may help to reverse those messages.

A second reason why prosecution may be the appropriate course is that some prosecutors have made changes in policy and procedure that demonstrate that the criminal courts can protect victims of abuse and can require batterers to change their behavior. Criminal justice officials have the power to take people into custody, deprive them of property, and require or prohibit certain behavior. Also, an arrest, a criminal charge or a conviction may have enormous symbolic impact, because of the stigma attached to criminal misconduct.

A third advantage of prosecution is that if family violence becomes a priority for prosecutors, police response to battered women may be greatly improved. Since the police are usually the first to be called for help, their action is critical. Police are often reluctant to make arrests or to file reports in domestic cases, in part because they believe that the offender will not be charged. If more batterers are prosecuted, police may be encouraged to make arrests where appropriate, and to provide victims with protection or referrals that may prevent subsequent violence.

Finally, unless prosecutors change their policies to take a more active role in protecting battered women, they may be subject to civil liability for denial of equal protection to battered women or for the wrongful death of battered women who have sought assistance from prosecutors and have been refused help. While most of the relevant case law holds that a prosecutor cannot be sued for failure to prosecute (because that decision is wholly within the discretion of the prosecutor), prosecutors may be vulnerable to liability for violation of constitutional rights, violation of a statutory duty, or for arbitrary, capricious or abusive conduct (Blum, 1980).

A more detailed examination of the major obstacles to effective prosecution of spouse abuse will provide a framework for understanding why the various innovations have been so effective.

## Traditional Views of the Family

In the early nineteenth century, a man in the United States was legally permitted to chastise his wife "without subjecting himself to vexatious prosecutions for assault and battery, resulting in the mutual discredit and shame of all parties concerned" (*Bradley v. State*, 1824). This rule was taken from English common law, under which the husband and wife were treated as one person (the husband) and under which the disciplinary authority of a man over members of the household was unquestioned. (Eisenberg & Micklow, 1977).

During the latter part of the century there was widespread protest against family violence by suffragists and others, and wife beating was declared illegal by courts and legislators around the country. By 1870, wife beating was illegal in most states (Pleck, 1979). However, few batterers were prosecuted, and no concerted effort to enforce criminal laws against batterers was made until the 1970s, a hundred years later.

Many of the historical reasons for nonintervention by criminal justice officials in family violence cases still influence current prosecutorial policy. Many prosecutors believe that spouse abuse is not serious or widespread and view cases involving family members or intimates as "minor disputes" or "disturbances." Most prosecutors avoid filing charges in family violence cases whenever possible (Miller, 1969).

Throughout the legal system, the family is treated as a sacred entity, as a stable social unit which must be preserved or at least left undisturbed (Dobash & Dobash, 1979). Viewed through this preconception, violence within families is minimized and treated as a minor disruption, a normal part of life.

Miller (1969), a former prosecutor, argues that "if prosecution were to be commenced in every case in which a drunken husband struck his wife, . . . the charging decision would place an additional strain on an inevitably continuing relationship" (p. 267). Some commentators who view family violence as caused by poverty or psychological problems believe that criminal action will worsen the economic plight of the parties, or at best will be an irrelevant remedy for a basically interpersonal problem (Subin, 1973).

Some prosecutors are disinclined to prosecute batterers because they believe that the violence is usually provoked by the victims. In explaining the minimal number of charges filed for spouse assault, Miller (1969) states that "in some cases the detective may determine that the infraction was minor and that both parties were equally guilty. . . . this normally is the result when a husband has assaulted his wife but the injury is not serious and it appears that there was 'good cause' for him to do so" (p. 269). This assumption that the victim probably provoked her abuser parallels outdated psychological literature in which women victims of domestic violence are characterized as masochistic (Snell, Rosenwald, & Robey, 1964).

For centuries prosecutors have assumed that domestic abuse is a minor problem, that for a man to strike his wife is a legitimate exercise of his authority to discipline her, that women provoke the beatings they receive, or that they enjoy them. The vitality of this tradition is one barrier to effective criminal intervention in violent families.

## Case Attrition and Other Problems

Traditional attitudes toward crime and family life that lead prosecutors to regard spouse abuse as outside of their jurisdiction are reinforced by negative experience in prosecuting spouse abuse cases. The prosecutor views a case from the point of view of its legal viability, and is concerned with the availability of the complainant, other witnesses and tangible evidence of the crime. In spouse abuse cases, witnesses and evidence are often less available than in stranger-to-stranger cases because police rarely make arrests, file reports, or thoroughly investigate spouse abuse cases.

The most pronounced problem reported by prosecutors is that victims of abuse who initially express interest in filing charges change their minds by the time of the arraignment of the preliminary hearing. A study of post-arrest procedure in the District of Columbia found that witness problems accounted for dismissal of 43% of the cases involving family members and 17% of the cases involving strangers (Forst, Lucianovic, & Cox, 1977). In examining reasons for dismissal of felony cases, the Vera Institute of Justice (1977) found that of the cases dismissed, victim noncooperation was the stated cause of dismissal in 92% of the prior relationship cases. Prosecutors from Philadelphia, Jacksonville, Florida, and Marin County, California, reported that approximately 80% of domestic cases in which charges are filed are dismissed prior to disposition. They all reported that cases were dropped because the victim requested dismissal or else failed to appear for a meeting with the prosecutor or for a court hearing.

Victims of abuse drop charges or fail to show up in court for a variety of reasons including ignorance about the justice system, fear of retaliation by or emotional attachment to the abuser, and inconvenience. Frank Cannavale (1976), an expert on crime victims, found that 28% of 922 witnesses surveyed expressed fear of retaliation by the defendants if they pursued criminal action. He noted that "witnesses in cases involving defendants known to them indicated more fear of reprisal than in cases when the defendant was a stranger" (p. 52). Nancy Sieh (1979), an assistant district attorney in Santa Barbara, California, observed that half of the victims of abuse who came to her office to drop charges were accompanied by their abusers, who had threatened them with further abuse unless they did so.

Many victims drop charges because they do not understand the criminal justice system, and receive little or no information about the steps in the process or the likely consequences of criminal action from either the prosecutor or the court (Cannavale, 1976). Many victims think that every criminal case goes to trial, that they will be required to testify and subjected to rigorous interrogation on the stand, and that if the abuser is convicted he will be given a lengthy jail sentence.

Prosecutors are in no position to give battered women the attention and the information they need because they are under tremendous case load pressure and are trained to focus their attention on proving the case, and not on the victim's needs. The National District Attorneys Association established a victim/witness assistance program because they concluded that "prosecutors are ill-equipped to handle, and have little information on, the very real problems of victims and witnesses with whom they must deal" (Cannavale, 1976, p. 16).

Prosecutors often suggest that the only reason victims drop charges is that the victim and the abuser have reconciled, that once "passions have cooled" the impulse to retaliate disappears, and the relationship returns to "normal." Reconciliation undoubtedly accounts for some withdrawal of charges by victims of abuse. Walker (1979) suggests that after an acute battering incident, there is a period of "loving respite" between the abuser and victim, during which the abuser is genuinely affectionate and apologetic. While many battered women are highly motivated to get help in stopping the violence immediately after an incident, some victims may later accept their mates' apologies and promises never to hit them again and withdraw from prosecution.

Another reason for withdrawal of charges is delay and inconvenience. Cannavale (1976) found that 619 out of 922 witnesses reported that their cases had been postponed, and over 50% said there had been more than one postponement. Marie Hegarty (personal communication, Nov. 1979), a paralegal with Women Against Abuse who works in the Philadelphia District Attorney's Office, believes that the primary reason why victims of abuse drop charges are that too much time would be lost from work or that child care would have to be arranged for too many court appearances. When a case takes months to process, the victim may lose confidence that the system has anything to offer her. She comes to court because of immediate danger and trauma and needs immediate protection.

Another reason for case attrition in nonstranger cases is that prosecutors anticipate the withdrawal of complaining witnesses who know their assailants and they discourage women from filing charges or following through with prosecution. Researchers found in one study (Cannavale, 1976) that victims are less likely to cooperate in prosecution if the prosecutor believes that they will not cooperate.

Family violence cases are difficult to prosecute. Often there are no witnesses except perhaps the children of the parties. There may be little or no evidence of the crime charged because the victim did not get immediate medical attention, no one took photos of the injuries, and bruises may have disappeared by the time the victim goes to court. Police reports are often inadequate or nonexistent. These factors increase prosecutors' reluctance to press charges and reduce the likelihood of conviction in cases which are brought to trial.

Most prosecutors rarely have an opportunity to take a domestic violence case to trial. Those who do report present yet another layer of practical problems. The batterer may appear in court looking respectable, confident, and collected. He may deny the occurrence of the alleged incident and urge that the victim was injured because she was drunk or took too many tranquilizers and fell down the stairs or ran into a door. He may claim that at the time of the alleged assault the victim became hysterical or violent and had to be restrained through the use of force. Some batterers claim that the assaults with which they were charged occurred accidentally. In one case a man took the stand and explained that his mate received two black eyes one day when he was stretching and she ran into his extended fists.

Where the proof of guilt turns on the credibility of witnesses, this pattern of denial can pose a substantial problem for the prosecution. The problem may be more acute if the victim takes the stand and is so frightened that she becomes unable to speak or to give coherent testimony.

Another set of obstacles to prosecution of spouse abuse cases, distinct from victim ambivalence and prosecutor behavior, relates to fiscal and practical constraints on the court system and the prosecutor's office to keep the case load down, and to focus on crimes designated as priorities. In part because of their numbers, and in part because of the attitudinal problems discussed earlier, family violence cases are usually rated as the lowest priority. This perspective is articulated in a report on felony prosecution in New York:

> Judges and prosecutors recognized that in many cases conviction and prison sentences are inappropriate responses. Because our society has not found adequate alternatives to arrest and adjudication for coping with interpersonal anger publicly expressed, we pay a price. . . . The congestion and drain on resources caused by an excessive number of such cases in the courts weakens the ability of the criminal justice system to deal quickly and decisively with "real" felons. (Vera Institute of Justice, 1977, p. xv)

Skolnick (1967) remarks that "if charging occurred in all of these cases, officials believe that an inordinate amount of resources would be expended in attempting to control infractions of a relatively minor nature" (pp. 57–58).

The case load in most prosecutors' offices is overwhelming and does not permit staff to spend extra time with reluctant victims in order to encourage cooperation with prosecutors. Priorities may be set based not on the seriousness of the crime charged or the likelihood of recurrence if no action is taken, but on the likelihood of conviction and potential benefit to the prosecutor's career.

The preceding discussion of obstacles to prosecution of family violence shows that the cases are not intrinsically impossible to prosecute successfully but rather that success is unlikely because of a wide array of attitudinal, practical, and institutional problems.

## Research on Case Processing

Recent studies show that at each stage of case processing in the criminal justice system, the number of domestic abuse cases drops dramatically.

In most cases the first criminal justice agency that a battered woman contacts is a police department. Though family abuse cases comprise a substantial percentage of police work (Parnas, 1971), research indicates that police responding to domestic calls rarely file reports on incidents of spouse abuse, and even more rarely make arrests. A survey of spousal violence against women in Kentucky conducted in 1979 by Louis Harris and Associates reports that 10% of the women interviewed had experienced some violence from their husbands during the preceding 12 months. The police had been called in less than one-tenth of these cases (Schulman, 1979). Of 155 police officers interviewed for a study in San Diego County, 83% stated that they filed reports for fewer than 20% of the domestic calls they answered (Pennell, 1980). In Cleveland, Ohio, during a nine-month period in 1979, the police received approximately 15,000 domestic violence calls (Kilbane, personal communication, 1981). Reports were filed on 700 of these calls, and arrests were made in 460 cases (Ohio Attorney General, 1979). These figures may reflect a higher than average rate of arrests and reporting because Ohio has new legislation allowing police to make warrantless arrests in misdemeanor domestic abuse cases.

Many times abusers are not arrested even where the violence is so serious that a homicide may be imminent. In analyzing homicides against family members in Kansas City in 1977, the Police Foundation found that in 85% of the cases, the police had been summoned to the residence at least once before, and in 50% of the cases the police had been called to the home of the victim five or more times before the killing (Police Foundation, 1977). In a recent case, a Washington, DC woman was acquitted of murder charges based on a self-defense argument. The defense introduced evidence that the police dispatcher had recorded 13 calls to the residence in the nine months before the homicide; several of the responding officers testified for the defense (Mann, 1981).

Several recent studies by the Vera Institute of Justice, the Police Executive Research Forum, and the Institute for Law and Social Research have examined factors that determine when police will make arrests. Police often impose a higher standard of probable cause to arrest in spouse abuse cases than on stranger cases. Injuries which would be considered to provide adequate basis for arrest of a stranger assailant are often found insufficient to justify arresting a man who beats his wife or girlfriend. Examining cases in which the New York City police made felony assault arrests, the Vera Institute of Justice (1977) found that there was a smaller percentage of arrests based on minor injuries, which were defined as those requiring medical attention, stitches, or hospitalization, in cases where the parties had a prior relationship than where the parties were strangers. Serious injury was present in 46% of the cases in which an arrest was made and the parties had some prior relationship, but in only 33% of the stranger cases. Police report that most domestic cases involve injuries not serious enough to justify making an arrest, and this suggests that police required more serious injuries to justify arrest in nonstranger cases.

In a recent study by the Police Executive Research Forum (Loving, 1980), 130 police officers in 17 police agencies in various parts of the country ranked in order of importance a list of factors that might lead them not to make an arrest. Factors listed as most important are listed below, with the percentage of officers who identified each factor as important in a decision not to arrest:

- refusal of victim to press charges (92%)
- victims' tendency to drop charges (72%)
- lack of serious injury (70%)
- availability of effective social service and civil alternatives (65%)
- commission of a misdemeanor (56%)
- participant's first encounter with the police (50%)
- frequent calls from household for police assistance (49%)
- no use of a weapon (48%)

In a cross-city comparison of felony case processing, the Institute for Law and Social Research (INSLAW) (Brosi, 1979) reported that only a few of the cases reported to the prosecutor by police officers and private citizens resulted in filing of charges. Where the parties to an assault case were married or intimate, prosecutors were less likely to file charges than where the parties were strangers.

Many of the domestic violence cases that reach the prosecutor's office have been screened by the police and judged to be serious. Even so, most family violence cases handled by prosecutors' offices are rejected before charges are filed or dropped prior to trial.

In the District of Columbia in 1972, according to Kristen Williams (1978) of INSLAW, assault cases had the highest rates of attrition at screening and subsequent stages of processing. Seventy-five percent of these cases involved family members, friends or acquaintances. Prosecutors declined to file charges in 39% of the simple assault cases in which an arrest had been made and in 30% of the arrests for felony assault. The INSLAW study also reports that of the assault cases in which an arrest was made, 45% of those charged were dismissed by the prosecutor.

The percentage of convictions in intrafamily cases that are prosecuted to disposition is, again, disproportionately low compared to the rate of conviction for assault charges in cases in which the parties are strangers. According to Brian Forst et al. (1977) at INSLAW: "Conviction rates in stranger-to-stranger violent offenses other than robbery in the District of Columbia are, on the whole, nearly twice as large as they are in the intrafamily violent episodes" (p. 26). In 1974 in the District of Columbia, 31% of arrests for aggravated assault involving strangers resulted in conviction, but only 18% of the arrests for aggravated assault resulted in conviction in intrafamily cases. Of arrests made for simple assault, 31% of the stranger cases and 8% of the intrafamily cases resulted in conviction (Forst et al., 1977, p. 27).

The 1977 Vera study of felony prosecution in New York produced a similar finding. Of the felony arrests in the sample, convictions (on any charge) were obtained in 71% of the cases involving strangers, but in only 46% of the cases in which the parties had some prior relationship. The rate of conviction for prior relationship cases was higher in the Vera study than in the INSLAW study. This could reflect the inclusion in the Vera study of not only family members but friends and acquaintances; it might also be related to the much smaller sample in the Vera study, which included a total of 67 cases, of which 46 involved parties with prior relationships and 21 involved strangers. The INSLAW study included a total of 1642 aggravated assault cases, of which 392 involved crimes against strangers, 239 involved crimes against family members, and 1011 cases in which the relationship of the parties was not recorded. One hundred ninety stranger cases involving simple assault were included in the INSLAW study, 73 intrafamily simple assaults, and 312 simple assaults that reflected no record of relationship.

Where convictions are obtained in family violence cases, the penalties imposed are lighter than those imposed in stranger cases. The Vera study states that of the felony assault arrests included in the sample, 5% of those involving strangers resulted in sentences of over one year in jail. None of those involving parties with a prior relationship received jail sentences of over one year.

The studies just discussed were conducted in several cities and examined different criminal justice agencies. While none had as a primary goal the gathering of information on domestic violence, each neverthe-less found that cases involving nonstrangers or family members are dropped from the criminal justice system at a much higher rate than stranger cases. This pattern suggests that in most places prosecution is seldom an available remedy for battered women.

## REDUCING CASE ATTRITION

A primary cause of case attrition in family violence cases is that prose-cutors, often unintentionally, discourage victims from following through with prosecution. The complaining witness is often made to feel personal-ly responsible for the prosecution of the case and for whatever penalty is ultimately imposed. She usually does not receive adequate information about the criminal justice system or about how to protect herself while charges are pending.

Most prosecutors discourage battered women from filing charges and freely permit ambivalent victims to back out after charges have been filed because they perceive that domestic violence cases involve only minor disputes which are impossible to prosecute successfully. Because other cases are easier to prosecute and are believed to be more serious, prose-cutors regard domestic cases as a waste of time. Many prosecutors also take the position that criminal action may jeopardize family relationships, and that the family is a sacred institution to be preserved at all costs.

A handful of prosecutors around the country have made spouse abuse cases a priority and have been aggressively prosecuting cases involving intimates. For example, prosecutors in Seattle, Santa Barbara, Los Angeles, Philadelphia, and Westchester County, New York, have examined reasons why battered women frequently drop charges, and adopted procedures to reduce pressures on the complainant.

Recognizing the victim's ambivalence about prosecution and the pres-sure on the victim to withdraw, these prosecutors attempt to relieve the complainant of responsibility for filing charges. Domestic violence pro-grams in these prosecutors' offices treat spouse abuse as a crime against the state and assert that the prosecutor, not the victim, is responsible for enforcing the law. In addition, the prosecutors have examined the reasons why battered women file charges—they looked at what these women want from the criminal court—and have set goals for prosecution that correspond with those of the complainants.

These programs have been effective in reducing case attrition. In 1979 in Santa Barbara, the rate of victim cooperation in cases in which charges were filed was 92% (D. Talmadge, personal communication, Nov. 1979)

Victim cooperation means that charges were not dismissed based on the request of the victim or on her refusal to testify. In Los Angeles, less than 10% of the family violence cases charged as misdemeanors are dismissed because of victim noncooperation (S. Kaplan, personal communication, Nov. 1979). In the Philadelphia District Attorney's Office, case attrition in spouse abuse cases was reduced to 20% during 1980 (B. Kivitz, personal communication, April 1981). In Westchester County, New York, during a six-month period in 1980, only 25% of the complaining witnesses in family violence cases withdrew charges prior to disposition (Westchester County District Attorney, 1980). In Seattle, during a two-year period, only 34% of the 1,116 family violence cases in which charges were filed resulted in acquittals because the victim refused to participate (Seattle City Attorney's Office, 1980).

These rates are impressive compared with those reported by other prosecutors. For example, in Jacksonville, Florida, the District Attorney's Office estimates that 80% of the complainants in spouse abuse cases drop charges prior to disposition. In Marin County, California, before their domestic violence diversion program was established, the rate of case attrition was estimated to be 70 to 80% (Lerman, 1980). Prosecutors interviewed in Miami, Florida, and in Cleveland, Ohio, were unable to supply data but were hard pressed to think of domestic cases which were *not* dismissed based on the victim's request.

Witness noncooperation accounts for dismissal of a significant number of criminal cases whether or not the parties are strangers. When the parties know each other, however, the likelihood that the complaining witness will not appear in court is much higher. The Institute of Law and Social Research (Williams, 1978) reports that in the District of Columbia in 1973, prosecutors dismissed 22% of the stranger cases and 54% of the nonstranger cases because of witness noncooperation. These figures indicate that a case attrition rate of 20% may be normal in stranger cases, but is an impressive achievement in family violence cases.

Domestic violence prosecution units have not only reduced case attrition, but have also obtained a high rate of convictions. Notably, the Seattle program reports that 83% of the domestic violence cases which go to court result in convictions (Seattle City Attorney's Office, 1980). In Westchester County (Westchester County District Attorney, 1980), 119 batterers were convicted during the first six months in 1980; only three were acquitted (Westchester County District Attorney, 1980). Although these programs developed independently of each other, they arrived at many similar conclusions about what can be done to encourage victim cooperation in spouse abuse cases.

## Identification of Wife Abuse Cases

Prosecutors generally accept as a given the pool of cases which are presented to them for screening, either as a result of arrests, police reports, or victim complaints. However, as indicated earlier, only a small percentage of the domestic cases in which the police are called to the scene result in either an arrest or a report. In order to have a significant impact on domestic abuse in any community, prosecutors must develop closer communication with police about domestic cases, so that all serious cases may be identified.

To enlarge the pool of domestic violence cases available to be screened for prosecution, prosecutors must solicit reports from police and from victims. One method is to have police report forms designed so that domestic cases can be quickly identified, and then to go through police reports daily and weekly and pull out the domestic violence cases. A second is to supply police with postcards and addresses to the prosecutor's office, and ask them to fill in the name and address of the victim every time they answer a disturbance call. A third method is to supply police with brochures describing the assistance available for battered women from the prosecutor's office and elsewhere and to ask that the brochures be distributed to battered women who call the police.

If the prosecutor identifies cases through reports or cards written by the police, victims can then be contacted to make them aware of available services. Regardless of the channel of communication, the goal is to make the cases available to the prosecutor and to make criminal action available to battered women.

All of these methods have been successfully used by programs designed to prosecute domestic violence. Their users report an enormous increase in the number of cases screened, charged and convicted. Likewise, they report that many of the cases in which no arrest was made are as serious and as appropriate for prosecution as those in which arrests are made.

In Seattle (Seattle City Attorney's Office, 1980) all police reports are screened by prosecutors to determine the appropriateness of prosecution. After the city attorney set up a Battered Women's Project, the police department was persuaded to modify the report form so that domestic violence cases could be identified by a checkmark at the top of the form. Cases thus identified are sent to the Battered Women's Project. Those in which an arrest was made are filed automatically; the project contacts victims in the other cases by phone or letter to determine whether they wish to prosecute. By screening police reports and contacting battered women, the project has more than doubled the number of domestic cases prosecuted by the city attorney. Since the rate of conviction in those cases which go to court is 83%, the increase in the caseload is considered a good service to the community and beneficial to the image of the prosecutor's office.

In Westchester County, New York, police reports are sent to the prosecutor's office only when an arrest is made. The primary channel by which the police inform the Domestic Violence Unit about calls answered is by sending postcards to the unit giving information about how to contact the victims. Then, as in Seattle, victims are contacted by the prosecutor's office and offered services. The unit gets calls from about 30% of the victims who are sent letters. According to Jeanine Pirro (personal communication, Sept. 1979), the Assistant District Attorney who directs the unit, police response has vastly improved because police "know they have a prosecutor who will back them up to the hilt."

Establishing such a system is no small task. The postcard may be simpler to sell than a request for increased reporting, however, because it involves less paperwork. The Westchester Domestic Violence Unit encourages use of postcards during personal visits to each of the 43 police departments in the county served by the prosecutor's office. These visits, usually made during roll call, are also used to encourage arrests in appropriate cases and to otherwise inform the police of the prosecutor's interest in family violence.

The most efficient means by which prosecutors may obtain information about domestic violence cases is through a direct report from the police, as in the systems described above. Where direct reporting cannot be implemented, however, police can refer victims interested in filing charges to the prosecutor's office.

In Philadelphia, for example, the District Attorney sponsored a domestic violence program which has received much publicity. The prosecutor's office assisted in drafting a new police directive on family violence, but the size of the city and the police force precludes systematic screening of reports. However, the domestic violence program supplies police with information cards to give to victims of abuse, and encourages police to pass out the cards and to refer victims to the prosecutor's office. Through this mechanism, the program has served over 4,000 battered women each year, more than almost any program in the country.

Some prosecutors are concerned that sending letters to victims based on police reports might place the victim at risk, because the abuser might open the letter and a violent incident might ensue. However, neither the Westchester nor the Seattle projects have had reports of violence precipitated by contact letters sent to victims. The project staff recognize the risk of the letters, but believe that the likelihood of subsequent violence is greater if no one intervenes than if services are offered.

The obligations of confidentiality that limit communications between mental health agencies or private attorneys and law enforcement officials are not at issue between police and prosecutors. The privacy of the parties is not violated by the sharing of information between one law enforcement agency and another.

Better working relationships between police and prosecutors regarding spouse abuse cases will not only increase prosecution, but also will encourage police to take family violence cases seriously. If practical considerations limit the number of cases that can be prosecuted, then selection should not be based on random self-identification. The prosecutor should screen as many cases as possible and prosecute the most serious.

## The Decision to Prosecute

Although sufficiency of evidence is a prominent consideration in any filing decision, various other criteria are often used in screening domestic violence cases. Some prosecutors extensively interview battered women about whether they feel any reluctance concerning the filing of charges. Others file charges against a batterer only if the victim has agreed to live apart from him or to file for separation or divorce. Some accept criminal complaints from battered women only where the injury is so severe that it would be inexcusable not to file charges. The use of such criteria limits the number of cases in which charges are filed, but does not help to identify the cases in which victims will cooperate. Improving the rate of victim cooperation depends *not* on weeding out ambivalent victims, but on setting up a system that will encourage victims to cooperate and will protect their interests.

The recent experience of family violence prosecutors reveals no correlation between any identifiable characteristics of the cases or the victims and the likelihood of cooperation. The probability of victim cooperation is in fact better predicted by the conduct of the prosecutor than by the conduct of either the victim or the defendant (Cannavale, 1976).

The domestic violence prosecution programs vary in their position as to whether the decision to file charges should be made by the victim or by the prosecutor. Some prosecutors believe that the victim must not be required to cooperate with the district attorney if, at the outset, she does not wish charges to be filed. Other prosecutors see themselves as advocates for the state and urge that the charging decision should be made by the prosecutor. They argue that the victim may not know what she wants or that she may shy away from prosecution because of fear of the batterer or of the criminal justice system. Knowing that without effective intervention the cycle of violence will escalate, they suggest that some cases should be prosecuted even if the victim objects.

Domestic violence units in the district attorney's offices in Santa Barbara, Philadelphia, and Westchester County file criminal charges only if evidence is sufficient *and* the victim wishes to participate. Victim advocates (persons who informally represent crime victims) discuss all available options with battered women to assist them in making informed decisions. The unit in the Los Angeles City Attorney's Office, on the other hand, takes the position that the "decision to prosecute a criminal case is the responsibility of a public prosecution agency, *not* the victim of the offense" (Los Angeles City Attorney, 1980, p. 23). The prosecutor's interest in enforcing the law is so strong that victims of abuse are obliged to cooperate.

The filing policy of the City Attorney's Office in Seattle combines that of Los Angeles with the approaches taken by the other programs. In domestic cases in which the abuser has been arrested, charges are filed automatically. Where no arrest is made and a victim reports an incident to the prosecutor, charges are filed only if the victim elects to participate. Separate statistics kept on the two groups of cases indicate no significant difference either in the rate of case attrition or in the conviction rate. This suggests that victim assistance and the policy against dismissal of charges (the project's other important innovation) are more influential than the screening policy in reducing case attrition (Seattle City Attorney's Office, 1980).

Prosecutors in Seattle and in Westchester County who keep data on domestic violence cases report that charges are filed in 39% of the cases referred to them, either by police or by battered women. Likewise, the units in Portland, Philadelphia, and Los Angeles report that charges are filed in about one-third of the cases referred to them. In Marin County, the percentage of reported domestic violence cases in which charges were filed rose from 14% to 25% when their domestic violence diversion program began in 1980.

Prosecutors evaluating their screening policies may wish to assess the impact that a change in policy may have on their case loads. The number of family violence cases charged may increase somewhat, but if other relevant changes discussed in this chapter are made, the number of cases dismissed or defendants acquitted may drop dramatically. This means fewer wasted resources and higher conviction rates.

## *The Decision to Drop Charges: Complainant Cooperation*

While prosecutors disagree about how much a victim's wishes should influence the decision *to file charges*, prosecutors who have succeeded in reducing case attrition agree that once a charge is filed, the decision *to go forward* rests with the prosecutor, not with the victim. They have developed several techniques to convince battered women that violent behavior is a crime against the state and to encourage them to cooperate with the prosecution.

When the prosecutor signs a complaint, it is the prosecutor's first opportunity to show the victim that she is a witness rather than a plaintiff. Though prosecutors frequently sign complaints in other types of cases, in spouse abuse cases many prosecutors ask victims to sign complaints as a test of their resolve to follow through with prosecution. Prosecutors in Santa Barbara and Los Angeles suggest that this places unnecessary pressure on the victim.

If the complainant is given control of and responsibility for the filing of a charge, she becomes a target for retaliation or pressure to withdraw by the abuser. If the prosecutor signs the complaint and explains to the victim that it is the state and not she who is filing the charge, she is less vulnerable to intimidation. Deborah Talmadge, a prosecutor in Santa Barbara, instructs the victim that if her mate tries to cajole or threaten her into dropping the charge, she should tell him that she has no power to do so because she did not file the charge and cannot tell the prosecutor how to do his job. Talmadge reports that this strategy is effective in making the victim more comfortable and reducing the likelihood of recrimination (D. Talmadge, personal communication, Nov. 1979).

In keeping with the policy that prosecution is not the responsibility of the victim, prosecutors in Seattle, Los Angeles, and Santa Barbara have instituted a policy of denying complainants' requests for dismissal once charges have been filed. This change in procedure is critical to the reduction of case attrition.

Parallel with policies on filing charges, prosecutors have adopted various approaches in order to implement no-drop policies. The Los Angeles City Attorney (1980) takes a hard line on withdrawal of charges and refuses to drop any case based on the victim's request, unless there are compelling circumstances. In Seattle, if a victim requests the city attorney to drop charges, the prosecutor asks her to defer her request and to appear in court on the date set for trial. She is encouraged to focus on the positive feelings toward prosecution which led her to make a complaint in the first place. If she still wants to drop the charge on the date of trial, the prosecutor will then request the judge to dismiss the case (S. Buckley, personal communication, Sept. 1980).

In Santa Barbara, victims are discouraged but not prohibited from dropping charges. The victim is informed at the outset that once charges are filed she will not be permitted to change her mind; the policy is presented as a rigid one to encourage cooperation. The battered woman is encouraged to call the District Attorney's Office anytime she has doubts about pursuing the charge. Usually the prosecutor is able to persuade her not to withdraw; only in a rare case is dismissal requested (D. Talmadge, personal communication, Nov. 1979).

An objection might be raised that even if the prosecutor wishes to go forward, a judge may defer to a battered woman's request for dismissal. A recent decision by an Ohio court of appeals held that a judge may not grant a defendant's motion to dismiss based on the victim's reluctance to go forward. The judge was held to have a duty to grant the plaintiff, the State of Ohio, a hearing on the controversy presented. The court held that the granting of defense counsel's motion to dismiss was not abuse of discretion but a violation of judicial duty, because the judge had no discretion (*City of Dayton v. Thomas*, 1980).

Another method of reducing the number of dismissals is to subpoena battered women before trial. This makes it clear that the victim is not the prime mover in the case, but is a witness for the state. It also may shield the victim from pressure from the abuser not to appear in court. If the abuser threatens retaliation if the victim testifies, she can show him that she is required by law to go to court. Some prosecutors feel that it is inappropriate to subpoena battered women, because if they fail to appear, they may be held in contempt of court. A few instances were identified in which battered women in North Carolina were jailed for refusal to testify. Unless the judge hearing a case is hostile toward battered women, issuance of a subpoena is more likely to prevent intimidation and to encourage a victim to appear than to result in inappropriate punitive measures.

When a victim fails to appear in court to testify, the case is usually considered lost. In Seattle, however, many domestic violence cases have been successfully prosecuted even when the victim is absent. Between 1978 and 1980, in 45% of the domestic cases charged by the Seattle City Attorney, the victim did not appear in court on the date of the trial. Rather than requesting dismissal, the prosecution proceeded without her. In 143 out of 420 (34%) cases in which this approach was taken, convictions were obtained, based either on the testimony of a police officer or another eyewitness or on photographs of injuries inflicted (Seattle City Attorney's

Office, 1980). The Philadelphia District Attorney's Office also reports an increasing number of domestic abuse convictions obtained based solely on eyewitness testimony.

## Matching the Prosecutor's Objectives with the Victim's Needs

The penalties imposed on the abuser after conviction may have an almost equal impact on the life of the victim. Many domestic violence complaints withdraw charges because they believe that criminal conviction will necessarily result in a jail sentence for the abuser, which they may not want and which may cause the victim to lose her only source of financial support.

In Santa Barbara, most of the women who file criminal charges want assistance from the court in stopping the abuse, but want to continue relationships with their mates. Many victims wish to avoid a courtroom confrontation with their mates. Therefore, the prosecutor tries to plea bargain as many cases as possible, and offers to recommend a sentence of probation with mandatory participation in counseling in exchange for a guilty plea. Talmadge explained that she is not so lenient in cases in which there has been serious injury. There, she stated, "it would be unconscionable" not to ask for a jail sentence (D. Talmadge, personal communication, Nov. 1979).

The Los Angeles City Attorney's (1980) program also aims for results that correspond to the complainant's desires. Attorneys do not request incarceration for a first offender unless the victim has been severely injured. Instead, the guidelines require prosecutors to recommend that the court require "[the defendant's] participation in a court-approved counseling program . . . as a condition of probation" (p. 23). A jail sentence is sought if the abuser has a prior criminal conviction on a domestic violence charge.

In Seattle, many cases are prosecuted as misdemeanors that, according to staff of the Battered Women's Project, could be classified as felonies. This is because the City Attorney's Office, which handles misdemeanors, has a highly visible advocacy unit for battered women; the County Attorney is reluctant to prosecute cases that are uncertain to result in conviction; and police perceive domestic abuse as a misdemeanor offense. So the charges filed and the penalties imposed in domestic cases in Seattle are often lower than those imposed for similar crimes between strangers. However, the result is that the penalties sought, most often probation and counseling, match the desires which led the victim to seek help from the courts (Seattle City Attorney's Office, 1980).

Some prosecutors who work with battered women are concerned that a systematic reduction of charges and penalties sought leads to treatment of spouse abuse cases as less serious crimes than assaults between strangers. Failure to request jail sentences for serious abuse may confirm the prejudices of criminal justice officials who treat domestic violence as a trivial matter. They, in turn, may refuse to treat decisively other cases in which stiffer penalties are sought. What happens to domestic violence cases in court then filters back to the police and reinforces their reluctance to make arrests or to take victims' requests for protection seriously.

Prosecutors should take care that, in a zealous effort to promote equal enforcement of the law against those who assault strangers and those who assault family members, victims are not overlooked. The prosecutor must be aware of whether the victim intends to continue her relationship with her abuser and of the reasons why she has come to court. He or she must then balance the complainant's goals and the need for cooperation against the promotion of equal enforcement of the law in stranger and nonstranger cases.

### Victim/Witness Assistance

Lack of communication between prosecutors and battered women is perhaps the biggest single cause of case attrition in domestic violence cases. Victims of abuse who file charges against their mates are often inadequately informed about the process of prosecuting a charge, about what is expected of them and what they should expect. Prosecutors' offices in Westchester County, Philadelphia, Seattle, Cleveland, and Santa Barbara have set up victim/witness assistance programs to provide information for and to maintain contact with victims and witnesses of crime. Some specific forms of assistance they have offered are discussed below.

*Information about prosecution.* Most people do not understand the criminal justice system. Crime victims need basic information about the functions of criminal courts and prosecutors, the steps in the criminal process between charging and disposition, the amount of time and number of hearings involved, and the possible results. At each step, the victim needs to be told what has happened and what the next step will be.

An advocate can explain how the court may use the possibility of conviction or jail as leverage to require that the abuser stop his violent behavior, stay away from the victim, or attend counseling, even if it is unlikely a jail sentence will be imposed. The advocate may learn the victim's objectives and in turn communicate them to the prosecutor.

An advocate can inform complainants of the limitations of criminal action, such as likely delays and the possibility of acquittal or an inappropriate sentence. He or she can estimate at the outset the amount of time victims may need to take off from work, and can prepare them if necessary for the experience of telling their stories many times to several prosecutors. Some battered women may be put off by a realistic description of what the criminal justice system offers, and what it demands; those who persist will be better prepared and less disappointed.

*Practical assistance.* Victim/witness assistance programs often provide a wide range of practical help to facilitate victim participation in prosecution. Some victims fail to appear in court because they have no money for bus fare to get to the courthouse or to pay a babysitter. An advocate can discover such problems and arrange assistance. Many advocates accompany victims to court to explain the process and to reduce the victims' fear of confronting the defendants.

Battered women filing criminal charges against men they live with are in a precarious position. If the situation is extremely volatile, a victim advocate can contact local shelters to find out if space is available or advise the victim to move out and stay with friends or family. If the victim does not wish to leave, she might be advised to alert the neighbors to the danger and ask them to call the police if they hear loud noises. The victim might visit the local police department to discuss the problem; this may result in quicker police response and increased willingness to provide protection, especially if the department is small.

If the parties do not live together or if the abuser is ordered out of the house, the victim should be encouraged to change the locks on the doors and to make sure that the windows fasten securely. Any weapons in the house should be removed.

Battered women should be instructed how to respond if the abuser threatens to become violent unless the victim drops charges or agrees to deny in court that she was beaten. The victim should insist that she has no choice but to proceed and to tell the truth in court. Deborah Talmadge (personal communication, Nov. 1979) in Santa Barbara reports that this tactic may make the abuser more cautious because it removes his power to keep the violence hidden. Also it may increase the likelihood that he will plead guilty.

Some victim/witness assistance programs provide services not directly related to criminal prosecution, such as information about other avenues of legal redress, referrals to shelters or counselors, and advice about how to obtain employment or public benefits. Because battered women often initiate criminal action during crises, it may be necessary to obtain counseling or other support services for them to ensure their cooperation with prosecutors. This broader assistance is important because the criminal courts are a major intake point for people with a variety of problems. While prosecution may be one step in intervening in a violent relationship, other forms of assistance may be equally useful in preventing subsequent violence.

*Protection of the victim*. Prosecutors cannot guarantee that a battered woman will not be assaulted while criminal charges are pending, unless the defendant is held in jail until trial. This is rarely an option (Lerman, 1980). There are, however, measures that can be taken by the prosecutor's office and by the victim to reduce the likelihood of violence.

The prosecutor can request that the abuser's release on bail be conditioned on his staying away from the victim and on his not threatening, assaulting or otherwise intimidating her (Lerman, 1980). Bail contracts or agreements should be modified to allow revocation if the victim is intimidated (American Bar Association, 1979). If the court system does not provide for police notification of such orders, a victim advocate can contact the police and request their cooperation in enforcement.

If the victim is threatened or assaulted, prosecutors should request a speedy trial of the pending charges to reduce the likelihood of subsequent intimidation. Also, care should be taken that the victim's address is not released to someone likely to threaten her.

Legislation on victim/witness intimidation, which makes it a crime to interfere with a citizen seeking redress through the criminal justice system (or with any witness to a crime), has been enacted in some states. However, this legislation is rarely enforced. In 1979, the American Bar Association proposed model legislation making it a felony to attempt to prevent or dissuade any witness from testifying in a trial through the use of force or threatened or attempted force against the witness or a family member of the witness. Under the model statute, any pretrial release is deemed to include a condition that no witness be intimidated. However, absence of such legislation does not preclude prosecution of victim/witness intimidation under existing criminal laws, nor is legislation needed to impose conditions on the release of the abuser.

If the judge does not impose conditions on release, complainants may be protected from intimidation by civil protection orders. Protection orders may be used in conjunction with criminal charges since most of the statutes expressly provide that the remedy is nonexclusive. Helen Smith, an Assistant District Attorney in Portland, Oregon, reports that no-contact orders are available from criminal court, but they are difficult to enforce. Therefore, she advises complainants in spouse abuse cases to petition also for a protection order (H. Smith, personal communication, Jan. 1980).

Many of the new statutes allow a judge to evict an abuser; they also provide detailed procedures for enforcement (Lerman & Livingston, 1983). In some places, victim advocates assist complainants in filing criminal charges and in filing petitions for protection orders. In Carson City, Nevada, prosecutors are willing to file protection order petitions for battered women. The Ventura County, California, District Attorney's Office has also set up a system to help battered women to file petitions for protection orders. If no one else in the community offers free assistance in preparing petitions, it may be important for staff in the prosecutor's office to assume this function.

### Victim Compensation

Many battered women who file criminal charges have suffered substantial losses as a result of the abuse. These may include extensive medical bills, attorneys' fees, property damage, or time lost from work. Few victims are in a position to seek compensation through a personal injury lawsuit because of the time and expense. A victim advocate may provide an important service to the victim and buttress her desire to cooperate with the prosecutor by informing her of available victim compensation programs and by helping her to obtain compensation.

Victims of domestic violence are ineligible for compensation under most of the 29 state statutes providing for compensation of crime victims (Carrow, 1980). Prosecutors concerned about reducing case attrition should urge expansion of programs created by these statutes to make battered women eligible for compensation. The domestic violence diversion program in Marin County, California, requires that abusers pay restitution to victims as a condition of their participation in diversion. The benefits of such programs may be more tangible to a victim than any other consequence of criminal prosecution.

### Case Assignment

Prosecutors' offices that handle large numbers of domestic abuse cases should consider assigning at least one full-time advocate to work exclusively on those cases. This would allow for the development of expertise to address the myriad problems which arise in spouse abuse cases.

Whether or not functions are specialized, staff should provide battered women with information and referrals, maintain contact while charges are pending, facilitate court appearances by arranging transport or child care, and help battered women who become criminal complainants obtain needed protection. Provision of these services in Santa Barbara, Westchester County, and Seattle has greatly reduced the number of domestic assault cases that are dismissed because of victim noncooperation.

## POST-CHARGE DIVERSION

Diversion (also referred to as deferred prosecution) is an alternative to traditional criminal case processing in which prosecution is suspended while a defendant completes a counseling program. Successful completion results in dismissal of charges. Diversion of domestic violence cases provides a means of obtaining control over a group of defendants who have largely eluded criminal justice intervention.* The leverage obtained over batterers admitted to a diversion program may be used to require participation in a counseling program focused on stopping violence and/or alcohol abuse. Few batterers voluntarily participate in counseling, but many accept treatment ordered by the courts.

Deferred prosecution is not new. During the last decade, many criminal courts made it a standard practice to divert offenders who have no criminal record. Most diversion programs do not admit persons charged with crimes of violence. However, prosecutors in Miami, Florida, in Marin County and Santa Barbara, California, and in Portland, Oregon, have found diversion to be a useful way of handling domestic violence cases. In several states, statutes have been enacted that lay out procedures for domestic abuse diversion programs.

Prosecution may be deferred after a defendant is charged with a crime at any point prior to a final adjudication of guilt. A defendant accepted by a diversion program makes a contract with the program to comply with certain requirements, such as attending counseling sessions and refraining from violence. If the defendant fulfills the requirements of the con-

---

*The National Association of Pretrial Services Agencies (1978) defines diversion to include any dispositional practice if 1) it offers persons charged with criminal offenses alternatives to traditional criminal justice or juvenile justice proceedings; 2) it permits participation by the accused only on a voluntary basis; 3) the accused has access to counsel prior to a decision to participate; 4) it occurs no sooner than the filing of formal charges and no later than a final adjudication of guilt; and 5) it results in dismissal of charges, or its equivalent, if the divertee successfully completes the diversion process.

tract for the period agreed upon, charges are dropped and the defendant's arrest record may be expunged. If the defendant fails to comply with the terms of his contract, prosecution is resumed.

Some diversion programs may be used as a dumping ground for cases regarded as inappropriate for serious treatment. Many critics lump diversion with mediation and suggest that both are inappropriate in domestic abuse cases because both mediation and diversion sidestep traditional criminal justice response. This critique of diversion is theoretically—and regarding many programs actually—an accurate assessment. Some diversion programs, however, treat domestic violence far more seriously than do many progressive prosecutors. The critical issue is not what the remedy is called but what actually happens to wife beaters against whom the remedy is sought. Described in this section are some of the possibilities for using diversion to stop violence.

Diversion may solve some of the practical and institutional problems confronted by prosecutors in handling domestic violence cases. Most charges filed against batterers are dismissed on the request of the victim or on her failure to appear in court. The few defendants who are convicted are most often given a short sentence of unsupervised probation. Admitting an abuser to a deferred prosecution program after charges are filed eliminates both the problems of complainant withdrawal and ineffectual sentencing.

A good diversion program can reduce the time prosecutors and judges spend on domestic violence cases. If a defendant successfully completes a diversion program, only two hearings occur—one when the batterer is formally accepted into the program and one when he completes the program and charges are dropped.

Deferred prosecution, however, may not be less expensive than processing a case in court. There must be staff to screen, refer, and track cases accepted for diversion. The state must pay for counseling of indigent defendants, and long-term counseling may be necessary to reduce the likelihood of subsequent violence. While the overall cost to the system may not drop, time and money may be more usefully spent on counseling programs for batterers than on charging cases which never reach disposition.

A diversion program may be established by statute, court rule, or administrative policy. While statutory authority is not needed to set up a diversion program, implementation of statewide programs may be facilitated by legislation which lays out procedures for diversion. Comprehensive legislation on diversion of domestic violence cases has been passed in California, Arizona, and Wisconsin (Lerman & Livingston, 1983).

## Planning for Abuse Counseling

If the court system processes large numbers of family violence cases, community mental health agencies must be encouraged to develop special programs for abusers, and to bring in therapists who have experience with abuser counseling to train those who will work in the program. Defendant batterers may then be referred to such programs. The field of abuser counseling is in its infancy, but many psychologists agree that the court system and the mental health system may be more effective in reducing family violence by collaboration than by separate effort.

Some therapists feel that group therapy for batterers is more effective in stopping violence than either individual or family therapy. Group therapy is an efficient use of counseling resources and less expensive than individual therapy. Group therapy provides a setting in which batterers may identify and articulate their feelings about their violent behavior. Many men who batter avoid dealing with their own violence in part by not talking about it with anyone. The group setting forces each man to confront his own violence because he sees similar behavior in others, to stop denying responsibility for it, and to begin to try solving problems by talking with other people about them. As some members of a therapy group gain control of their behavior, they become models for the others (Ganley & Harris, 1978).

Use of family therapy to treat the abuser and his family is criticized by many psychologists because family therapists tend to treat problems as a function of the relationship, and not as the responsibility of one member of the group. Although it is true that abused family members may not know how to deal effectively with the abuser, in order to stop the violence it is necessary to focus on the abuser, who is solely responsible for his violent behavior toward his family. In many violent relationships, both the victim and the abuser blame the victim for the violence. Some family therapists reinforce this dynamic by asking each party what he or she did to contribute to the problem, and by asking each to accept some responsibility for taking steps to stop the violence within the context of the relationship. The victim might in such circumstances take steps to avoid the types of conduct (e.g., not having dinner prepared on time) that the abuser alleged had "caused" the violence. The abuser would be more likely to interpret his wife's adjustments as further evidence that she had "caused" him to become violent.

There are other problems with family therapy. One is that many family therapists are biased in favor of reconciling difficulties rather than terminating marital relationships; in some violent relationships this conciliation process is unproductive or dangerous. Many family therapists see couples together most or all of the time. Many victims of abuse are unable to speak about the violence in the presence of their abusers; in such cases the therapist might never learn of the violence. Finally, the structure of a couple counseling session suggests that the nature of the problem is interactional rather than one of criminal conduct and the individual responsibility of the perpetrator. To stop domestic violence it is necessary to treat it as a crime and to hold the abuser responsible.

Therapists report that batterers are most susceptible to treatment immediately after a violent incident because the batterer is unable to deny or minimize his behavior when the memory is so recent, and because he may be very afraid that his wife will leave him because of the beating. Counseling may be effective then, when initiated early in the criminal process. For example, Domestic Intervention Program staff in Miami, who see many abusers within 24 hours of an assault that led to arrest, report that communication between the batterer and therapist is more difficult when they meet after a delay of even a few days than when they meet immediately after the abuse occurs (Miami State Attorney, 1980). In setting up a system for handling spouse abuse cases, prosecutors should keep in mind the importance of immediate intervention, and design a system that will minimize the time required for processing a case.

*Admission Criteria*

Historically, many diversion programs have admitted only nonviolent first offenders on the premise that those who commit violent offenses should be prosecuted to the full extent of the law. Even though spouse abuse cases involve violent crimes, they are good candidates for diversion because successful prosecution of these cases is so rare. Even convicted batterers are more often sentenced to counseling than to jail. In light of the fact that batterers can be placed more quickly in counseling through diversion, some advocates prefer diversion over prosecution on grounds of expediency.

Though traditional prosecution may not be useful or necessary in all such cases, batterers charged with assault must be carefully screened for admission to a diversion program to exclude cases in which the violence is extreme or in which the batterer has a long criminal record. The Miami domestic intervention program (Miami State Attorney, 1980) allows abusers to participate in diversion if:

- there has been no prior arrest for a violent crime. Batterers who have had prior experience with the criminal justice system may recognize diversion as an easy way out and use the program to avoid more serious consequences. They tend to be less receptive to counseling and to take other demands of the program less seriously than abusers who have not been arrested before.
- the defendant consents to participate. Because diversion usually occurs before any adjudication of guilt, the protection of the defendant's rights requires that his participation be voluntary. The defendant has a right to have the offense adjudicated, and the courts have no power to impose penalties for an offense charged unless a conviction is obtained. Because the conditions of diversion are the same as some of the sanctions that might be imposed after conviction, the protection of the abuser's rights requires that his consent be obtained.
- the victim consents to the abuser's participation in the diversion program. Diversion should not occur if a victim of abuse feels that prosecution and incarceration is more appropriate or if she is afraid for her safety and does not want the abuser to be released. The option to veto diversion gives the victim, perhaps for the first time, control over the conduct of the abuser. This changes the balance of power between the parties, gives the abuser a clear message that he has violated the victim's rights, and encourages the victim to make decisions about her life.
- The counselor who initially interviews the abuser feels confident that the abuser's participation in the program would be sincere, that he is motivated to change, and that he is unlikely to injure the victim during diversion.

During 1979 and 1980, 169 batterers were accepted by the Miami Post-Arrest Unit. Abusers who satisfy the criteria for admission are accepted if the counselors in the Unit have space in their case loads. Screening is a critical element of any diversion program, both because many abusers may not be responsive to treatment and because treatment may be more effective if each counselor has some control over the size of his or her caseload (National Association of Pretrial Services Agencies, 1978).

## Protecting the Defendant's Rights

In planning a diversion program, careful consideration must be given to the defendant's constitutional rights. While protection of these rights may be at odds with considerations of efficiency and minimizing the cost of the program, constitutional mandates should be carefully observed. Each defendant who participates in a diversion program must waive certain constitutional rights, including "his right to have the government prove his guilt beyond a reasonable doubt, his right to confront his accusers, and his right to a speedy trial" (*Brady v. United States*, 1970). In *McMann v. Richardson* (1970), the Supreme Court stated that "waivers of constitutional rights not only must be voluntary, but must be knowing, intelligent acts done with sufficient awareness of relevant circumstances and likely consequences" (p. 766).

In *Brady v. United States* (1970), the Court set standards for what constitutes a voluntary waiver of rights in negotiating a guilty plea. The court held that waiver of rights for the purpose of obtaining a lesser penalty is not involuntary, as long as it is knowing and intelligent. One primary consideration in the finding that the waiver in question was voluntary was that the defendant had had the assistance of competent counsel (National Advisory Commission on Criminal Justice Standards and Goals, 1973).

A batterer admitted to a diversion program should have an opportunity to consult an attorney before prosecution is suspended. To ensure that counsel will be available, diversion must be initiated at a point considered to be a "critical stage" of prosecution. Whether a proceeding is a critical stage depends on "whether potential substantial prejudice to a defendant's rights inheres in the . . . confrontation, and (on) the ability of counsel to help avoid that prejudice" (*Coleman v. Alabama*, 1970, p. 9).

Diversion should not be initiated until after charges are filed. This ensures that the defendant will not waive his rights without knowing what charges he faces; also it protects his right to consult a lawyer about whether it is in his best interest to waive his rights.

Another reason that charges should be filed prior to diversion is to protect the defendant's fourth amendment right to a "judicial determination of probable cause as prerequisite to extended restraint of liberty following arrest" (*Gerstein v. Pugh*, 1975, p. 114). In *Gerstein v. Pugh*, the Court found that imposing conditions on release of a defendant following arrest could constitute "a significant restraint on liberty." In such cases, where a charge is initiated by a warrantless arrest, *Gerstein* could be interpreted to require filing of charges prior to diversion.

By giving a defendant an opportunity to discuss options with an attorney prior to diversion, and by deferring admission to a diversion program until after charges have been filed, program planners can protect the defendant's constitutional rights. This protection will prevent inappropriate or coercive uses of diversion and is important to the development of a sound program.

*Admission Process*

Admission of criminal defendants to a diversion program involves four steps: 1) identification of candidates, 2) interviews to determine their eligibility, 3) review of the charges by a judge who releases them to a diversion program, and 4) meeting of program staff and defendants to fill out written waivers of certain rights, draw up contracts specifying the terms of participation, and arrange referrals to counseling.

Staff of the Miami Domestic Intervention Program (DIP) identify domestic violence cases by screening police arrest reports and by attending preliminary hearings. A DIP staff member goes to the jail each morning and reads the list of persons arrested the night before. Generally, aggravated assault and burglary charges are examined to determine the relationship of the parties. Persons arrested for family violence and held overnight are interviewed in jail before the bond hearings that morning to determine their eligibility for diversion. Other cases are identified by a DIP staff member who attends the felony and the misdemeanor bond hearings each day. Judges are asked to release selected cases to the family violence programs. Some misdemeanor cases reach the Post-Arrest Unit (which is mainly concerned with services to victims) through complaints it receives from victims. If charges are filed, the batterer may be admitted to the diversion program after he is arrested or summoned to court (Miami State Attorney, 1980).

During the jail interview, the DIP staff member determines the seriousness of the violence that led to arrest and whether the defendant has a prior record or is experienced in evading the criminal justice system. An assessment is made of the arrestee's attitude toward counseling, whether he would use the program as an easy way out of the charge or make a commitment to deal with his violence. During the interview, the staff person calls the victim to ask whether she consents to the batterer's participation in the program.

In their first year annual report, the DIP Program reported that the "jail interview procedure continues to represent the greatest impact upon defendants at a time when their motivation for behavioral change is at its peak" (Miami State Attorney, 1980).

After the bail hearing, at which the defendant is released into the program, the offender returns to the DIP office to sign waivers of his right to speedy trial and of the statute of limitations. Once each week the counselors in the post-arrest unit meet to discuss acceptance of new clients and to assign each client to one of four therapists who work in the unit.

Some batterers who are arrested are released from jail on bail before they can be interviewed by DIP staff. After release, the next stage at which defendants eligible for diversion can be identified by DIP staff is at a pretrial conference between the victim and an assistant state attorney. DIP staff often attend these meetings. Eligible defendants identified at this stage are diverted at the arraignment. Diversion after arraignment, which takes place two weeks after the arrest, is less effective than after a bond hearing because, as discussed earlier, abusers are observed to be most receptive to treatment if counseling begins immediately after a battering incident.

## Conditions of Participation

There is general agreement on some basic requirements that should be imposed on batterers admitted to a diversion program. Defendants admitted to a program should identify goals to be accomplished during the period of diversion and should participate in developing a plan by which those goals may be attained. During the period of diversion, regular and frequent contact between the participants and the program staff must be maintained.

Requirements of some diversion programs include:

1) that the abuser participate in weekly counseling focused on stopping the violence for 6 months to 1 year;
2) that he avoid conduct which could lead to rearrest;
3) that the abuser avoid all contact or communication with his victim during the period of diversion;
4) that he visit his children only at times specified by the court; and
5) that he repay the victim for any medical expenses incurred, wages lost or property damaged as a result of the battering incident which led to filing of charges.

The Miami diversion program requires participants to attend weekly therapy, which is conducted either with individuals, couples, or groups. In all cases the victim is invited to visit the program and offered counseling (most often separate from the abuser). Of the abusers admitted to the

Post-Arrest Unit, 90% receive counseling from one of the four therapists in the unit; the other 10% are referred to outside therapists. Where a batterer also has drug or alcohol abuse problems, he is referred to a counseling program that specializes in substance abuse, either instead of or in addition to the abuser counseling program.

The duration of the counseling is determined by the therapist's assessment of the abuser's progress. Eleven percent of the abusers admitted during 1980 received counseling for one to three months, 31% for three to six months, 25% for six to nine months, and 29% for over nine months. Four percent received counseling for less than one month. After release, abusers are offered follow-up counseling for three months (Miami State Attorney, 1980). To be discharged successfully from the program, the abuser must attend counseling sessions and, in the view of his counselor, must make a sincere effort to deal with his violent behavior.

### Tracking

Careful supervision of batterers is critical to the success of family violence diversion programs. In many diversion programs, screening, referral, and tracking are conducted by one agency, often part of the court system or the prosecutor's office, and counseling is handled by community mental health agencies. Others, such as the Miami program, both provide services to defendants and follow their individual progress with the court system.

There are good arguments to support both models. It may be desirable to separate functions to use the expertise of an agency that specializes in tracking large numbers of cases. If no such agency is present or if the caseload is not so large as to require separation of functions, it may be preferable to delegate the tracking function to a counseling agency, which will have regular contact with participants.

The Miami program staff who work with batterers handle both counseling and tracking. Batterers see a therapist or participate in a therapy group each week. Also, DIP staff maintain contact with the victims, even if they are seeing counselors outside the program. Victims are strongly encouraged to report any violation of conditions of diversion or any violent incidents. In addition, the program works closely with a special police unit in Miami and maintains regular contact with problematic cases.

Another diversion program in which tracking and counseling functions are separated is NEXUS, a program in Philadelphia that tracks about 700 clients referred by the courts for counseling on alcohol or drug problems. The NEXUS system may be useful to family violence programs.

NEXUS staff obtain information about whether the defendants have been rearrested from computer records kept by the court. To track participation in counseling, NEXUS staff keep lists of defendants referred to each participating mental health agency, and make weekly calls to each agency to check client attendance. If a defendant misses an appointment, his name is tagged by the tracking staff. If a second session is missed, NEXUS staff attempt to contact the delinquent defendant to find out why he has not appeared. If the nonattendance persists, the offender is returned to court for a hearing on violation of the terms of his diversion.

If counseling and tracking are handled by different agencies, monitoring may be facilitated by making referrals to a few mental health agencies that have expertise in working with violent families or with alcoholics. Counselors at these agencies should be asked to make available attendance reports on court-referred clients at a designated time each week. Attendance reports may then be collected by diversion program staff during phone calls to each agency at the times agreed upon (M. Bencivengo, personal communication, July 1980).

## Terminating Diversion

A batterer's participation in a diversion program may be terminated with the dismissal of charges if he successfully completes the terms of his agreement with the program. If a batterer fails to appear for counseling or violates other terms of his agreement, diversion is terminated and prosecution is resumed. It is critical that when a defendant is dismissed from a diversion program, prosecution be carried through. Prosecutors should be acquainted with techniques for ensuring victim cooperation to facilitate successful prosecution where diversion is unsuccessful. The diversion program should follow cases dropped from the program through the criminal justice system to ensure that those cases receive proper attention.

Defendants should be informed at the time of admission to a diversion program of conduct which will lead to resumption of prosecution. Those returned to the State Attorney should be given written reasons for their termination; these statements should not, however, be admissible as evidence against them.

If an abuser participating in the Miami program fails to keep an appointment with his therapist, he is sent a warning letter and asked to come to the DIP office. If he fails to appear, diversion is terminated and prosecution is resumed. Similarly, if he is arrested, if he commits further abuse, or if he violates an agreement to avoid contact with the victim, the batterer may be dropped from the program, and the case returned to the State Attorney.

In Miami, when an abuser successfully completes the diversion program, a hearing is scheduled at which DIP staff request that criminal charges be dismissed and, if the charge was initiated by arrest, that the abuser's arrest record be expunged. According to DIP staff, record expungement is a significant motivating factor for abusers who have no prior criminal record.

The Miami criminal justice system pays careful attention to batterers admitted to the diversion program. However, many of the cases that are initially rejected by or dropped from the program are never prosecuted to disposition. The State Attorney's Office does not keep systematic data on domestic violence cases, but several prosecutors in the State Attorney's Office stated that the vast majority of criminal cases that are not diverted are dropped prior to disposition at the request of the victim. This discrepancy between the conduct of one office and another is typical. In most communities in which initiatives are taken to prosecute spouse abuse, different levels of cooperation are received from different agencies. In Miami, even though the State Attorney is DIP's sponsor, the prosecutorial function is the problematic link in the system.

## Confidentiality

Therapists who work with batterers referred to them by courts cannot win the trust of their clients unless the confidentiality of the counseling relationship is protected. Yet, if prosecution is resumed after a batterer is dropped from a diversion program, either the prosecution or the defense may subpoena records kept on a defendant during diversion.

In many states the confidentiality of communications between therapists and clients is protected by statute. Some of these statutes cover psychiatrists and psychologists but do not privilege social worker/client communications. Relevant state law should be carefully examined when a diversion program is designed, so that new law or informal agreements can protect the confidentiality of those communications not covered by the existing law.

Even if the communications between a counselor and a defendant are protected, other records kept by the diversion program, such as notes taken during intake interviews, may be subject to court subpoena.

If diversion is established by statute, the law should provide that program records be kept confidential and not be released without the defendant's consent. If it is necessary for the diversion program to share information with a mental health or other agency, clients should be asked to give written permission to release information (National Association of Pretrial Services Agencies, 1978).

If a diversion program is set up without a statute, agreements should be made with both prosecutors and defense attorneys that, to protect the credibility of the diversion program, records will not be subpoenaed for use in prosecution or defense of persons who have participated in the diversion program. In Miami, such an informal agreement with prosecutors and defense attorneys has protected program records from court subpoena. In New Jersey the confidentiality of diversion records is protected by a court rule which states that "during the conduct of hearings subsequent to an order returning the defendant to prosecution in the ordinary course, no program records, investigative reports, reports made for a court or prosecuting attorney, or statements made by the defendant to program staff shall be admissible in evidence against such defendant" (National Association of Pretrial Services Agencies, 1978, p. 98).

## An Assessment of Diversion

Participants in an LEAA-sponsored conference on programs for men who batter agreed that therapy groups for men who batter are effective in reducing violence. Although many mental health practitioners believe that counseling is ineffective unless the client's participation is voluntary, experience during the last few years with court-mandated treatment for abusers suggests that the opposite may be the case (Mott-McDonald Associates, 1980). It is characteristic of batterers to deny responsibility for their abusive behavior and be unwilling to seek help. Also, batterers are often externally motivated and do what is required of them more readily than they take steps by themselves to change their behavior. Without a court order, few batterers seek treatment; where counseling is ordered by a court, a majority are receptive to therapy. Vicki Boyd, a psychologist in Seattle, cautions that while violent behavior may change, it is difficult to bring about extensive psychic changes through court-mandated counseling (V. Boyd, personal communication, Nov. 1980).

There are several characteristics of diversion which make it effective in domestic violence cases. First, a diversion program may be structured to maximize the impact of counseling. In Miami, the abuser is placed in a counseling program within 24 hours of the battering incident. If he has just spent the night in jail and is released based on his admission to the program, then he identifies the program as the agency which got him out of jail. This may increase his trust of the therapist because the program has done him a favor. Also, the therapist may provide some stability during the crisis which so often follows an acute battering incident and at which time the batterer is fearful about his mate leaving him and feels guilty about his violence.

Second, diversion eliminates the long delay between charge and disposition that is likely if the case is prosecuted. Most men arrested for wife beating are released on bail and asked to appear for an arraignment two weeks later. During those two weeks, the defendant's normal life resumes; the disruption caused by the criminal charge and the threat of prosecution diminish with each delay. After the arraignment, months may pass prior to trial. In the meantime, the batterer may reconcile with his mate or discourage her from prosecuting, either by courting her or by threatening injury if charges are not dropped.

While the Miami program does not conduct any systematic follow-up to determine how many of the batterers who have participated in the program continue to be violent, the program has gathered some useful information. Of 260 cases closed by the program during 1979 and 1980, only 11 defendants were unsuccessfully terminated because they were rearrested. This includes those rearrested during the 1980 riots in Miami. Of 260 cases closed by the Domestic Intervention Project during its first two years, 196 cases were successfully terminated. At least during the period of diversion, the vast majority of abusers participating were not violent toward their mates.

Only six cases were terminated because the victim withdrew charges after diversion had been initiated. This suggests that the primary problem with prosecuting spouse abuse, that of victims dropping charges, is virtually nonexistent if prosecution is deferred and the abuser is ordered into counseling (Miami State Attorney, 1980).

Another diversion program run by the District Attorney in Portland, Oregon, likewise reports few incidents of violence committed by participants. As in Miami, abusers admitted to the program participate in weekly counseling for an average of six months. Only three out of 39 batterers accepted into the diversion program during the first ten months of 1980 committed any act of violence while in the program. Two of those incidents involved violence against a mate or family member of the abuser (C. Howard, personal communication, Nov. 1980). It is impossible to determine how many of the abusers participating in these diversion programs would have, but for the program, committed another assault against their mates. Nevertheless, the low levels of recurrence of violence among participants suggest that these programs may deter a significant number of assaults.

## RECOMMENDATIONS

Violence in families continues partly because it is ignored or tacitly accepted by the institutions from which battered women seek help. By taking a firm stand that battering is a crime that will be punished, prosecutors can provide victims with an enforceable right not to be beaten and communicate to abusers that family violence will no longer be treated as a private matter. Also, by prosecuting spouse abuse cases, prosecutors may influence other criminal justice and social service agencies which still treat wife beating as a characteristic behavior of the "multiproblem family" and fail to respond in a useful way.

The experience of prosecutors who have established programs or units to handle battering cases suggests that these cases can be prosecuted. While further empirical study is needed to determine the effectiveness of various procedures in preventing witness intimidation or in preventing subsequent violence, the practical experience of prosecutors in Seattle, Westchester, Santa Barbara, Miami, and other areas throughout the country, may guide others who wish to take initiatives in prosecuting crimes between intimates. The relative uniformity in their experience that certain procedures reduce case attrition and increase conviction rates forms a basis for the following recommendations:

- To reduce case attrition, prosecutors should adopt a policy that once charges have been filed in spouse abuse cases, victims' requests for dismissal will be denied. Battering should be treated as a crime against the state.
- To make a no-drop policy effective, victim advocates must be placed in the prosecutor's office to provide battered women with information about the criminal process, maintain contact while charges are pending, see that victims obtain adequate protection from intimidation, and field calls from those who wish to drop charges. This assistance will greatly reduce case attrition. If funding for new staff positions is unavailable, prosecutors should approach advocates who work in shelters or crisis centers about coordinating these activities.
- Charges should be filed in spouse abuse cases based on the sufficiency of available evidence, regardless of whether the parties are still married or living together.
- Prosecutors should relieve battered women of responsibility for filing charges by signing complaints rather than asking victims to sign, and by sending subpoenas to victims prior to trial. This deprives the batterer of his power to manipulate the criminal justice system by intimidating the victim.
- To prevent intimidation of battered women who become complaining witnesses, prosecutors should request that the pretrial release of suspected batterers be conditioned on a no-contact or-

der. This order should specify, in writing, that the defendant vacate a shared residence, avoid personal, telephone or written contact with the victim, not assault or harass her, and that visitation with children shall be at specified times in the presence of a third party. The defendant, the victim, and the police should receive copies of the order.

- Where violence has been serious and chronic, prosecutors may have no choice but to recommend incarceration. In less serious cases, sentencing recommendations should be based at least in part on the goals of the victim in making a complaint. In many cases this will lead to a recommendation of probation or a suspended jail sentence conditioned on participation in counseling.
- Post-charge diversion may be used in cases where the abuser has no prior criminal record. A diversion program should include intensive treatment focused on the violence. If possible, treatment should be initiated within a day of the beating that formed the basis for the charge. Diversion should be conditioned on the victim's approval; if there is any abuse during diversion, prosecution should be resumed and jail recommended.
- Prosecutors should work with mental health agencies to make training on treating men who batter available to therapists. Sentencing recommendations may then request that defendants in domestic cases be ordered into treatment focused on their violent behavior. Batterers ordered into counseling should be closely tracked by a bail agency, a probation department, or if prosecution is deferred, by a prosecutor's office.
- Police should arrest batterers whenever probable cause and statutory requirements are met, and they should detain persons arrested for domestic assault overnight if the victim would be endangered by the defendant's immediate release, or if she was seriously injured and remains in a common residence. Police should file reports on spouse abuse cases whether or not an arrest is made. The report will guide the police in responding to subsequent calls, and will be available for use as evidence if the prosecutor or the victim takes legal action to prevent subsequent abuse.
- Staff in the prosecutor's office should identify spouse abuse cases by reviewing police reports and should contact victims by telephone or letter to inform them of the option of filing criminal charges.
- Prosecutors may prevent subsequent abuse in spouse abuse cases in which no charges are filed by sending warning letters to batter-

ers or by meeting with batterers to inform them of the criminality of violent assault and the likely consequences of subsequent violence.

Implementation of changes in prosecutorial policy and practice may be slowed by a variety of political, fiscal, and bureaucratic obstacles. When the programs described in this chapter sought to improve access to criminal court for battered women, all encountered objections from chief prosecutors, resistance to change from judges, or problems in persuading police to file reports more frequently. Overcoming or circumventing these problems is the first and most difficult step in changing prosecutorial policy on domestic violence cases. Prosecutors who make clear to their communities that battering is a law enforcement problem and that wife beaters will be treated as criminals can play a major role in stopping domestic violence.

## REFERENCES

American Bar Association. (1979). *Reducing victim-witness intimidation*. Chicago: Author.

Blum, J. (1980). *Draft memorandum on prosecutorial discretion*. The National Center on Women and Family Law, New York, NY.

Bradley v. State, 2 Miss 156, 158 (1 Walker 1824).

Brady v. United States, 397 U.S. 742, 748 (1970).

Brosi, K. (1979). *A cross-city comparison of felony case processing*. The Institute for Law and Social Research, Washington, DC.

Cannavale, F. (1976). *Witness cooperation*. New York: Lexington Press.

Carrow, D. (1980). *Crime victim compensation*. The National Criminal Justice Reference Service, U.S. Department of Justice, Washington, DC.

City of Dayton v. Thomas, 17 *Ohio Opinions* 3d 255 (1980).

Coleman v. Alabama, 399 U.S. 1 (1970).

Dobash, R., & Dobash, R. (1979). *Violence against wives: A case against the patriarchy*. New York: The Free Press.

Eisenberg, S., & Micklow, P. (1977). The assaulted wife: Catch—22 revisited. *Women's Rights Law Reporter, 3*, 138–160.

Federal Bureau of Investigation (1980). *Crime in the U.S. 1979*, pp. 10–11. Washington, DC: U.S. Gov't. Printing Office.

Field, M., & Field, H. (1973). Marital violence and the criminal process: Neither justice nor peace. *Social Service Review, 42*, 221–240.

Fields, M. (1978). Wife beating: Government intervention policies and practices. In *Battered women: Issues of public policy*. U.S. Commission on Civil Rights, Washington, DC.

Forst, B., Lucianovic, J., & Cox, S. (1977). *What happens after arrest?* Institute for Law and Social Research, Washington, DC.

Fromson, T. (1980). *Prosecutor's responsibility in spouse abuse cases*. Washington, DC: U.S. Department of Justice.

Ganley, A., & Harris, L. (1978). *Domestic violence: Issues in designing and implementing programs for male batterers*. Unpublished paper presented at the Annual Meeting of the American Psychological Association.

Gerstein v. Pugh, 420 U.S. 103, 105 (1975).

Lerman, L. (1980). *Prosecution of spouse abuse: Innovations in criminal justice response*.

Washington, DC: Center for Women Policy Studies.

Lerman, L. (1984a). Mediation of wife abuse: The adverse impact of alternative dispute resolution on women. *Harvard Women's Law Journal, 7,* 57.

Lerman, L. (1984b). A model state act: Remedies for domestic abuse. *Harvard Journal on Legislation, 21,* 61.

Lerman, L., & Livingston, F. (1983). State Legislation on Domestic Violence, Response to Family Violence and Sexual Assault, September–October.

Los Angeles City Attorney (1980). *Domestic violence program manual.* Los Angeles.

Loving, N. (1980). *Responding to spouse abuse and wife beating: A guide for police.* Washington, DC: Police Executive Research Forum.

Mann, J. (1981, May 13). Spouse abuse: A problem that cries for answers. *The Washington Post.*

McMann v. Richardson, 397 U.S. 759, 766 (1970).

Miami State Attorney, Domestic Intervention Program. (1980). Statistical summary of post-arrest unit. In L. Lerman (Ed.), *Prosecution of spouse abuse: Innovations in criminal justice response.* Washington, DC: Center for Women Policy Studies.

Miller, F. (1969). *Prosecution: The decision to charge a suspect with crime.* Boston: Little, Brown.

Mott-McDonald Associates. (1980). The report from the conference on intervention programs for men who batter. The Center for Women Policy Studies, Washington, DC.

National Advisory Commission on Criminal Justice Standards and Goals (1973). Report on Courts, Washington, DC.

National Association of Pretrial Services Agencies (1978). *Performance standards and goals pretrial release and diversion,* Washington, DC.

Ohio Attorney General (1979). *The Ohio report on domestic violence.* Columbus, Ohio.

Parnas, R. (1971). Police discretion and diversion of incidence of family violence. *Law and Contemporary Problems, 36,* 539–540.

Parnas, R. (1973). Prosecutorial and judicial handling of family violence. *Criminal Law Bulletin, 9,* 733–769.

Pennell, S. (1980). *Preliminary evaluation: Social assault projects.* Available from the Comprehensive Planning Organization, San Diego, CA.

Pleck, E. (1979). Wife beating in nineteenth century America. *Victimology, 4,* 60–71.

Police Foundation (1977). *Domestic violence and the police: Studies in Detroit and Kansas City.* Washington, DC.

Schecter, S. (1982). Women and male violence: The visions and struggles of the battered women's movement. Boston: South End Press.

Schulman, M. (1979). *A survey of spousal violence against women in Kentucky.* Washington DC: U.S. Gov't. Printing Office.

Seattle City Attorney's Office (1980). Battered women's project: Statistical summary. In L. Lerman (Ed.), *Prosecution of spouse abuse: Innovations in criminal justice response.* Washington, DC: Center for Women Policy Studies.

Sherman, L., & Berk, R. (1983). *Police responses to domestic assault: Preliminary findings.* Washington, DC: Police Foundation.

Sieh, N. (1979). *Family violence: The prosecutor's challenge.* Unpublished paper, Center for Women Policy Studies, Washington, DC.

Skolnick, J. (1967). Social control in the adversary system. *Journal of Conflict Resolution, 11,* 52, 57–58.

Snell, J., Rosenwald, R., & Robey, A. (1964). The wifebeater's wife: A study of family interaction. *Archives of General Psychiatry, 11,* 107.

Stark, E., Flitcraft, A., et al. (1981). *Wife abuse in the medical setting: An introduction for health personnel.* Washington, DC: Center for Women Policy Studies.

Straus, M. (1977–78). Wife beating: How common and why? *Victimology, 2,* 443.

Subin, H. (1973). *Criminal justice in the metropolitan court.* New York: DaCapo Press.

U.S. Commission on Civil Rights (1982). *Under the rule of thumb: Battered Women and the administration of justice.* Washington, DC: U.S. Government Printing Office.

Vera Institute of Justice. (1977). *Felony arrests: Their prosecution and disposition in New York City's courts*. New York: Author.

Walker, L. (1979). *The battered woman*. New York: Harper & Row.

Westchester County District Attorney. (1980). Domestic violence unit: Statistical summary. In L. Lerman (Ed.), *Prosecution of spouse abuse: Innovations in criminal justice response*. Washington, DC: Center for Women Policy Studies.

Williams, K. (1978). *The role of the victim in the prosecution of violent crimes*. Available from the Institute for Law and Social Research, Washington, DC.

# 12

# *Prevention Approaches to Child Sexual Abuse*

## David Finkelhor

Sexual abuse in the family is a form of family violence whose large scope we have only recently recognized. In a random sample survey of 334 women in the Boston metropolitan area, 5% revealed that they had been a victim of sexual abuse at the hands of a relative (Finkelhor, 1984). Diana Russell (1983) reported even higher rates: In a random sample of 930 adult San Francisco women, 16% had been victimized by a family member before the age of 18. Such surveys give a sense of the large percentage of children who may be at risk for sexual abuse in the family, and they have prompted major interest in strategies for reducing this risk.

However, the nature of the problem of sexual abuse has posed some dilemmas for those concerned about prevention. In the case of other types of child abuse, prevention has been implemented primarily by targeting programs at potential abusers. Groups of parents who are particularly high risk abusers, such as teenage parents or parents of unhealthy children, have been offered education and supportive services. They have been taught parenting skills and gotten involved in self-help programs, such as Parents Anonymous, to give them assistance in dealing with the stresses of parenting.

However, several factors have restricted an equivalent approach to the prevention of sexual abuse. First, less is known at this time about who is at risk of becoming a sexual abuser (Finkelhor, 1984). Thus, it is hard

---

This article was made possible thanks to a grant from the National Center on the Prevention and Control of Rape. The author would like to thank Ruth Miller and Kathy Hersh for help in preparing the manuscript. Cordelia Anderson, Linda Sanford and Rich Snowden gave valuable insights in the course of research. This article is one of a series on the subject of sexual abuse available from the Family Violence Research Program.

to target particular groups with prevention services. Second, many sexual abusers are not parents, but include older siblings, members of the extended family, as well as neighbors, babysitters, and even strangers (Finkelhor, 1984). Thus, the potential target group for prevention is very dispersed and heterogeneous. Third, it may be very hard to interest sexual abusers in services and education that would reduce their likelihood to abuse. Most sexual abusers are men (Finkelhor, 1984) who are traditionally much more resistant to offers of assistance or self-help groups such as Parents Anonymous. Moreover, sexual abusers characteristically rationalize about and deny their behavior, and tend to be amenable to change only when under substantial pressure (Groth, Hobson, & Gary, 1982). Thus, even if they can be targeted, they may not respond easily to positive prevention efforts.

All this is not to say that prevention aimed at potential sexual abusers is impossible and fruitless. Even if difficult, it may be very important to pursue. Suggestions have been made for approaches such as eliminating child pornography (Rush, 1980), deterring abusers with stiffer criminal penalties (Armstrong, 1983), or even making men less abusive by letting them have more responsibility for the early care of children (Herman, 1981). These are all broad social policy interventions, not targeted to any particular group, that may have a tangible effect on the problem. However, their potential for immediate effectiveness is difficult to gauge. They all require rather large-scale social and political changes. Moreover, they may not be rapidly forthcoming.

Thus, in trying to formulate prevention approaches to sexual abuse that can be readily translated into community programs, prevention advocates have tended to focus on potential victims rather than potential offenders. Rather than deter offenders directly, they have made it their goal to make children more resistant to abuse. Here again, some differences with physical abuse make this kind of strategy particularly appropriate to sexual abuse.

For one thing, sexual abuse victims are generally somewhat older than victims of child abuse and neglect. Thus, they may be more capable, knowledgeable and effective as allies in the prevention of their own abuse. For another thing, much sexual abuse seems to capitalize on the ignorance and naivete of children. Those who work with victims seem convinced that many children could have been spared if they had been informed, for example, about their right to refuse sexual advances or about the inappropriateness of the abuser's behavior. Some abuse may be relatively easy for a child to avoid if he or she has better information at an earlier age. This has encouraged a strategy of directing prevention to children.

## VARIETY OF SEXUAL ABUSE PREVENTION APPROACHES

Many prevention efforts are targeted directly at children through a variety of media. Programs like the Illusion Theater of Minneapolis (Anderson, 1979) and the Child Assault Prevention (CAP) program of Columbus (Cooper, Lutter, & Phelps, 1983) go directly into schools, where their trained staff conduct workshops for children at all grade levels (Brassard, Tyler, & Kehle, 1983). Children's authors have written storybooks and coloring books with titles like *Red Flag, Green Flag People* (Williams, 1980) to teach children how to avoid being sexually abused. A number of films like *Who Do You Tell* or *No More Secrets* have been produced primarily for use in the schools (Deitrich, 1981). In Seattle, ad campaigns with famous people such as basketball star Bill Russell have been used to teach children to identify possible child molesters (D. James, personal communication, 1984).

Prevention efforts have been aimed at a very broad spectrum of children. This strategy has been reinforced by two important facts emerging from contemporary research on sexual abuse. First, it is apparent that boys are subject to victimization as well as girls. Current estimates are that one boy is victimized for every three girls (Finkelhor, 1984). Thus prevention education is usually conducted in mixed classrooms and both boys and girls are used as models in the media. Second, children are victimized at an alarmingly early age. Estimates from some research indicate that a quarter of all abuse occurs before age 7 (Finkelhor, 1984). This highlights the need to bring prevention to very young children.

Some prevention educators have also recognized that there are special populations of children who need special approaches, including children who are handicapped and children who have already suffered victimization. For example, the Minnesota Program for Victims of Sexual Assault has developed a prevention curriculum specifically for disabled adolescents that tries to take into account the fact that parents and the rest of society give such children less basic sex information (O'Day, 1983).

As for children who have already suffered victimization, many treatment programs have started to offer prevention education after they became aware that previously abused children were at high risk for re-abuse and that prevention skills could be an excellent vehicle for restoring their sense of security and self-esteem (L. Berliner, personal communication, 1983; Snowden, 1983). However, since some victimized children will be present in any audience, all prevention programs have to take their special needs into account. Illustrating these special needs, Linda Sanford (personal communication, 1983), one leading prevention educator, cautions against formulating concepts, such as "never keep a secret," in a way that will make already victimized children feel worse because they did something they shouldn't have. She favors dealing with this problem by presenting children with options rather than absolutes.

## NEEDS OF PARENTS

As an alternative or supplement to direct approaches to children, some prevention education has been aimed at parents. This education has taken the form of parent groups or commercially published books such as Linda Sanford's *The Silent Children* (1980).

Prevention education directed toward parents has some distinct advantages. If parents learned to educate children themselves, children might receive repeated exposures to information from a trusted source, something that a classroom presentation cannot parallel.

However, it is clear at the present time that parents are a long way from providing such information in an accurate and useful way. Some of the inadequacies of current parental handling of sexual abuse prevention became apparent in a recent survey (Finkelhor, 1984) of 521 parents of children ages six to 14 in the Boston metropolitan area:

1) Only 29% of the parents said they had had a discussion with their child specifically related to the topic of sexual abuse.
2) Even when such discussions had occurred, in many cases they failed to mention important aspects of the problem. Only 53% of discussions, for example, included the possibility of abuse by an adult acquaintance, only 22% by a family member. Only 65% mentioned the possibility of someone trying to take off the child's clothes.
3) The discussions that did occur often occurred too late. Most parents believed the optimal age for discussing sexual abuse with a child was around age nine. Evidence from the parents own childhood experiences revealed, however, that over a third of all victims of sexual abuse would be victimized before age 9.

Why do parents have such difficulty teaching their children about child sexual abuse? The survey and the discussions with parents suggested some answers. Some parents simply did not visualize sexual abuse as a serious risk to their child. They tended to think of their own child as well supervised, as able to avoid danger. Sixty-one percent thought their neighborhood was safer than average and only 4% thought their neighborhood less safe.

Another reason parents often gave for not telling children about sexual abuse was the fear of unnecessarily frightening the child. They said they were afraid both of creating additional anxiety for a child and of possibly making the child suspicious of adults. While these parents are certainly sincere in their concern, prevention educators point out that parents warn children about strange animals without worrying that it will make them afraid of all animals or about cars without worrying that they may never want to learn to drive (Sanford, 1980). It is particularly curious that virtually all parents warn children about the possibility of kidnapping, too. The idea that someone might try to take the child away must certainly be a far more frightening idea to a child than the idea that someone might try to fondle his or her genitals, particularly since children have a very keen awareness of separation but rather a vague one of sex. The contrast is particularly ironic because although kidnapping is a far less likely event in a child's life than sexual abuse, most parents warn children about it. It suggests that the anxiety that parents are trying to avoid is not their child's but their own.

Kidnapping may be much easier to talk about than sexual abuse because parents have ready-made formulas for discussing the subject. Every parent has heard phrases like "don't get in a car with (or take candy from) a stranger," which he or she can repeat. Similar formulas have not existed in the past concerning sexual abuse. So a parent, confronted with the need to mention something about sexual abuse, has to improvise, using his or her own confused knowledge about the subject, and this prospect has probably deterred many. Now efforts are being made by prevention educators such as Linda Sanford and Cordelia Anderson to provide formulas for parents, and these may make the process easier.

A more profound problem for parents in talking about sexual abuse, and a feature of sexual abuse that differentiates it from kidnapping, is that it concerns sex. Parents have a notoriously difficult time talking to their children about sexual topics of all sorts, and this difficulty generalizes to sexual abuse (Roberts, Kline, & Gagnon, 1978). First, parents often feel they lack the knowledge, vocabulary and practice to speak about sexual matters. They fear embarrassing themselves in front of their children by appearing ignorant, tongue-tied or confused. Second, sexual topics trigger strong emotional feelings for parents, reminders of sexual embarrassments, traumas, or disappointments in their own lives. Third, parents are unsure of their own values about sexual matters, and are aware that sexual discussions may oblige them to talk about matters of value, opinion or even personal experience. All these concerns may be triggered when parents contemplate a discussion of sexual abuse with a child.

A question of some importance for parent education efforts is whether there are particularly high risk children whose parents should be specially targeted. One consistent finding about risk is that children who live in stepfamilies are unusually vulnerable (Finkelhor, 1980; Giles-Sims & Finkelhor, 1984; Russell, 1983). This suggests some special sexual abuse awareness information directed to parents who are remarrying, and who have children.

Another group of parents with some special needs may be those parents who were themselves victimized when they were children. Many workers in the field are of the opinion that children of such parents are at high risk, although no good research data have yet confirmed this point. Some of these parents undoubtedly have an extraordinarily difficult time raising the issue of sexual abuse with their children because of the painful memories it triggers.

Undoubtedly parents from different ethnic backgrounds and different social classes need to be educated in a manner and with concepts that are consistent with their own specific backgrounds and needs. In a diverse country like the United States, this makes it more difficult to design a single approach that can be effective with everyone. One interesting finding from the Boston study (Finkelhor, 1984), however, was the uniformity with which parents of all classes and ethnic groups abdicated their responsibility. Parents who had more education or high occupational status definitely did not do a better job than poorly educated and lower social class parents. There were also no differences along racial, ethnic or religious lines as to the likelihood of parents educating their children about sexual abuse. This does suggest that equivalent if not identical problems confront parents in all social groups, and that no group should be assumed to be superior.

## CURRENT CONCEPTS IN PREVENTION

Despite some disagreements among the variety of groups offering approaches to sexual abuse prevention, for the most part their approaches are similar. These educators have had to confront a common set of challenges, and have resolved them in common fashion.

The nature of the common challenges might be outlined as follows:

1) Sexual abuse, as adults generally talk about it, is a complicated issue, involving concepts of appropriate sexual behavior, appro-

priate sexual partners, ethics, and social obligations. These concepts are not ones that are necessarily readily grasped by children,
especially young children. Prevention programs need to translate
the notion of sexual abuse into concepts that make sense in the
world of the child.

2) The notion of sexual abuse is also one that has large and frightening overtones for adults. But as CAP educators point out (Cooper et al., 1983), children who are simply made to feel frightened
and powerless may be even less capable of avoiding abuse. Prevention programs have wanted to find some way to avoid or
moderate the potentially fearsome overtones of the issue.

3) Sex education is a controversial matter in many communities in
this country. As a result, teachers and particularly school admin-
istrators, who in most American communities are politically vulnerable officials, are very reluctant to permit inclusion of anything
that appears controversial in regard to sex in the educational
curriculum.

Prevention programs have used very creative solutions to confront
these challenges. For example, how can sexual abuse be made meaningful
to younger children? For the most part, educational programs have tried
to relate the problem of sexual abuse to other kinds of problems that
children do readily grasp (Crisci, 1983; Hutchinson & Chevalier, 1982).
The CAP programs start their explanations of sexual abuse by talking about
bullies; they illustrate with a skit of an older child trying to force a younger
child to give him his money. Being the victim of a bully is a kind of experience presumably all children can relate to. In this context, the explanation of sexual abuse, illustrated by a role play of an uncle trying to coerce
a little girl to kiss him, is readily understood.

The Illusion Theater makes sexual abuse comprehensible by putting it
in the context of what they call the Touch Continuum. They start out by
discussing the differences between touching that feels good (also called
"nurturant" or "positive" touch), illustrated by hugs, pats, snuggles, etc.,
and touch that feels bad (also called "exploitative," "manipulated," or
"forced" touch), illustrated by hitting, bullying, and trapping. Illusion also
has a category of what they call "confusing" touch ("touch that mixes
you up or makes you feel funny"), which are touches that convey double messages. In this context, Illusion Theater introduces sexual abuse as
a form of touch that feels either bad or confusing (Anderson [Kent], 1979).

The Touch Continuum has been borrowed and adapted, often being
illustrated as a dichotomy between good touch and bad touch, or as one

adaptation puts it, "red flag vs. green flag touches" (Williams, 1980). Obviously, good and bad touch is a vocabulary very readily understood even by small children.

The use of metaphors about bullies and touching has another effect: it makes the discussion of sexual abuse seem less like sex education. Prevention programs usually talk about their goals as ones of personal safety or assault prevention or empowerment, not sex education. Although it varies from program to program and setting to setting depending on the community's sensitivities, most programs are designed so that the subject of sex is implied. Words generally associated with sexual activities or sex education do not have to be explicitly used. In some programs, sexual organs are not referred to by name. Instead references are made to such things as "private zones" (Dayee, 1982), "molestation," "touching in private areas," "touching all over," "touching under the panties," and "places usually covered by a bathing suit." With some important exceptions, the formal curricula of most programs do not usually try to provide children with other kinds of sex education, such as sexual terms or information about sexual anatomy.

Another device common to almost all programs has been the use of humor and entertainment. They have usually utilized either theater, role playing, puppets, or coloring books. They have also been very participatory, asking children to get involved. This entertainment format creates a light tone that has allayed anxieties that adults have about sexual abuse education frightening children.

Programs have also relied on other devices to undercut the potentially frightening element of discussions of sexual abuse. For one thing, they have not tended to illustrate, although sometimes they are mentioned in passing, the more frightening forms of sexual abuse, ones that go on over extended periods of time or that involve great amounts of violence. The kinds of illustrations that are given in a variety of programs include such things as an older brother who always comes into the bathroom when a little girl is showering, an uncle who wants a highly sexual kiss, or a man who wants to put his hands into a child's pants (Hutchinson & Chevalier, 1982; Williams, 1980).

The programs have also tried to deal with the potentially frightening nature of sexual abuse by emphasizing positive actions children can take to handle such situations. They encourage children to believe that they have "rights": the right to control their own bodies, the right to be "safe, strong and free" (Cooper et al., 1983), the right not to have someone touch them in a way that feels bad, the right to privacy of their private parts.

Armed with these notions about rights, programs instruct children to say no to abusers. In more methodical programs, they are also taught how to be assertive of their rights and their safety, even in the face of adults who insist otherwise. In the CAP program, they act out situations to help one another find ways to say no. They brainstorm strategies for getting away from or out of dangerous situations. Some programs teach certain self-defense techniques, such as yelling and getting assistance from a friend. The CAP program has a special yell, which they practice with all their classes.

All programs place a very strong emphasis on the idea that if abused, children must tell someone right away. This special emphasis reflects the reality that in the past most children have not told. To encourage children's talking about it, these programs warn them that offenders will usually intimidate them from telling, but that they should ignore this. One of the concepts that has gained great popularity in prevention education is the distinction between a secret and a surprise (Sanford, 1980). Secrets, which you are never supposed to tell, are a bad idea, but surprises, which you will tell someone later in order to make them happy, are OK. Also, sometimes children are alerted that not all adults will necessarily believe them but that they should continue telling until someone does. These avoidance, resistance and help-seeking techniques are intended to help children avoid victimization and develop in themselves feelings of empowerment rather than of fright and helplessness.

## ORGANIZATIONAL ISSUES

Most prevention programs have devoted serious attention to their approach to communities. Although this is not always an aspect of the programs that is easy to communicate or transfer to other communities as a package, it is a crucial part of the current prevention efforts. As in our earlier discussion of concepts, although a variety of organizational frameworks exist, one can find consensus about certain common organizational elements that are seen as indispensable to prevention.

First, it is clear that the successful prevention programs define what they are doing not merely in terms of developing an educational program, but in terms of community organization. They have thought through political and organizational issues, and although their ultimate goal may be the education of children, much of their initial effort is directed to the community.

Successful prevention programs generally do a great deal of work to create the proper climate for gaining entree into a community. This includes developing a cadre of influential people who support the use of the program and who can lobby on its behalf. Of course, for long-established programs this is made easier by the reputations the programs may have developed based on their prior accomplishments.

Once school systems are interested in the program, one of the first steps in most programs that work within the schools is to present the material to parents and professionals in advance of any presentation to children themselves. The advance presentation can be used not only as a way of defusing any opposition and allaying anxieties about the program, but also as a way of educating this important audience.

In addition to presenting material to professionals, prevention programs usually recruit some local individuals to receive intensive training. This serves a number of functions: These individuals can assist the leaders in presenting the program to the children. They are more likely to know the children (often they are teachers or other school personnel) and thus give the program additional credibility. They are also instrumental in helping the program to have a sustained effect. These are individuals within the system who will continue to convey prevention concepts long after the trainers from the prevention program leave.

Another practice of responsible prevention programs is to prepare the community for the influx of reports of sexual abuse, which are inevitably produced by training. In some communities referral resources need to be developed by contacting professionals and agencies and assessing who have and who do not have the skills to receive reports. Then any professionals who are going to be involved in the prevention program or its follow-up, including classroom teachers or school guidance counselors, need to be trained in how to deal with reports from children. Some of the prevention programs like CAP make their own staff available to receive reports by scheduling time after the program when children who have special questions can come and talk privately.

There appears to be some difference of opinion in the field over the advisability of getting prevention education incorporated directly into school curriculum. In Seattle, trainers for the Committee for Children train regular classroom teachers who in turn present the material to children. The trainers themselves only rarely appear in front of classes. Committee member Donna James (personal communication, 1984) feels that this method is efficient because trainers do not need to go back to a school each year, and effective because students can get ongoing instruction from a person they already know and trust, their teacher.

Other educators, such as Rich Snowden (1983) of San Francisco, prefer a model in which outside trainers come into schools and work with the children. This model ensures that the trainers will be true specialists in the field. Snowden also worries that schools will not give support and encouragement to their own staff who specialize in sexual abuse prevention and that these programs will suffer in times of budget cutbacks.

## CONCEPTUAL DILEMMAS

Solutions to some problems sometimes create other problems. While the concepts developed by prevention programs demonstrate a great deal of creativity, they also create dilemmas.

Perhaps the most troublesome dilemma concerns the relationship between sex education and sexual abuse prevention. As we mentioned earlier, in order to deal with public squeamishness about sex education in schools, prevention programs have devised various ways for avoiding direct sexual references and discussions. Programs often can and do bring in more sexual content (two that seem to make a particular effort to do so include *Childproof for Sexual Abuse* [1981] from Washington state and *Sexuality and Sexual Assault: A Disabled Perspective* [Stuart & Stuart 1983] from Minnesota) but they do not require it. The tendency to avoid may be particularly great when less experienced trainers selectively borrow concepts from other programs, or when the education is done in a setting where sexual topics could be particularly controversial.

There are a number of possible negative consequences to sexual abuse prevention that avoids explicit sexual content. First, there is some question about whether under such conditions children truly learn what sexual abuse is. The problem is particularly acute in some of the less graphic media where stick figures are used or where abuse is described as "touching all over" or the "uh-oh feeling." (Uh-oh feelings are referred to in the Renton, Washington sexual abuse prevention program [Renton School District No. 403, 1981].)

Second, children may not be getting enough practice in using words and phrases to talk about sexual activity. There has been a general consensus among professionals in the field for a long time, emphasized quite clearly in Sanford's (1980) book, *The Silent Children*, that children are inhibited from talking about abuse when they do not have a vocabulary for or experience in discussing sex-related matters.

Third, the avoidance of explicit sexual content may be conspicuous and confusing to the children. They hear adults saying they want to discuss sex, while using vague euphemisms and circumlocution in talking about it. The message behind the message for some children may be that in spite of what adults say, they still do not want to talk in plain terms about sex.

And last, it is worth being concerned about other inferences children may draw when sexual abuse is talked about in isolation from other aspects of human sexuality. It is possible that when adults talk to children only about avoiding the coercive forms of sexuality, this leaves children with the impression that sex is primarily negative. For example, one wonders what underlying message is conveyed by the heroes of one program whose names are "Hands Off Bill and the Untouchables" (Martin & Haddad, 1981). It would not be too hard for children to misinterpret the message and come to feel guilty about their childhood sex play. Programs often try to leaven their approach by talking about positive touch, affection or assertive behavior, but almost never do they discuss what might be positive and age-appropriate sexuality.

To their credit, professionals in the field of sexual abuse prevention are aware of these dilemmas. We have not encountered one who was not in favor of more general sex education in schools. The Illusion Theater has even implemented this awareness with a new play, *No Easy Answers*, aimed at the junior and senior high school audience, and which explores the full range of adolescent sexual concerns. Some educators like Cordelia Anderson and Rich Snowden see sexual abuse prevention as the vehicle through which sex education will ultimately be accepted by school systems.

However, most sexual abuse prevention educators also are very realistic. They acknowledge that if sexual abuse prevention were to be too closely linked to a sex education focus, fewer schools would adopt it and fewer children, especially young children, would be exposed to it. Most feel that prevention education could be improved with more sex education, but that under present circumstances children at least get valuable if not exhaustive or complete knowledge.

Nonetheless, the relationship between sexual abuse prevention and sex education is an important one that needs further exploration, especially when evaluation research is done (Wall, 1983). We are inclined to believe that lack of sex education is an important component of the sexual abuse problem. Children cannot get adequate information about sexual abuse in a climate where adults who have contact with the child feel constrained from ever talking about sex. People working in the sexual abuse prevention field need to confront this. One way they can do it is to bring pressure, influence, and opinion to bear where they can, on behalf of more and better sex education. As their programs gain in reputation and credibility, such educators may come to be trusted enough to initiate more sex education. By seeing their responsibilities lying in the sex education area too, they may make sure that they are not reinforcing, albeit unwittingly, the idea that children can be well protected from sexual abuse in a setting where adults are fearful of talking with children about sex.

## REFERENCES

Adams, C., & Fay, J. (1981). *No more secrets*. San Luis Obispo, CA: Impact.

Anderson (Kent), C. (1979). *Child sexual abuse project: An educational program for children*. Minneapolis, MN: Hennepin County Attorney's Office Sexual Assault Services.

Armstrong, I. (1983). *The home front*. New York: McGraw-Hill.

Brassard, M. R., Tyler, A. H., & Kehle, T. J. (1983). School programs to prevent intrafamilial child sexual abuse. *Child Abuse and Neglect, 31*, 241–245.

*Childproof for sexual abuse*. (1981). Yakima, WA: Parent Education Center.

Cooper, S., Lutter, Y., & Phelps, C. (1983). *Strategies for free children*. Columbus, OH: Child Assault Prevention Project.

Crisci, G. (1983). *Personal safety curriculum for the prevention of child sexual abuse*. Hadley, MA: Personal Safety Program.

Dayee, F. S. (1982). *Private zone*. Edmonds, WA: Chas. Franklin Press.

Deitrich, G. (1981). Audiovisual materials with critique. In P. B. Mrazek & C. H. Kempe (Eds.), *Sexually abused children and their families* (pp. 257–259). New York: Pergamon Press.

Finkelhor, D. (1979). *Sexually victimized children*. New York: Free Press.

Finkelhor, D. (1980). Risk factors in the sexual victimization of children. *Child Abuse and Neglect, 4*, 265–273.

Finkelhor, D. (1984). *Child sexual abuse: New theory and research*. New York: Free Press.

Giles-Sims, J., & Finkelhor, D. (1984). Child abuse in stepfamilies. *Family Relations, 33*, 407–414.

Groth, N. A., Hobson, W., & Gary, T. (1982). The child molester: Clinical observations. In J. Conte & D. Shore (Eds.), *Social work and child sexual abuse*. New York: Haworth.

Herman, J. (1981). *Father-daughter incest*. Cambridge: Harvard.

Hutchinson, B., & Chevalier, E. A. (1982). *My personal safety book*. Fridley, MN: Fridley Police Department.

Martin, L., & Haddad, J. (1981). *What if I say no?* Bakersfield, CA: M. H. Cap & Co.

O'Day, B. (1983). *Preventing sexual abuse of persons with disabilities*. St. Paul, MN: Minnesota Program for Victims of Sexual Assault, Minnesota Department of Corrections.

Renton School District No. 403. (1981). *Sexual abuse prevention: A unit in safety*. Renton, WA: Department of Curriculum Instruction.

Roberts, E., Kline, D., & Gagnon, J. (1978). *Family life and sexual learning*. Cambridge, MA: Project on Human Sexual Development.

Rush, F. (1980). *The best kept secret*. New York: Prentice-Hall.

Russell, D. E. H. (1983). The incidence and prevalence of intrafamilial and extrafamilial sexual abuse of children. *Child Abuse and Neglect, 7*, 133–146.

Sanford, L. (1980). *The silent children: A parent's guide to the prevention of child sexual abuse*. New York: Anchor Press/Doubleday.

Snowden, R. (1983). *Boys and child sexual assault prevention project*. Unpublished paper, CAP Training Center of Northern California, San Francisco, CA.

Stuart, V., & Stuart, C. K. (1983). *Sexuality and sexual assault: A disabled perspective*. Marshall, MN: Southwest State University.

Wall, H. (1983). *Child assault/abuse prevention project: Pilot program evaluation*. Concord, CA: Mt. Diablo Unified School.

Williams, J. (1980). *Red flag, green flag people*. Fargo, ND: Rape and Abuse Crisis Center of Fargo-Moorehead.

# Name Index

# Subject Index

316